Billionaire Puppet-masters: The Evil Empire

President Trump and Elon Musk, Today's George Washington and Thomas Jefferson

Volume I

INTENSIVE PSYCHOTHERAPY AND GENETIC RESEARCH PROVES THE ENVIRONMENT RULES

RONALD VASU, M.D.

The Billionaire-Communist China Axis agenda seeks the destruction of Western Culture, of America as a sovereign nation and of individual liberty. Their goal is one-world of puppets in a conspiracy to control money. The middle class and working class are subjected to unrelenting propaganda because they are the only remaining power block left still capable of resisting the evolving dictatorship. The billionaires pretend solidarity with minorities. They are fascist wolves dressed-up in socialist sheep's clothing. Human relationships are under siege because they resist brainwashing and lock-step obedience to tyrannical dictates. Expression of one's personal identity is now deemed a menace to the "Greater Good."(puppetry). History, education, speech, all manifestations of individuality both psychologic and biologic are being policed. In truth we are the product of life experience starting in childhood. We are not Big Business hard-wired puppets.

Dedicated to the memory of Henry Ruehr,
M.D. Acknowledgement of the invaluable technical help and
suggestions of Paul Christ
In memory of Arthur Lipman, M.D.

Table of Contents

Volume I

Part I	**Psychiatry and Culture**	**1**
Chapter 1	The Role of Economic Factors, Unbridled Profit Motive and the Ultimate Dehumanization of the Person: Historical Perspective	3
Chapter 2	The Psychology of Unbridled Capitalism: Its Sociopathic Roots	8
Chapter 3	Psychiatry is influenced by the Culture in which it is Embedded Who Controls Present Day American Culture?	10
Chapter 4	How the Economic Pie is Divided Between Rich, Poor and Middle-Class: A History (Remember, Costs for Healthcare must be Slashed !)	24
Chapter 5	The Ethics of Unbridled Capitalism: Its Goals And Ultimate Consequences. Is the Public Fully Aware of the Extent to which America has been Hijacked?	34
Chapter 6	How the Plutocracy Masters Propaganda	41
Chapter 7	A History of Killing Americans for Profit: The Leopard Never Changes its Spots	46
Chapter 8	Unbridled Capitalism in the Armament Industry	52
Chapter 9	Unbridled Capitalism's Corruption of the Political Process: Selling out the Country	59
Chapter 10	Globalization – Free Trade	67
Chapter 11	Unbridled Capitalism in the Market place of Medicine	71
Chapter 12	The Cost of Mental Illness and Treatment, the Efficacy of Psychotherapy	79
Chapter 13	Managed Care Compromised the Quality of Care: The Case for Criminal Racketeering	87
Chapter 14	"No Money for Medicare" – "Health Care Costs Out of Control!" "You Cannot Tax the Plutocrats. Rape the Middle Class and Poor Instead."	100
Chapter 15	Unbridled Capitalism and the Corruption of Medical Research, Academia and Psychiatric Practice, A History	123
Chapter 16	Media, and Mind Control. Psychiatry and the Fundamentals of Propaganda	141

Part II	**Dehumanization of the Individual**	**157**
Chapter 17	The Plutocrat Puppet-Master's Agenda	159
Chapter 18	The Dehumanized Arts The Bread and Circuses	182
Chapter 19	Don't Think – Obey! "1984" Refined for the 21st Century	192
Chapter 20	Psychiatry Dehumanized	211

"For the corruption of the mind is a pest far worse than any such miasma and vitiation of the air which we breathe around us. The latter is a pestilence for living creatures and affects their life, the former for human beings and affects their humanity."

"and pass through the remainder of thy days as one that with his whole soul has given all his in trust to the Gods, and has made of himself neither a tyrant nor a slave to any man." [Marcus Aurelius Antoninus, Emperor of Rome, Meditations, Books IX and IV]

Introduction and Overview ix-xc1

In the real world, human relationships, starting with the family, are the foundation for what we become in life and underlie both mental health and mental illness. How we treat ourselves and others, sexually and otherwise, is related to how we were valued as children. At present, however, a parallel virtual universe is being fabricated and it has little to do with string theory or physics. In this virtual world, emotional problems, if not our basic identity as human beings, are a product of inborn, independent brain factors. Economic forces, masquerading as scientific advancement, and controlled by the billionaire-Communist China agenda, have orchestrated this dehumanizing rupture with the real world in which we live. The profound psychological impact of life experience and its unconscious childhood roots are denied. This work investigates the culture in which psychiatry and our culture is currently embedded, (in depth clinical case studies, and research on the brain and heritability will be addressed in a second book). Navigating life's at times treacherous seas in our Odyssey toward self-realization, we encounter manipulative forces that, for clandestine motives, seek to deter us from our own best interests and obscure our true nature. If we are to reach the homeland of a fulfilled life, we must recognize the "born that way" agenda for what it is: the siren-call of a brainwashing machine that aims for cookie – cutter compliant puppets. In these pages, we will consider at several levels the depth of the human condition. We will rely on an analysis of the psychological forces at play in our culture, clinical expertise, scientific research, and common sense. As for common sense, we can ask whether it is really rational to conclude that those suffering from the great majority of serious emotional problems are "born that way?" Are African-American children who cannot read or write "born that way?" Are the poor "born that way?" To discern the face of present-day psychiatry one must bring to light the all-powerful influence of the plutocrat agenda across the entire spectrum of American culture.

The plutocracy-billionaires control all aspects of the culture

The plutocracy-billionaires, our Orwellian puppet-masters, define themselves by a simple credo that has nothing to do with ideology: the control of money. Money is power. History shows that they will sacrifice any citizen and the welfare of any nation in pursuit of that end. Our culture is increasingly shaped by the power of American multinational corporations who anoint themselves "citizens of the world" and disavow any particular responsibility to the American people. The Billionaire-Communist Chinese agenda seeks the destruction of America as a sovereign nation, the destruction of Western Culture and the destruction of individual liberty, including the curtailment of small business and individual property rights. Their goal is money and power, one globalized world of puppets where they control everything. Scratching the surface beneath the loudly broadcast assertion that the new Democrat party (the real Democrat party is extinct) is driven by Socialism or Marxism, avoids the real truth: Fascism. Big Business is the engine behind an evolving dictatorship. Wall Street and Big Business are not Marxists. Of course, the Republican establishment can't hold the real menace responsible because they also count on the billionaire's money spigot. The toxic wealth disparity had reached a tipping point such that the billionaires could now openly resort to curtailment of democratic liberties, all the while pretending concern for the downtrodden. Our Founding Fathers realized that the foundation of democracy and a humanistic state rests upon The First Amendment, upholding free speech. On the ancient temple in Delphi of the god Apollo, son of Zeus, is the inscription "Know Thyself," the first acknowledgment in recorded history that recognized the value of the individual, not Caesar or Siva, but the individual. Free speech was recognized by Sigmund Freud to be the cornerstone of psychotherapy and essential if one is to understand the origin and treatment of emotional problems. Psychoanalysis is vilified because Big Business seeks mind control and recognizes that free-thinking individuals resist enslavement. The billionaires seek the destruction of human relationships as evidenced by the increasing mayhem in American society. The mentally ill are shoveled under the rug until violence inevitably erupts. Official psychiatry, taken over by Big Business, no longer mentions human relationships or "talk therapy." The billionaires, with one or two prominent exceptions (President Trump, Elon Musk) aim to destroy our freedom to consider our own best interests. They control the organs of propaganda (lifting from the pages of Joseph Goebbels and Stalin) and recently attempted to install a "Ministry of Truth" under the auspices of their lackey in the White House, Biden, Pravda anyone? President Biden, under massive pressure from the billionaires has since stepped aside, clarifying who is really in charge. "Hate speech" is defined as any opinion that runs counter to prevailing Tech-Titan propaganda. Inculcating white school children with the message that they are inherently racists is "good speech." Nazis and Communists have a right to express their views as long as they do not themselves incite violence.

There are only a handful of very wealthy powerful individuals in recorded history who were not corrupted by money/power and never forgot the highest value of a life, that being human relationships and the worth of the individual. Among them, hopefully, is President Donald Trump. Elon Musk so far also seems to be one of those people. He has built his companies out of thin air (a simplification of course), in itself a remarkable feat, but he values the liberty of the person, the bedrock of democracy and of civilization. His avowed goal is to establish a public forum for free speech. He bought "Twitter" which up to now has served the totalitarian interests of the establishment-billionaires. As a consequence, he has stirred up hysterical recriminations from the mind-control contingent fearful as they are that if one free voice can escape their blanket censorship the dictatorship's house of cards will collapse. [Yahoo News "Elon Musk says he wants Twitter to be the WeChat of the Western World]. President Trump and Elon Musk are today's George Washington and Thomas Jefferson.

Totalitarians always use the same tried and true tactics, Hitler, Mao and Stalin for example. Adolf Hitler's crystallized strategies are as follows accompanied by the BidenBig Business current parallels:

1. Eliminate Freedom of Speech
2. Destabilize the nation through mob violence (the S.A. brownshirts, The Red Guard); destroy a nation's history (Die Neue Ordnung).
   Current parallel: unleashing unprecedented mob violence, destruction of revered figures of America's past (Abraham Lincoln. Our Founding Fathers). Nullifying the constitution.
3. Create a fictitious enemy of the state, Jews, confiscate their property, replace them.
   Current parallel: Claim that "white supremacy", white racism, is the #1 menace, eclipsing Al Qaida. Replace them with 3rd world puppets. (and yet Black on white murders are more than twice white on black murders, FBI 2018).
4. The Nazis set The Reichstag fire, blaming the Communists, and used it to institute a police state.
   Current parallel: The new Democrat-billionaire dictatorship-in-the-making labels a Jan 6 riot of two hundred unarmed Trump supporters who breached the Capital an insurrection worse than Pearl Harbor and are using it to justify a police state. One young unarmed woman, a Trump supporter, was shot to death.
5. The Nazi state and the Fuehrer become the only valued entity.
   Current parallel: Destroy individuality and human relationships. All priorities other than those endorsed by the controlling billionaires are treasonous.
6. Hitler instituted his own party secret police, The Gestapo
   Current parallel: The F.B.I arrests political opponents, putting them in leg irons, Invading and ransacking their homes, solitary confinement.
7. The Nazi / Stalinist state controls the news, the organs of propaganda Current Parallel: The Biden administration institutes the Ministry of Truth.
   Big Business news all parrot the same script, the exact same adjectives the same wording and bias. Big Tech censors political opponents so they have no forum.

Under orders from Biden's Justice Department in 2022, former President Trump's home was ransacked by 30 gun wielding F.B.I agents for 12 hours, the first time in the nation's history that anything like that has ever occurred. Big Tech's propaganda organs talk of "espionage and nuclear secrets" just as they lied for three years about the disproven Trump / Russia collusion hoax. The real motive was to dig up dirt that could eliminate Trump from running again for the Presidency.

The F.B.I. acting as the personal Gestapo of the Biden administration has feverishly worked to lend validity to the claim that white supremacy (Trump voters) is the # 1 threat to America. LI, Mary Chaistain [8/23/22. "Two Michigan Men Convicted…"] writes that F.B.I. informants infiltrating a group of white men whom they accused of plotting to kidnap the Michigan governor were more than passive observers and allegedly orchestrated every step in the contrived plot, to entrap the defendants. The judge in the case limited cross-examination and told the jurors the defense lawyers employed "crap." As for the F.B.I., How come they have shown zero interest in infiltrating Antifa or Black Lives Matter who fueled hundreds of violent riots in 2020 and current mayhem replete with arson, murder, unchecked looting, skyrocketing carjackings, killing of policemen, burning of police stations ? The D.A. in New York has decreed that holding up stores with guns must be considered only "petty larceny." His mantra is empty the jails. In Philadelphia young car jacking criminals can have their record expunged if they sign up for one month of violin lessons. Tell that to a grandmother whose car was carjacked and she was dragged along until her arm was severed. She bled to death.

Mark Zuckerberg in a Joe Rogan podcast before the 2020 Presidential election stated that the F.B.I. warned him to be on the look-out for "Russian propaganda," causing him to suppress the New York Post factual story about Hunter Biden's incriminating laptop. President Biden's worry about a white backlash may well stem from a legitimate concern that whites may someday get fed up with being relentlessly humiliated and brutalized. Criminals should be convicted and go to jail whatever their skin color. If underage, several years of workcamps are in order.

Again, the new Democrat party is a front for the one-world globalization agenda. But the Republican establishment likewise shows little real concern for the American people. Former President Trump and Governor Ron DeSantis etc. are exceptions. Senator M. McConnell, in contrast,+ has other priorities such as his wife's Chinese ship building interests.

Ever wonder about the oft repeated refrain that the current social mayhem is Marxist/ socialist inspired ? Are Wall Street, Multinational Corporations, Big Tech. Big Business billionaires all of whom fuel the anti-America 1st movement Marxists? No, not really. They are fascists out to control the world for power and money. Western Culture blocks their way because it values the individual and the billionaires want puppets. No mention is ever made anymore of taxing the billionaires.

The decline of America mirrors the decline of Ancient Rome and for the same reasons.

The Roman Republic was destroyed by an oligarchy that over time got control of the wealth and bought off the people with bread and circuses. Liberty gave way to increasingly despotic dictatorships motivated by power and money. Rome fell from within as the people lost their moral fiber. America is also succumbing to the toxic wealth disparity that undermined Rome. Individual freedom is rapidly eroding in a devolving dictatorship. Biden has spent trillions on "clean energy," thereby enriching our enemy Communist China and absurdly making America's energy needs dependent on windmills. Printing money by trillions debases the dollar. Rome debased its currency as well.

"Already long ago, from when we sold our vote to no man, the People have abdicated our duties; for the People who once upon a time handed out military command, high civil office, legions, everything, now restrains itself and anxiously hopes for just two things: bread and circuses." Juvenal, Roman poet.

The agenda of unbridled capitalism to control money is multi-layered: current examples

We see, for example, that the decline of America on the global stage and the powerful rise of an adversary is a consequence of globalization trade policies that, in exchange for imagined access to a billion Chinese consumers (access that China blocks), allows American multinational corporations, hat in hand, to divulge Silicon Valley technology secrets to a Chinese dictatorship. Current attempts to reset unfair Chinese/American trade imbalances that continue to funnel almost $400 billion annually to China elicits howls from both American parties, orchestrated by American plutocrats: "It's going to cause a suicidal trade war!! The stock market will drop!!" "China will not back down!" (Hitler and The Imperial Japanese Government wouldn't back down either, as is the pattern with totalitarian regimes.) Pseudo-leftist pundits who support American multinational corporations in the trade war warn that prices will rise for the American consumer. [Newsweek 12/10/21, "The US Has Mismanaged Trade Policy for 20 Years.."; The New York Times, 1/20/2008] Scott Paul, Director, Alliance for American Manufacturing, points out that any benefit accrued by cheaper prices of imported goods was more than offset by the economic activity that wages, business, and profits contributed to the economy when jobs remain in the U.S.

Absurd trade treaties put the interests of multinational corporations above the interests of the nation, allowing sanguine China to impose 25% tariff s on new cars imported from the US while the US tariff on imported cars is 2.5%. Tesla founder, Elon Musk, tweeted that no US auto company owns even 50% of their own factory in China but there are five 100% China-owned electric vehicle companies in the US [The Verge Twitter 3/8/18 by Sean O'Kane "Elon Musk pushes Trump on China tariffs…]. China has embedded itself deeply in American business and academic research. The flood of its exchange students, fully funded by their government (no crippling student loans here), hold sway over many American universities ($$$) while young Americans languish. Taking advantage of an "open and collaborative university atmosphere," Ruopeng Liu, a Chinese citizen and student at Duke, worked on a cloak that shields objects from a broad spectrum of wave frequencies at a Pentagon funded lab. In that process, he collaborated with colleagues in China, photographed cutting-edge technology, returned to China where he founded an institute and played host to Chinese President Xi Jinping. Regulations to restrict Chinese incursion into American university research would be "tragic" according to Chinese-American front organizations [The New York Times, 5/1/18 "White House Considers Restricting Chinese Researchers Over Espionage Fears" Ana Swanson et al] U.S. Sen. Marco Rubio states that the cost to the United States from China's theft of U.S. intellectual property is $600 billion annually: the value of the technological research that American companies handover to Chinese "partners" as the price of doing business in China [The New York Times, 3/28/22, "Marco Rubio leads GOP push for a more combative stance 0n China"by B. Hounshell].

The CNN pay-television news channel reports that five million American manufacturing jobs were lost since the year 2000 due to outsourcing. It isn't that there are not enough Americans trained in sophisticated computer technology. Even highly educated Americans lose employment security as jobs move to India. The New York Times, however, computes the situation differently ["As Trump Punishes China, Detroit Braces for the Pain," 7/13/18 by Ana Swanson]. It quotes extensively from the Detroit auto and related industries that view Chinese business investments there as just plain healthy for America. China has invested billions in Detroit and its floundering companies. Globalization is the life's-blood of American big business, we are told, and fear of undue Chinese leverage in the American economy is just so-much paranoia. But where did the Chinese billions come from we might ask? Perhaps from the above quoted trillion a year (or is it $600 billion?) that American multinational corporations have invested in a totalitarian Chinese dictatorship? What would such vast sums of money have done had they been invested in the public's welfare? The New York Times has run ongoing articles purporting to bemoan the consequences to Americans of a trade war with China. It is, of course, beholden to its big business advertisers. Its editorial board is a mouthpiece for the grand scheme of multinational corporations. Mark Levin has researched the history of The New York Times with dictators (Fox News).

The billionaire Koch brothers have given vast sums to a Republican establishment whose sole function seems to be as a conduit for the interests of the billionaire class. Needless to say, the Koch brothers are champions of unbridled immigration (cheap labor) and find tariffs on Chinese imports an anathema (multinational corporate profits are at risk).

Big bank profits take precedence over the nation's best interests

["Meetings in Beijing aim to strengthen financial ties between 2 nations," NYT 9/17/18 Alexandra Stevenson et al]. Executives from Goldman Sachs Group, Morgan Stanley and the Blackstone Group etc. planned to meet with Vice President Wang Qishan, President Xi Jinping right hand man in a hastily convened meeting: "Even as they win tax cuts and regulatory rollbacks from the Trump administration and the then Republican controlled congress, they [the banks] appear to be able to do little to stop the trade war." It should be remembered that it was Wall Street pleading Beijing's case to President Clinton that loosened trade barriers against China, catapulting China from the backwaters to a threatening American adversary.

Or, [The New York Times 9/21/15, "Drug goes from $13.50 a tablet to $750, overnight" Andrew Pollack] on the local front, the rapacious behavior of the pharmaceutical industry and the newly minted robber-baron-parasites who buy up a sixty-two year old drug patent and then raise the price from $13.50 a tablet to $750, overnight. Unscrupulous pharmaceutical companies, taking advantage of the healthcare system, acquire drugs that have been off patent for decades and drive up the price to stratospheric levels. Mallinckrodt PLC is the present-day maker of H.P.Acthar gel, a 1950s vintage off-patent drug that went from $40 a vial in 2001 to $38,000 in 2016 [The New York Times 12/25/16 "A costly drug missing dose of disclosure" Gretchen Morganson].

The final destination for the plutocrats is a "virtual" world where they control everything. In league with politicians of both American parties, whom they also control, they spy on our every movement and predilection in their pursuit of mind-control and profit.

At present, the plutocrat's juggernaut is operating on all levels of our culture to crush individuality. They now seduce the masses into playing little Big Brothers too, spying on fellow citizens with cameras, Google Glasses and intrusive online snooping. Google offers spyware apps that, equipped with little more than a phone number, can secretly embed in a victim's mobile phone to track their step by step whereabouts, including, in some cases, video recording. Google's A.I. aims to replace human phone callers with robots refined to mimic the nuance of the human voice. In fact, beyond those isolated examples, Google, a $685 billion behemoth, is tracking your every move. It knows where you are going during the day, what time and where you stopped off, whom you called, the choices you make, and then selling that information to advertisers. Seeking answers from Amazon's Alexa? It was recently reported that the software secretly recorded conversations from users and that, by virtue of wifi, a third party can secretly listen in on conversations of others even when they are not present. The company states that this is a very rare occurrence. Smart TVs can be accessed remotely to spy on you in your living room. Facebook gathers comprehensive data on all your activities and thoughts even if you don't have a Facebook account.

Brian X. Chen writing in The New York Times, "How To Delete Facebook" 4/12/18], rarely posts on his Facebook account or clicks on ads, yet, when he downloaded a copy of his file, he was dumbfounded to find out that about 500 advertisers, many of whom he had never heard of, like "Bad Dad," a motor-cycle parts store, had his contact information including his entire phone book, email, the number to ring his apartment buzzer. Facebook had a permanent record of the 100 friend's list he had deleted over the past fourteen years. Learning from their history with police states, the European Union recently enacted the world's toughest rules to protect people's online data, the General Data Protection Regulation. The law lets people request their online data and restricts how businesses obtain and handle the information [NYT 5/25/18 "GDPR A New Privacy Law Makes Europe World's Leading Tech Watchdog" Adam Satariano]. The EU resists the claim of the billionaires to be judge, jury, and executioner regarding privacy. In the following pages, my esteemed reader will sense the ominous portent of facial recognition tools that the Chinese dictatorship already employs to perfect the police state. It has a score on everyone that determines what they may do, if they can travel etc.. At the cutting edge of this technology, Facebook and Google are helping to forge our own police state, controlled by the plutocrats, right here at home. It was also reported that Google is now collaborating with a Chinese company that is involved in intelligence operations, the same Google unit that formerly had worked with American intelligence.

The billionaires brainwash the young into feeling like pariahs who risk character assassination if they don't blend in. "We're all connected," as I will later show, is the technology titan's mantra to facilitate the addiction and transformation of our abandoned youth, their ultimate goal being a society of lobotomized puppets. Seduced by the seeming magic of controlling life's stressors through machines, the failure in really getting to know another human being is circumvented by thousands of virtual electron-friends and obsessive, dumbed-down, web-entertainment. Taking a page from the 1950's when the cigarette companies manipulated nicotine cigarette levels to addict smokers, the tech monopolies aim to supplant our ability to think independently with brainwashing software and millions of phone apps to addict the young into obeying algorithm directives to make all life-decisions, thus ensuring the elimination of personal identity. Inevitable isolation ensues and with that isolation, depression, growing anxiety, rage, and, ultimately, the breakdown of civilization. Personal identity, reflective solitude, privacy, freedom of speech, in short, the essential foundation of a humanistic civilization is being undermined by an unscrupulous oligarchy, an oligarchy that, like a wolf in sheep's clothing, professes phony concern for the downtrodden. And this is merely the tip of the oncoming iceberg. Exploiting technology to marginalize the thinking individual, the technology titans advance the "Singularity Movement," the goal to "merge mind and technology in a new post – human species." "Singularity" is fitting word choice: the center of a black hole where all individuality in nature is obliterated. Heralded as "the next step in evolution," it would be comical were it not an all-too-realizable blueprint to eliminate our identity and that most precious of human emotions, our ability to care about one another. Individuals that value human relationships stand squarely in the plutocracy's way because they think critically, resist enslavement, and cannot be bought off by bread and circuses.

There is much soul-searching regarding the looming threat of a "1984" style dictatorship. Few seem to recognize, however, that it is the multinational corporations and their friends, the tech-titan brainwashing manipulators who are the real modern-day equivalent to Orwell's "1984." It is they who control the media and subvert education. This work investigates the origin and treatment of emotional problems. It raises the iron curtain on psychiatry forged by plutocratic propaganda and exposes their economically motivated stranglehold on all aspects of our culture, psychiatry included.

Systematic propaganda aims to further globalization and erase America as a nation. Ridiculous lies refashion personal identity, making ventriloquist dummies out of a proud people:

The totalitarian media feigns dismay at the alarming prevalence of white supremacy in America. Every Big Business news outlet inserts obligatory marketing assertions that trumpet how concerned they are about (white) racism They force their white staff to undergo reeducation courses to root out their alleged inherent racism. Universities have made white racism their # one priority (Communist Chinese money might otherwise be jeopardized). Racism does exist but the most defamatory publicized racism is leveled against whites. The underlying agenda is to replace white Americans with 3rd world peoples who will obey their billionaire masters.

Wiping out America as a sovereign nation requires instituting mind control from the ground up. Reality is replaced by whatever politicians say it is regardless of how crazy. The goal is to police independent thinking and wipe out personal identity. The billionaires are out to fashion a colony of puppets. If you don't go along you will be arrested as an enemy of the state. The biological scientific definition of the sexes, man and woman, are subjugated to political redefinition such that reality is determined and policed by whatever politicians say it is. If a biologic man says he is a woman, he can compete successfully in women's sports even if women's sports are thereby destroyed. Or an impressionable male toddler is subjected to homosexual teachers who inculcate gender politics in the curriculum and foster homosexual outcomes. The Biden administration will withhold Federal lunch money unless gender politics is a standard part of the school curriculum. Big Business directly profits by Frankenstein doctors who subject helpless children to chemical castration and mutilating surgery. Speech is policed because if one cannot speak the truth, one cannot think the truth. International pronoun day teams up with the billionaire's agenda to wipe out the individual by forbidding the use of "boy" "girl" "mother" "father" "pregnant women" etc. The individual is to be transformed into a puppet.

Climate Control is the universal top priority of the billionaires, but not of the people. It pretends to have a very virtuous moral underpinning but its real aim is to transfer control of energy and food production to an oligarchy. Western Europe and the U.S. have been forced to succumb to this crazy farce because their politicians play footsy with Big

Business. Fossil fuels including clean natural gas and nuclear power are demonized. A universal rating scale, the ESG rating, gives high points to countries that eliminate nitrogen fertilizers from agriculture. Sri Lanka complied causing food prices to double and toppling the government. One suspects that the billionaires were involved. The Netherlands banned fertilizers dooming 30% of Dutch farms leading to widespread protests. Bill Gates gave 600 million to the brother of the Dutch Premier for his online grocery company. Of course China and India are exempt from climate control.

A plutocrat persona for the 21st century

One of the newly hatched billionaires tells the public with a straight face that he "just wants to promote friendship. It's not about money primarily," all the while secretly selling the public's personal information to corporate advertisers. This same Mark Zuckerberg makes a media-splash, by announcing that he will "give away" $45 billion in Facebook stock over his lifetime. However, Jesse Eisinger [NYT 12/3/15 "How Mark Zuckerberg's Altruism Helps Himself"] clarifies that this is not a non-profit charitable foundation but an LLC investment vehicle that allows Mr. Zuckerberg to do whatever he wants with his money including buying up for-profit companies, all the while being excused of allocating a percentage of his assets annually as would be the case were it a charitable foundation. If he donates appreciated shares of Facebook to charity, he doesn't have to pay taxes on the donation and can write it off as a tax deduction. True to the conceit that American multinational corporations are citizens of the world, Mr. Zuckerberg has explored (fruitlessly) every avenue to gain entry into the Chinese market. [The Daily Mail, "Unfriended: Snubbed…" Khaleda Ramen, 10/4/2015] He has "wined and dined Chinese politicians, showed off his newly acquired Chinese language skills….and talked with a potential Chinese partner about pushing his social network into the market…." At a White House dinner in 2015, he asked the Chinese president, Xi Jinping, the honor of offering a Chinese name for his soon-to-be-born first child. Mr. Xi declined. A New York Times editorial [6/6/18] rightfully condemns Facebook's surreptitious efforts to forge deals with the Chinese dictatorship regardless of the risks to American security. Money is at stake. "Facebook shared data with at least four Chinese electronic firms, including one flagged by American officials as a national security threat [Huawei]. We learned earlier this week, thanks to a Times investigation, that it allowed phone and other device makers, including Amazon, Apple, Samsung, and Microsoft, to see vast amounts of your personal information without your knowledge." Facebook made repeated changes to its privacy settings that allowed it to transfer user data without bothering to inform the users. Its partners include 60 device makers that have helped themselves to your information. A Times reporter was able to retrieve information on 260,000 Facebook users using a five-year old BlackBerry. Of course, The New York Times is right: Facebook is today's Standard Oil and should be broken up.

Google that pretends to be at the helm of patriotic values, diversity, and a champion of the downtrodden, had planned to launch a censored version of its search engine in China called "Dragonfly" which would allow China's Communist Party dictatoship to blacklist information about political dissidents, block free speech and discussion of human rights. The blacklisting would have been operative when people enter certain words or phrases according to confidential Google documents. The Chinese dictatorship, of course, will know who entered those key words or phrases and that could be a death sentence. China, has set up concentration camps for a million Chinese Muslims, and persecuted Chinese Christians. The individual is a non-entity, collateral damage, when Big Business seeks profits. Wouldn't Google bend its ethics here as well given the opportunity? Owing to protests by Google employees, Dragonfly was terminated [see The Intercept "Google Dragonfly" 5/14/2019 Ryan Gallagher].

The public is being diverted from the real issues. No one needs more than $500 million or a billion. There is an urgent demand for a special assessment so that the government, elected by the people, can use that money for the betterment of its people.

The globalization agenda: homogenize personal identity

At a societal level, the plutocracy aims to be the sole authority, the sole and only point of reference. Their agenda: The commerce of unbridled globalization profits. As a consequence, nations and their people, including The United States and its people, are headed for the blender. Priorities other than the global priorities of Big Business are vilified. All cultures are equal, we are told, and "nationalism" (devotion to the interests of one's own nation and its people) is bad.

At a personal level, the plutocracy is at work to replace the thinking individual with a faceless sea of one-size-fits-all brain factors (the new psychiatry), thus ensuring the obliteration of each and everyone's personal voice. No real protest except that condoned by unbridled capitalism will be permitted.

Through their brainwashing machines, they are fabricating pseudo-identities for both the individual and the culture as a whole. Already, legions of the young are seduced into believing that they will be dismissed as irrelevant unless they look to the plutocrat controlled social media for validation: "Tell me what I want? Tell me what I should think?" The old Roman formula for expansion of the Empire, "divida et impera" (divide and rule), has been a very successful ongoing tool for the plutocrats. Women are pitted against men, minorities against the white middle-class, racial anxieties on all sides stoked, all the while the super-rich titans on their private ocean liners have more trillions than they can possibly spend. Their foot-soldiers in the media and congress foam at the mouth (war on business!! class warfare!!) at any attempt to tax them at an equitable sixty to ninety percent rate that common decency and logic would justify. Equitable taxation is not only an indispensable tool for raising the quality of life for the common man, it is instrumental in removing the incentive for criminal greed. Dramatically taxing the 0.01% super-rich while lowering taxes on the middle class would ensure an unparalleled increase in productivity. But neither logic nor justice have a voice in Congress where only money talks. Consider Pfizer Pharmaceutical's $150 billion proposed takeover of Allergen Pharma to avoid U.S. corporate tax rates by setting up phony residence oversees. We were assured by Pfizer that what's good for Pfizer is good for the country. The venture was subsequently scuttled. Individuality and critical thinking are in the plutocracy's cross-hairs.

The multi-layered plutocrat agenda: homogenizing sex/gender

While idealistically there must be equal opportunity for all in a true democracy and traditional gender roles are not sacrosanct, neither is it true that historical male/female role models are merely a patriarchal power play. Gender roles are basically culturally determined, but there are fundamental differences between the sexes (women are biologically built and emotionally endowed to care for children and men are influenced by their own biology, hormones). Nevertheless, the culture does indeed influence role-playing profoundly, and those that control a culture have routinely sought to inculcate attitudes that will ensure consolidation of their control. The plutocrats who now control American society aim to wipe the cultural slate clean by undermining all cultural tradition and manipulating mass behavior in such a way as to fashion a world more malleable and friendly to their master blueprint. No other power block should be discernable on the cultural horizon. Everyone is in the homogenizer. Globalization profits are at stake.

Girls are made to feel weak unless they embrace masculinization. The plutocrat media, pretending honest concern for equality, lets girls know that quarterbacking the boy's high school football team is really plausible. Young women, even little girls, should take up boxing, weight lifting, wear jackboots, excel in military combat, or, the ultimate achievement, vie with the sociopathic despots that run the monopolies, even though despots, regardless of their sex, are despots. Echoing "Brave New World," women are told that motherhood is a relic of a bygone era of servitude (Gustave Courbet, however, in his famous painting "L'Origine du monde," gave motherhood cosmic importance). Of course, not all women, and, in particular, not all younger women, are buying into masculinization. Data from a Vanderbilt University study shows that female graduates of elite schools (with superior earning potential) work far fewer hours than their counterparts from less selective schools. The presence of children strongly influences how much a women works [NYT 4/8/13 "Women with Elite Education Opting Out of Full-Time Careers" Joni Hersch]. Some, including the silent majority of women, would argue that nurturing the identity of another human being from birth on is of greater significance to humanity and more rewarding than struggling for a cut-throat edge as C.E.O. of a conglomerate.

Flying in the face of biology and common sense, there are no real sex differences either according to the pseudo-liberal media. Individuality is bad and, we are told, the plutocrat's homogenizer will right wrongs. The armament billionaires have profited from engineered wars that have snuffed out the lives of hundreds of thousands of American young men for nothing. Nevertheless, a strong military is the nation's backbone. The plutocrats' politicians, however, aim to enhance their pretended concern for equality even if they undermine the Marine Corps in the process. Women are to be cheered into combat, sleep in the same barracks as the men, use the same latrines, and are told by the media-ventriloquists that they are just as strong physically as men even if they aren't. The bonds created between soldiers in warfare are interpersonal, not a consequence of love for the flag. Aside from politics, might it be realistically difficult for a corps of young Marines to identify with a transgender officer? A letter in response to a politically-correct editorial in The New York Times [12/13/15] states the issue realistically: "Your emphasis on sexual equality is irrelevant to combat, where physical strength and agility can be the difference between life and death. If you were in an eight-soldier squad on patrol in Iraq wouldn't you rather have all men with you? If not, I suggest you go watch a professional football game." Few women want to become fighter pilots.

As for changing one's biologic sex, the clinical evidence strongly indicates that a transgender outcome in a child is the consequence of abnormal, dysfunctional parenting and is not, in itself, a reason for celebration. There is no evidence whatsoever that the emergence of transgender conflicts is biologic in origin. Treating emotional problems through mutilating surgery and hormone treatments cannot change the facts: every cell in the human body has either the female XX or the male XY chromosome. Does gender reassignment surgery solve or even ameliorate the emotional pain of those suffering from sexual identity conflicts? For answers we turn to a rigorous Swedish population-based matched cohort study carried out by the Karolinska Institutet [Dhejne C. et al. "Long-Term Follow-Up of Transsexual Persons Undergoing Sex Reassignment Surgery: Cohort Study in Sweden; PLOS one, 2/22/11]. 324 post-surgical sex-reassigned persons who were also assigned a new legal sex (191male-to-female, 133 female-to-male) were followed from 1973-2003 along with matched controls. The results: deaths from suicide were 19.1 times higher in the post-surgery group than in the matched controls. Suicide attempts were 4.9 times higher and psychiatric hospitalizations 2.8 times higher. Previous studies whose results were inconclusive had far fewer participants and were of short duration (4-6 years). The present study showed increased mortality beginning 10 years post-reassignment. The authors conclude that sex-reassignment "may not suffice as treatment of transsexualism, and should inspire improved psychiatric and somatic care after sex-reassignment for this patient group." Of course, the editorial board of The New York Times isn't in depth analysis of the facts. The across-the board shredding of sexual and cultural roles is politically motivated.

Shaming males into hanging themselves

As a physician, I am always amused by the warning leveled at the medical profession by politicians that, "if you don't co-operate, they'll do it without you." In other words, if you don't hang yourself first, they'll do it for you.

The ordinary male, a countervailing power block to the big business globalization agenda, is very much in the way, and therefore subject to unrestrained media attacks. Young men are depicted as mindless brutish cogs for whom gradual emasculation is the only cure. They aren't college material anymore we are told and don't even want to go to college unless they win the equivalent of the lottery, a football scholarship ($$$). Already a minority in college, they should always cheerfully take a back seat to further diversity, even though no group ends up ahead in a culture that consists of only two classes the super-rich and the underclass. True, males have been unfairly favored in the past and females unfairly restricted, but that is history. Media propaganda suggests that no sensitive males exist (they are from Mars) and they are always ruthless in their relationships with women, who are always victims. In the real world, men have also been victims: hundreds of thousands of young men are dead or maimed, herded into wars hatched by the captains of industry and their politician-allies; thousands of young men, the poor, are routinely raped in prisons but no one seems to care because they are not celebrities vying to make their power-mark in Hollywood and corporate America. To smoothly facilitate the plutocrat globalization agenda, the male in our society, the traditional bedrock of authority, is being targeted, the pretended pretext being that traditional female/male roles are bad.

Even The Boy Scouts are under attack. After 100 years, no longer "The Boy Scouts of America," the politician-administrators in charge now promote the inclusion of girls and delete the word "Boy" from the organization. Membership declined after the exodus of church sponsored participation in part due to allowing openly "gay" adults to serve as scout masters. While being gay, in and of itself, should not prohibit adults from serving, are adults who publicize being gay really good role models for susceptible young boys? Boys, apparently, are not to be allowed a boyhood anymore. They are to be pressured into a premature adulthood and their male identity formation undermined. The Girl Scouts of America are opposed to these changes.

In Sweden's pre-schools, a drive has been underway to eradicate the acknowledgement of gender differences [NYT 3/24/18 "In Sweden's Preschool, Boy's Learn to Dance and Girls to Yell"; Ellen Barry] and it is finding a receptive chorus among American university politician/bureaucrats. Initially promoted by a Swedish man who "wanted to breakdown the norm of stoic, unemotional, Swedish masculinity," the policy entails vacating the terminology that distinguishes sexual differences. "Boys" and "girls" words are to be replaced with "friends." Girls are told to shout "No" and boys assigned to the kitchen. A gender neutral pronoun is to be used. Girls are not supposed to draw girls with eyelashes and makeup "because boys have eyelashes too." Boys cannot sort themselves by gender. Otto, "a sturdy three year old" was wearing a dress. His mother wants this to continue" (a homosexual outcome and sexual identity confusion in accordance with the mother's and the schools message is not unlikely). Boys are to massage one another's feet and girls to throw open the window and scream. A teacher, Ms. Sandberg, says: "This is what we do here and it is not going to stop." Tanja Bergkvist, a columnist, says Swedes are afraid to criticize it in public. In the United States, politicians are actively joining this campaign to control the use of pronouns, speech, and thinking. This campaign is calculated to divert the public from the real issue: where all the money is going.

This is not "liberal" brainwashing, it is totalitarian brainwashing. Screaming girls is a code word for chaos. The elimination of a father rooted in reality is the end-goal. And, as I think back to elementary school, I don't recall girls "whimpering" all the time. Men who are hyper-masculine caricatures (and reflect a power-oriented culture) hardly justifies turning all men into obedient drones.

Historical resentments

"Penis envy," as conceptualized by Sigmund Freud, does have psychological symbolic validity. It has its origin in families where the male child is more highly valued and granted opportunities denied the female child, leading to resentment. Women should be free and encouraged to have any career within their capacities. No one should be forced to have children. Unwanted children will suffer. On the other hand, that only 20% of the Silicon Valley employed are women does not in and of itself prove discrimination. Women often seem more relationship oriented than men who, in turn, appear to gravitate more to technology and abstraction. Of course, such issues cannot be oversimplified and upbringing plays an important role. I must add that when I think back to elementary school, a number of girls I knew handled math with aplomb. Be that as it may, women currently obtain 65% of all graduate certificates, 52.2% of doctorates, and graduate in equal numbers to men in medicine and law. Such is not the case, however, in engineering and math. Of those who obtain a degree in engineering only 20% are women and, of those, 40% leave the field after graduation. Of those obtaining a doctorate in physics, only 19% are women. The American Institute of Physics concluded that these numbers were not the result of bias [Huffpost Science 7/2313 "Women in physics: no hiring bias..." by M. Cooper=White] In a British study, The Economist reported that when women's pay starts to fall behind men's, it tracks having their first child [The NYT "The 10 year baby window..." by Claire Miller, 4/8/18] Again, women should be encouraged to express their interest in any valid field they so desire, but men and women do not have to be carbon copies of one another nor are their differences necessarily proof of discrimination.

Lost boys

Currently, boys are being increasingly abandoned. In our society, a controlling oligarchy (interested only in money and basically sexless) is intent upon eliminating all human relationships. Add to this the fact that masculinity is under special attack, and we have a situation where boys and young men are in trouble. The plutocrats need to brainwash males early on so that they obey and co-operate with the agenda of multi-national corporations. Plutocrat media exploits feminist-activists who think they are furthering women's rights and opine a pretended level-headed objectivity in the service of equality: fathers should be side-lined and boys civilized (feminized) by putting feminists in the driver's seat, notwithstanding the fact that feminists are as irrational when it comes to understanding their rage at the opposite sex as machismo oriented males are toward women. Healthy self-assertiveness in a boy's spirit is, indeed, healthy and that includes expression of their inner sensitivity. In the Renaissance, men expressed their poignant feelings openly. Boys need fathers actively involved in their upbringing.

The facts are alarming. The Centers for Disease Control and Prevention showed increasing suicides for teenage boys: in 2015, for ages 15-19, there were 1,537 suicides among young men as opposed to 524 for young women. In 2017 it was 5016 suicides for boys and 1225 for girls. 43% of U.S. children live without their fathers (US Dept. of Census). 63% of youth suicides are from fatherless homes (US Dept. of Health/Census). 90% of all homeless and runaway children are from fatherless homes. 85% of all children who show behavior disorders are from fatherless homes. 71% of all high school dropouts come from fatherless homes. 75% of all adolescent patients in chemical abuse centers, 80% of all rapists, 71% of all pregnant teenagers come from fatherless homes.

A strong father is an obstacle to dismantling nations

Any authority, any power-block, that might jeopardize the plutocrat's total control of all the money is subject to stealth attack. Currently, their prime target is the middle class, in particular, the middle class father, the keystone of the family. Both the mother and father introduce the child to the world and aid the child in becoming an independent being. As Heinz Kohut ("self-psychology") once told me, it is the mother behind the chair that makes the chair real. But the father, the traditional authority figure, is the other lynchpin. A society without the guiding hand of a father is a society without structure and presages chaos. The Father is the first relationship and first step away from the Mother as the child strives for independence and attempts to connect with the world beyond. If the child's attempt to separate and individuate from the maternal figure is blocked, as it can be in the course of troubled mothering, the child will never become a person in its own right. There is a reason why research studies measure communication deviance from a disturbed mother to determine the risk for schizophrenia in the child. Schizophrenia represents, among other things, a break with reality, i.e. the real world. Extrapolating from the family unit, a society that has depreciated the role of the father is a society without moorings where the individual and individuality are likewise cast adrift. Our symbolic fathers, The Founding Fathers, are also under attack. Currently, with much exaggerated ballyhoo, a rap-musical with a cast of Hispanics and African-Americans, "Hamilton," depicts The Founding Fathers, Thomas Jefferson and George Washington as little more than conniving slave owners, but Alexander Hamilton, proponent of The U.S. Bank and an elitist, as having a heart of gold (a coin he greatly valued). As for Thomas Jefferson, were it not for him ("All men are created equal") and The Father of Our Country, Washington, there might not be a United States. With the accelerating demise of the middle class, the destruction of the unions, and a rudderless poor, any organized opposition to the outsourcing of jobs, whether industrial or high-tech, is effectively emasculated.

We can see the consequences of fatherless families in the black inner-city. Breaking up the black family during the era of slavery was a key to eliminating blacks as economic competitors and a key to maintaining subjugation. Presently, strong echoes of that strategy are at work undermining the middle class family. The white male father-figure, formerly a bulwark of the middle class, is an object of ridicule in the plutocrat controlled pseudo-liberal media. Big Business advertisements not infrequently depict white males, in the presence of women or minorities, as feckless weaklings. "Stupid white men" do exist but the dumbing-down of every faction of our society including women and minorities is a work in progress. Big Business cloaks their motives with pretended concern for the down-trodden. News then becomes propaganda. To be fair, white males are not the only perpetrators of racism, sexism, and hate crimes but they are a thorn in the side of the billionaire's globalization agenda, and, as such, need a good public whipping to teach them who really holds the reins of power. White male racists who murder innocent blacks are criminals. But blacks who have a history of racist hatred and murder innocent whites seem to be more thoughtfully characterized by The New York Times as products of mental illness (true). En suite the reportage shifts to the need for rational gun control (also true). The label "hate crimes," however, seems to be reserved for white males only. Racism unfortunately exists among all races. The recent episode of a sniper who gunned down five policemen and was quoted as saying that he "wanted to kill white people," for example.

As noted, the mother fixes reality for the child and the father reinforces independence. Most women, not all, want to rear children born of them. Few want to bec ome Navy SEALS or fighter pilots, while men seek self-assertion. Men fuel armies and revolutions. This poses a problem for the billionaire-China power-money goal of creating puppets that can further their unbridled commerce agenda. In the East, individual freedom is not historically valued as is the case in Western Culture. The puppet-masters see subjugation of the

American working class, particularly the whites, as the solution. The whites are too independent and have to learn to heel. Reeducation is necessary using Pavlovian dog methods. The billionaire companies and universities subject them to forced brainwashing under the pretext that they are Nazi racists. The goal is to emasculate and replace them with puppets.

Now enter the new Disney. Star Wars was a creative wildly popular series with a mostly white male cast depicting both Good and Evil. Disney bought the plot from Lucus Films and assumed that the white male Jedi were political dead meat. The last Jedi became a woman and all the white males were decrepit or eliminated. The female Jedi try to ape male warrior grim resoluteness. It was laughable. Next Disney's dead hand tries "The Acolyte". Now white males are completely eliminated by minorities, homosexuals and women. It flopped. Politics is death to the arts. The white male didn't feel it was ready for the museum. Inclusivity and diversity spawn parasites, rewarding merit, independence.

Children and childhood will not escape the plutocrat's purge of innocence. Brainwashing is most effective when started early in development [The New York Times, "Picture Books Try Giving Children a Taste of Kerouac and Capote," 12/19 16 by Alexandra After]. To be in compliance with the federal Education Department's Common Core testing program, schools must promote nonfiction over fiction. The rational for this is that baby must learn early how to compete in a global economy and maximize the chance of being admitted to elite schools. Of course, "nonfiction" does not necessarily insure critical thinking and it is the perfect vehicle for political propaganda. Creativity is fueled by the imagination and childhood is its fertile matrix. Robbing children of a secure childhood by exposing them to adult novels and political propaganda that they could not possibly understand is a corruption. Is present-day propaganda really morally superior to the propaganda of yesteryear? Who is selecting these works and what is their motivation in making the interpretations they choose to make? The end result will be puppets without imagination groomed to obey.

The plutocrat's academic arm

The elite educators appointed presidents of vaunted American universities have become the foot soldiers of plutocrat controlled educational priorities. Commanding multimillion dollar salaries and "earning" (a nice way of depicting a corrupt quid pro quo axis) millions more sitting on corporate boards curiously unrelated to education, they decree, by fiat, new rules governing morality and "inclusiveness" in the student-body, while the humanities and classics disappear from the curriculum and getting a job on Wall Street become the #1 motivation for getting an education. The average middle class young person, of course, won't make it to Wall Street, nor will poor minorities, unless one among them has the good luck to be appointed a corporate figurehead. The classics, formerly a fundamental component of a liberal arts education that valued critical thinking in the realm of the arts, ethics and society, no longer merit official academia's unreserved respect because they are deemed the product of a biased white male establishment. Of course, it is true that women were, for hundreds of years, not allowed a contributing voice. Nevertheless, the classics have endured because they reveal eternal truths above and beyond propaganda. Instead, we are led to believe, the student body must be politically indoctrinated in the only issues truly worthy of a forum: gender, gay-rights, white bigotry, and multiculturalism. Censorship and thought control are deemed morally justified in spite of the fact that The First Amendment, guaranteeing freedom of speech, is, above all, the one safeguard that protects us from dictatorship. Exaggerated attention is paid to mediocre, if not inferior, oeuvre by politically correct writers. The plutocrat's academic arm waves aside the "luddites" who call into question the inexorable march toward globalization and the dissolution of nations. Current diversionary news tells us that future automation and artificial intelligence are the real problem. No, there has always been ongoing automation (Charlie Chaplin's movie "Modern Times").In the past, however, the public's vision for their place in the future was encouraged. Today, brainwashing takes precedence over independent thinking.

College administrators are forcing young men to comply with a political agenda that denigrates masculine identity [Tucker Carlson Fox news]: Ohio State opines that masculinity is used to justify certain kinds of violence by men. Men are required to consult a male privilege check list. Duke University requires a nine week workshop: "Masculinity and Maleness." In Washington State, a women teacher banned boys from playing with legos. Wheaton College states: "We need to do a better job of addressing issues around toxic masculinity." Banning alcohol, not masculinity, at fraternity parties, might be a better solution to keeping both young men and women out of trouble. Valuing human relationships for both sexes is the only true foundation of true civilization.

Diverting the public from the real issues

We are led to believe that the public needs to be reeducated in order to fully appreciate the wisdom of multinational corporate agendas. This necessitates dismantling an independent middle class and working class power base. The billionaire's propaganda machines limit the news to topics that divert attention from the monstrous wealth disparities that are poisoning the nation, all the while pretending grave concern for morality. The so-called "left" is in fact a far cry from a true "left." They are merely another tentacle of the superrich. The plutocrats thrive on chaos.

The goal of the Billionaires is the elimination of individual property rights and ultimate enslavement of the individual

The climate control agenda: The global control of food production and the transfer of property from individual farmers to giant collective corporate farms or worse, synthetic food conglomerates. the EU (a pawn of Big Business) has been a willing tool along with the Dutch Prime Minister, to force the sale of thirty % or more of small farms in the Netherlands in order to comply with meaningless nitrogen/ammonia emission rules (China and India are exempt). Those farmers who resist will lose their farms. Police have shot at demonstrators. The Netherlands is the largest exporter of meat in the EU. These farms and cows have been in these families for hundreds of years. [USAA 7/8/22 "Dutch farmers protest climate policies that could drive them out of business…" by M. Nevradakis]. Eva Vlaardingerbroeck exposed a 600 million $ gift from Bill Gates to the brother of the Dutch Prime Minister who owns "Picnic" an online grocery company. She highlights corruption. Bill Gates has a goal to replace real meat with synthetic meat and plans to expand his control into the rest of Europe. Robert F. Kennedy Jr. hosted Christian Westbrook as they targeted the real goal of the climate control billionaires: the control of global food production. This has not been an isolated phenomenon.[BPR business and politics 7/9/22 "He owns 270000 acres" Ashley Hill] The Charlie Kirk Show. Here in the U.S. Bill Gates has been very active. Multiple sources reveal that he now has become the largest owner of U.S. farmland at one % total of American farmland, having recently won a legal battle in North Dakota to add to his 270,000 acres. He and the governor of North Dakota are reported to be good friends. Not far behind is Communist China that now owns 190,000 acres of U.S. farmland (as of 2020).

The ultimate aim to destroy single family home ownership, historically the #one means by which the middle class and working class could accumulate financial security.

[The New York Post 7/18/20 "How corporations are buying up houses, robbing families of the American dream" by Larry Gitlan] Ryan Dezember writes in his book "Underwater: How Our Dream of Homeownership Became a Nightmare" details in the aftermath of the subprime 2008 debacle and the massive foreclosures of 2011 how corporations swooped in to feast on distressed real estate. It was an opportunity, as Morgan Stanley termed it, to take advantage of "a rentership society." Corporate landlords raise rents by hundreds of dollars with little notice, care little about maintenance and shut out the middle class from ever owning a home. As of 2020, corporate giants like Blackstone Group owned 300.000 homes of what would become the tip of an iceberg.

[The Western Journal "Report indicates the devastating impact of covid 19 lockdowns on small business" by Steven Hall 6/16/21]. And [The Desert Review 6/14/21 "The number of small businesses destroyed by covid 19 lockdowns will astound you" Victoria Taft]. [The New York Post 7/5/21 by Carol Roth "Lockdowns were a gift to Big Business designed to kill small biz"] Nearly 40 % of small businesses were destroyed and closed as a result of lockdown policies. Big Businesses box stores thrived. Small business employs in total 50 million Americans. As is apparent, the new Democrat party isn't "leftist" at all. It is a tool of the billionaires to destroy the economic power of America and further their one world global control agenda. Just look below the phony "liberal" surface.

Turning to dehumanizing power in human relationships

In Das Rheingold, the first opera of Richard Wagner's Ring cycle, we see the Nibelung, Alberich, ridiculed and spurned by the Rhein maidens from whom he sought love. Only after being rejected does he espy the glint of the Rheingold....power.

We are the product of our life experiences as my clinical case p; in a second book will show. Men and women who control and dehumanize others are themselves products of parental neglect. They were never valued as persons in their own right. As a consequence, they turn to power instead of mutual intimacy. Unfortunately, true civilization, based on humanism, has yet to make its debut on the world stage.

It is hardly news that some men sadistically abuse women and dehumanize them sexually. Furthermore, it isn't a surprise that exploitation is common-place in pseudo-liberal Hollywood or the corridors of Big Business and Congress, where everything lis filtered through the prism of money and power. In my clinical practice, I have successfully treated women who acted out a self-destructive masochistic pattern vis á vis the worst kinds of men and were abused over and over again. Women caught in this trap suffer from low self-esteem and grew up in a family where their mothers denied them maternal support. Sex becomes a way to make contact at any price. The origin of these problems isn't limited to the father-daughter relationship as simplistic psychology would suggest. Recently I talked to a successful young women in her forties who told me that she has been living for many years with a man who doesn't want marriage. She said she loves him very much but was startled at a recent get together with "friends" when her partner told his "friend" to give her a sexually suggestive pat on her thigh, which the other man took him up on. In this initial session, she told me that she was starting to wonder if the relationship was what she had told herself it was. She also noted life-long depression and associated to an angry volatile mother who was an alcoholic. "My father was reliable and solid." "It looks like I'm involved with a man whose more my mother than my father." In short order it was revealed that this partner was involved in sado-masochistic relationships with several women and lied about it. She had been fooling herself all along, a consequence of her low self-esteem.

She had a dream that she gave her male partner a dress that she treasured whereupon he proceeded to refashion it by cutting and sewing. He returned it to her and at first glance it fit well until she noticed that he had removed the ruffle, the most beautiful part of the dress. The refashioned dress fit the role of a corrupted sex object. He was bent upon altering her identity. (Mozart's "Don Giovanni" in the character of Donna Elvira clearly recognizes this psychological problem). I read in The New York Times theatre review [1/30/18 "Liliom" Jon Sobel] of the play that the musical "Carousel" is based on: Molnar's "Liliom" whose last line spoken by the mother to her teenage daughter is: "It is possible, dear, that someone may beat you and beat you and beat you – and not hurt you at all."

But there is a current propaganda campaign that is aimed at all men. Curiously, only men, as a group, seem to be held accountable for moral lapses by Big Business media. All men apparently have the mark of Cain in the form of "toxic masculinity" and feminists are cheered for leading the way toward acknowledging long suppressed truths regarding feminine victimhood. In what is touted as an exposé, page after page of "The Times" is devoted to what is purported to be the nation's #1 moral lapse: sexual harassment. Propaganda makes it simple: Only men are predators and women are always victims. Unwanted flirting, touching, groping, and rape are seen as intertwined, all part of an evil spectrum in which women are victims. Big Business in its overarching concern for the bottom line, dismisses immediately any man so accused, regardless of the right to due process. But is touching the same as groping? Is flirting sexual harassment? It could be, of course, if a women's employment or career is on the line, but I am also aware of the fact that money and power create ruthless environments, not just for women but for the average man as well. Are women ever seductive to further their power and ambitions? Can women be manipulative? Controlling? Sadistic? Lie? I read of a male celebrity who tried to kiss a women in the 1990s (unsuccessfully). She recently brought this shocking episode to light. Title IX university trials of students accused of sexual misconduct are particularly stacked against the accused. Although they are not criminal proceedings, decisions are made that carry the weight of criminal convictions and ruin lives forever. The accused have no right to cross examine their accusers and decisions are rendered regardless of the right to due process. The accuser can appeal a decision until the sought for outcome is realized. Keith Mumphrey, an African-American student at Michigan State, was twice cleared, first by the police, then by a university trial, only to be tried a second time by the university without his knowledge, subsequent to which he was expelled from the school. When the Houston Texans found out, he was released from the football team and his career in pro football finished. The Duke lacrosse scandal damaged the lives of innocent men who were accused of rape, accusations that later proved to be lies. As we know from history, innocent people have been victimized. Alfred Dreyfuss was convicted in 1894 because of an underlying agenda: he was a Jew. The presumption of innocence for the accused is a fundamental right of Western Civilization.

Is it any news that a number of politicians could exploit the "sexual harassment" issue for political gain? In 2018, New York State's powerful attorney general was long celebrated by feminists as a super-hero, a self-styled feminist icon, who decried the mistreatment of women at the hands of men. He was quoted thusly: "We have never seen recently anything as despicable as what we are seeing here" and, "the challenges facing survivors are part of a larger system of discrimination and really a long overdue reckoning with our culture of violence and silence, manifestation of a culture of male supremacy." In his private life, however, he was exposed by four women as a man who sadistically slapped, beat and strangled them, sending women to the emergency room with bleeding from the ears and bruises. He also threatened them with punishment, adding "I am the law." He excused his behavior as "role playing." He recently resigned his office.

Leaving aside those at the helms of power who are mostly male, the average man is no more predatory than the average woman (and women who are in a position of power in powerful companies can be just as abusive as their male counterparts). Men and women are equally prone to opting out for controlling power-oriented partners (see my case studies that show both sides of the same coin). In Puccini's opera, Calaf abandons poor Liu for a grotesque Turandot while women fall victim to men like Picasso who viewed women as "machines for suffering." Women are no more victims in our culture than men and playing the helpless martyred role is not necessarily evidence of weakness. In some cases it has also been lucrative. The New York Times reports "How Some in the Finance Industry Are Trying to Cash In on #Me Too" 1/29/2018." By Matthew Goldstein et al. Through television advertisements and online, "Companies that offer money to plaintiffs in anticipation of future legal settlements are racing to capitalize on sexual harassment lawsuits," often charging 100 percent interest on their "advancement." In other words, it has become a way to make money. Working males still command influence in the work sphere, unions etc. and may need to be emasculated to give free reign to the unbridled globalization profit agenda as it reduces labor costs through cheap and slave labor.

As ordinary individuals, it is doubtful that men are of lesser character than women or women more righteous than men. It seems that many feminists cloak themselves in the mantel of the unassailable perfect mother (fathers are merely mortal). Far from the sanctimonious sarcastic cliché that "it's always the mother," in our culture, holding the mother accountable is the greatest of all taboos. How does it go....flag, apple pie, and ....? The mother is not a powerless martyr as the childhood game of "mother may I?.." attests. Recently, a feminist classicist's new novel makes Circe, the witch from Homer's Odyssey, who turned men into swine, a heroine. She, according to The New York Times, noted that Circe was created by men (Homer) who were prejudiced, victimized women, and failed to understand a women's psychology. I do recall, however, that men also created Aphrodite, Athena (for whom Athens was named), Demeter, Penelope who was loyal to Odysseus, and Psyche. Some years ago, I was in Tübingen Germany with a friend and was about to enter a feminist bookstore. A hostile female employee forbad my entry because I was a man.

The creative arts are the next target of the plutocrat homogenization agenda to emasculate male self-assertion. New Hollywood screenplay software tells you whether or not your script accords the same number of words for female characters as male characters in spite of the fact that the arts, above all, should be free of implicit censorship even if they do not conform to politics. David Leonhardt, NYT columnist, is a proponent of software that shows, in various fields, how many women are quoted in articles as opposed to men. He will strive, he says, to correct this imbalance. That is his right. What is not right, however, is to suppress freedom of speech and abet politicians, scrounging for the imagined women's vote, to pass legislation that installs political gender mandates in the arts and journalism. Censoring the heritage of the past according to some kind of gender scale will ensure a cultural graveyard. Creativity and thought control cannot co-exist even if politicians call it "Pravda." Will Titian/Georgione's beautiful "Sacred and Profane Love" and "Fête champêtre" be relegated to a forthcoming political Entartung? At the Manchester Art gallery, a Pre-Raphaelite painting, "Hylas and the Nymphs" by the Victorian artist John William Waterhouse that depicted Hylas, a companion of the mythological hero Heracles, being lured into a lily pond by several naked young women (he did not survive) was altogether removed from public view. A female artist and the gallery's administration appealed to the righteous need for a cultural critique of current gender priorities. She stated that "power" was in play because people feel entitled to view particular works. But whose power, the people's or that of tunnel vision feminist-activists and bureaucrats? The beautiful painting was eventually restored [NYT 2/7/18,"A Barometer of Public Taste" J.Fortin]. "Sexual harassment," put in context, can be directly tied to the devaluing of human relationships in a power-driven culture where both men and women opt out for simply "hooking up." True sexual harassment is a matter for the police. The lives of a number of young men have been tarnished if not ruined by university politicians for political reasons. Women are being used as foils to play their part in dismantling a supposed male powerstructure. The real power, however, resides with the plutocrats whose media apparatus orchestrates a divide and rule agenda.

Political correctness and censorship are one and the same. The National Gallery of Art, the nation's museum, has cancelled an exhibition of the painter Chuck Close's work because of sexual harassment allegations in his personal life. Banishing artistic expression because of alleged misconduct in the artist's personal life, is more chilling and a greater threat to our democracy than the alleged personal indiscretions. Totalitarian regimes have always claimed the right to "protect" the public from artistic expression they deemed unsuitable. There is always an underlying political agenda and it is thought control. The Nazis burned books by Jews and others and censored the exhibition of German expressionists (Die Entartung). Is it wrong to censor art because of current politics. Should the reading of T.S.Eliot be banned because he was an anti-Semite?

The multi-layered agenda and the politics of unrestrained immigration

The people are branded as racists by the plutocrat media unless they welcome a tidal wave of illegal immigrants, many of whom are rejecting of and fundamentally hostile to Western culture, Western Culture where the value of the individual was first recognized. No doubt the Ancient Greeks would have been branded far-right extremists/xenophobes by the plutocrat-media for resisting the Persian onslaught. As a matter of fact, we come upon "Making

Museums Moral Again" [Holland Cotter; The New York Times, 3/17/16] in which The Times anointed art critic sanctimoniously enlightens us with his exposé of corporate money's influence on art museums, along with the "truth" about the Vietnam War, historical white-on-black exploitation, anti-fossil fuel protesters throwing muck in the Louvre etc.. He allows that we can appreciate beautiful objects but should be informed of how the benefactors of a beautiful object were often immoral plutocrats. Is he telling us something we don't know? His rear-view insights are 20:20 but he is hardly independent of current politics. Having validated his pseudo-liberal veneer of politically correct credentials, he gets to the newspaper's real point, that being the politics of globalization. Thus, the Ancient Greeks, the cradle of nascent democracy and Western civilization, were really racists who "[conjured] an image of populations outside Greece's borders – Persians, for example – as dark, disease-carrying agents of chaos, an image often applied in many cultures to immigrants today." He finds Greek classical art admirable "but it is also an assertion of ethnic exceptionalism in a barbaric, Other-filled world." Even the term "classical," he implies, connotes a power-conspiracy because it implies a qualitative ranking of objects and ideas as superior or less-than. The politics of Globalization necessitates homogenization in support of a nationless one-world agenda (otherwise there could be resistance to outsourcing). If the art critic had independent insight, he could honestly fault the corporate largess for dumbing down the public and the museums with dehumanizing junk masquerading as high art. The Met is succumbing, the Frick never. No, you do not have to believe that all cultures are equal. As for labeling those who oppose opening the floodgates to immigrants from opposing cultures, "racists," the premise is that witnessing one's own culture washed away is little more than a trifle. Apparently, if an American working class family were transported to China and forced to live there, they shouldn't have any feelings about it.

Aside from cheap labor for the plutocrats, is it really in the cultural interests of Western countries to open wide the floodgates for global immigration? In the name of Islam, for example, countless terrorist acts have taken place around the world. While the majority of Muslims are tolerant, including those who have been in this country for generations, many of the stricter religious doctrines of radical Islam are intolerant, leading to fanatic repression of women, persecution of homosexuals, violence against Christians and even other Muslims. If their fundamental religious orthodoxy is operative, representation of the human figure in the plastic arts (aniconism) is prohibited. Logically, an ideology based on those principles has some fundamental differences with the heritage of Western humanism. Yes, the Papal armies of Alexander VI led by his murderous son Cesare Borgia were gangsters, not to mention the Inquisition, but Jesus preached compassion for the individual. Muhammed led armies for political and territorial conquest. A case in point: Italian politicians recently boxed-up the classical nudes of the Capitoline Museum in Rome so as not to offend a visiting Islamic dignitary. Big business supports illegal and wholesale immigration for the same reason that they outsource American jobs, namely cheap/slave labor for the plutocrat mills.

"The "greater good" and the best interests of the individual

In the name of "self-sacrifice" the individual has been exploited since the beginning of time. Self-sacrifice "for the greater-good" has always been the directive the totalitarians employed to further their pursuit of power and money. They, of course, are exempt from self-sacrifice. Currently, the plutocrat media tells us we are supposed to be ashamed if we don't celebrate the dissolution of Western Culture by the "all cultures are equal" globalization agenda. Realistically, however, the eventual take-over of existing Western nations by a tidal wave of the impoverished from third world countries could have disadvantages for the existing inhabitants of Western nations even though multinational corporations and certain politicians will profit. The principles of Humanism and The Golden Rule do not demand that one self-sacrifice one's own best interests. Clinically, every major emotional disorder has its origin when the child is forced to give up their own best interests and their identity in order to get along with dysfunctional parents.

A conservative, Mark Krikorian [The Wall Street Journal, 3/25-26/2017 "The Immigration Dodge"] writes that an authoritative study published in 2016 by the National Academies of Sciences, Engineering and Medicine (NAS) found that immigration creates a small net economic benefit by lowering the wages of Americans competing with immigrants by $500 billion but in turn benefiting businesses by $550 billion. The nativeborn disenfranchised working class have the most to lose from the politics of unbridled immigration. Low-skilled immigrants command low wages, pay little in the way of taxes, yet are the recipient of extensive government medical and welfare benefits. The NAS examined the balance between services used by immigrants and taxes paid and found that the fiscal drain to be as large as $299 billion a year. Mr. Krikorian also points out the need in any culture for stability, cohesion, a sense of solidarity and fundamental affection for our fellow citizens that we do not share with those of other countries. An unbridled influx of immigrants who have little interest in integrating Western values leads to cultural instability and chaos [see also the epidemiological studies in Part V that show an increased incidence of stress and serious mental illness when the culture with which one identifies becomes fragmented and foreign].

All races are equal as human beings, but not all cultures are equal. Ancient Greece for the first time in recorded history upheld the value of the individual, the cornerstone of a potentially true civilization and the foundation of Western Culture: "Know Thyself" the inscription on the Temple of Apollo, Delphi. Democracy, and for the first time, the depiction of man whole and unabstracted, attests to the value Greece placed on the individual. Our Founding Fathers echoed these truths in the Constitution and The Bill of Rights. Confucius prioritized our obligations to society and the state but the rights of the individual were ignored. The further East you go, the more corrupt it is. That all cultures are equal is billionaire politics for dismantling Western Culture to favor their economic alliance with Communist China. Is the Parthenon superior to backward culture's junk? Yes, it is Unbridled immigration composed of illiterate, impoverished 3rd world illegal aliens that will soon replace the white American majority is deemed a "gift" to America, states current President Biden. Clearly the one world economic agenda of the billionaires will be gifted as will Communist China as America is destroyed. The problem is that the narcotized white working class is not organized. Were it to openly exercise their robust political might, forcing them to roll over and get raped would be history. The propaganda of the tech-giants of course would smear any resistance to their agenda to emasculate the white working class as "racism" and "white supremacy." Replacing the majority of Americans with hostile cultures from around the world is a "gift" and "good" according to the politician puppets of the billionaires. Good for whom? Americans and America come first, not billionaire's blood money. America is sliding into chaos by design. Encouraging mob violence lawlessness, arson, looting, as justified reparations for slavery that occurred 200 years ago is the means by which the billionaires consolidate their dictatorship. White sociopaths lend a helping hand too, eager to find an excuse for mayhem. Politicians nod their approval. They are "The Lord of the Flies." Prison is the obvious solution for those who revel in violence.

The billionaires are not egalitarians. Empires seek riches by relying on slave labor and subjugation. The classics and liberal arts that promote critical thinking have been eliminated from education. Western culture, that validates the worth of the individual, stands in the way of globalization and the limitless profits thereby envisioned by the super-rich. A cauldron of constant change and insecurity (a critical tool for effective brainwashing) in a culture that stifles critical thinking, leaves only one authority, the plutocracy. The Apollonian principle of order and moderation is valued throughout history because it is the foundation of civilization. Nobel prize winning economist Angus Deaton and economist Anne Case recently published a paper showing that mortality rates among middle-aged white Americans has been rising since 1969 while death rates among other groups has been falling. The cause?: marked increase in suicides, drug poisoning and alcoholism. Martin Gillins of Princeton University and Benjamin Page of Northwestern University examined 1,779 policy issues and found that attitudes of wealthy groups and business groups mattered a great deal to the final outcome, but that preferences of average citizens were almost irrelevant [Nicholas Kristof, NYT 1/21/16 "America the Unfair?"]. The middle-class, lacking both organization and shrill political activists, has become the number one political minority, smoothing the way for plutocrat totalitarian control.

What then is the solution? Tax the plutocrats at sixty to ninety percent and give that money back to the people.

Dehumanization: Wiping out memory and personal history

Totalitarian forces predictably aim to scrub our minds clean of any memory of the past. In so doing, they refashion reality according to the politics that furthers their current ambitions and power. A culture that revers other loyalties, and individuals that remember their personal history threaten the mindless allegiance to those who seek absolute control. The Nazis solemnly proclaimed "Die Neue Ordnung," Mao manipulated the youth and created The Red Guard that destroyed China's heritage, and, as of this writing, The Islamic State is destroying all art and artifacts of ancient cultures and killing those who think independently. The plutocrats have a parallel aim. Peddling their money, they have corrupted official psychiatry, academia, and the political apparatus. Their mouthpieces say that all emotional problems and all motivating predilections are inborn and genetically determined.

Our memories of past experiences that have shaped us have curiously disappeared from the literature, both "scientific" and popular. The fundamental influence of life experiences, parenting, and interpersonal relationships are never mentioned anymore. Eliminating our personal history erases our identity as individuals and ends in puppetry. And, by the way, the plutocrat media is not above ignoring violence if it fits their political agenda.

"Inundated with information"?

It is apparent that those who style themselves of "the right" (don't tax the super-rich) or "the left" (tax the super-rich a little bit but censor first amendment rights in education) rely on propaganda (the manipulation of politically motivated half-truths/lies) rather than a balanced presentation of the facts. Politics and, yes, money, affects the scientific community as well. Invoking the word "Science" and "studies show" does not in itself guarantee objectivity. Who is funding the "research" and what is their underlying agenda? For example, [NYT 3/18/18 "NIH to Investigate Outreach to Alcohol Companies" Roni Rabin] The National Institute of Health, a government agency, is currently launching a $100 million research project to determine whether moderate amounts of alcohol have certain health benefits. A Harvard University academician is overseeing this research but executives from the alcohol industry are intimate partners in the project and funding the research. The National Institute of Mental Health, receives outright grants from the pharmaceutical industry to fund "research." Do you think money influences the findings? Researchers are beholden to grant money: no grant money, no job. How will an academician rise in academia without the big business/government grant money? At present, as part of the plutocrat agenda to eliminate the importance of the mind and human relationships, all current research aims to emphasize primary brain/gene factors in spite of incontrovertible scientific and clinical to the contrary.

In humans, the environment is primary and, in turn, changes the brain and controls genetic expression. The pretext for dismissing the accumulated in-depth clinical findings of trained experts, who have worked in the real world with patients, is the assertion that these findings are not backed up by randomized controlled trials, the so-called gold standard for scientific research. In defense of expertise, Jamie Homes [NYT Sympathy For the Dentist; 11/27/16] quoted a spoof scientific article that maintained that we don't know if parachutes really work because we have no randomized controlled trials of them. Follow the money.

Divide and rule through propaganda

A strong and independent middle class and working class could thwart the plutocrat's globalization profit agenda. The stagnating incomes of the ninety-five % struggling with the high cost of raising a family ("there is NO inflation!!") will someday lead to calls for a redistribution of wealth. The outsourcing of jobs will also be jeopardized. The plutocrat's have a solution: whittle down the middle class and working class power structure rendering them ineffectual. And if they complain about it, accuse them of racism and fascism. It is crucial as well to demonize the male in our society because they assert themselves too much. They need to obey!

"At his best, man is the noblest of all animals. Separated from law and justice, he is the worst," Aristotle, 384-322 B.C.

Law: Let's illustrate an example of propaganda used to burnish the media's (pretended left-wing) concern for the down-trodden and divert attention from their fundamental support of the plutocrat establishment, their financial benefactors: the reportage concerning the greater percentage of African-Americans incarcerated in American prisons versus other races. Prominent self-styled liberal newspapers label that statistic proof of blatant racism. A balanced presentation of the data, however, should also include the fact that African-Americans, who constitute 13% of the population, commit 50% of all the murders in the U.S.. On average, blacks murder more than twice as many whites as white on black murder [FBI statistics for 2018]. It is also irresponsible to convict anybody in the public media without a trial or a full discovery of the facts. The ACLU, in the past, rightfully supported the right of any political group to peacefully demonstrate, including Nazis and Communists.

Violence, arson and looting, however, is against the law and not compatible with a civilized society. According to official statistics, some fifty police officers were shot to death in 2014 [NYT 12/31/14 "Number of Police Officers Killed on the Job Climbs" Timothy Williams]. In 2016, by July 28, 66 police were shot to death [NYT 7/28/16 "Deaths So Far This Year" N. Chokshi] (equally divided between black and white perpetrators according to Fox News).62 police were murdered in 2021. Roland G. Freyer, a professor of economics at Harvard and an African-American, author of a new study, found that there was no evidence of racial bias in police shootings or use of lethal force [NYT 7/12/16 "Surprising New Evidence Shows Bias in the Police Use of Force but Not in Shootings" Q. Bui et al]. Relentless editorials in the NYT decry stationing police in inner-city public schools but ignore the classroom conditions that mirror the societal conditions in the inner-city which necessitate such measures. Even one rebellious student in a classroom where needed discipline is lacking, makes learning to read and write impossible. Propaganda fuels "studies" that claim that black students are being unfairly disciplined in schools compared to white or Hispanic students. Lies will not, however, improve the circumstances of African-Americans. It may be an inconvenient truth, but a higher percentage of blacks are disruptive in the classroom than other groups (ask any teacher). Former President Clinton's 1994 crime bill added 100,000 cops on the beat, that, along with "broken windows" policing, led to mass incarceration but also a 33 year low in the murder rate.

Justice: The above observations may be true, but African Americans are indeed subjected to racism. Blacks are herded into prison for drug addiction (one-fifth of those entering prison since the 1990's according to John F. Pfaff of Fordham University) rather than treated as human beings with measures that recognize the need for treatment. The poor, in general, are brutalized in an incredibly barbaric prison system. Why aren't humane efforts made toward rehabilitation as is the case in Germany where rehabilitation is the top priority?

Inner-city African-Americans are destitute because jobs at decent wages are unavailable and families are broken. There is a profound disparity in the quality of education among the different classes that giving each child a computer cannot correct. The legacy of slavery and the callous neglect of the economically impoverished is ongoing. Should the police be allowed to force DNA sampling when no charges have been filed, or confiscate cars, houses and bank accounts without convicting or even charging someone with a crime and then dispersing these funds to the local police organizations? No question that there exists chaotic conditions in the black inner city but all of us are equal as human beings and are born with the same potential, so what is the origin of this chaos? No efforts are made to stop black on black violence or provide productive stability. Slavery was instituted by plutocratic forces for money. It is an ongoing legacy. The dishonest super-rich aren't losing any sleep over it. The New York Times claims a liberal cachet, but, aside from spotty veneers, it has been less than sincere when it comes to fighting for the political changes that would create a more humanistic culture. I don't recall any headlines demanding the appropriate taxation of the plutocrats in a manner that would address the toxic wealth disparity in this country, taxation that would go a long way, through job creation and education, to uplift the impoverished poor and aid a true middle class recovery. Perhaps a December 30, 2015 near-headline represented a turning point in the paper's politics: "By Molding Tax System, Wealthiest Save Billions – Hiring an Army of Lobbyists and Lawyers to Exploit Loopholes and Steer Laws" by Noam Scheiber and Patricia Cohen.

But, for example, the paper's stance leading up to the 2016 presidential election hardly reflects run-away liberalism. The Times officially endorsed Wall Street's choice for the

Democratic nomination while depicting the alternative Democratic candidate, Senator Bernie Sanders, a knowledgeable and courageous champion of the working class and middle class, as little short of looney. His lunacy? He embraces a social-support network concept that has been successfully in place in Europe for decades (free college tuition, medical care etc.) to be paid for by appropriately taxing the Wall Street billionaires. Of course, he might not have been able to achieve all of his goals had he been elected, but he unflinchingly looked the enemy in the eye. As for his frequently invoking the problem that is "Wall Street," The Times wondered if the citizenry didn't find it all a little too "esoteric." Appallingly, The Times three key columnists curiously fell into line, supposed liberals who champion gay activism, African-American rights, and a Nobel Prize winning economist. To a man, they denigrated Senator Sanders as a manipulative, if not dangerous, fool. The Republican establishment was also fearful. Donald Trump, who put America first, like Senator Sanders, had a groundswell of popular support and, back then, the Republicans weren't so sure that he could be counted upon to support the unbridled profit agenda of giant corporations, including the outsourcing of American jobs. His speeches rightfully questioned whether the American public should feel gratified that outsourcing had lifted some of the Chinese from dirt-poor poverty at the cost of the well-being of the American middle class.

The middle class and blue collar working class, economically foundering, elected President Trump causing consternation and alarm among the billionaires. Would globalization be jeopardized? The Times publishes: "In Trump, Tech Leaders Fear a Challenge to Their Vision"; 11/19/16. Regarding Amazon, Apple, Facebook, Google and Microsoft, the paper states: "Leaders of these behemoths have long spoken in ambitious, gauzy sentimentalities about a broadly progressive future. Their goals weren't simply financial but, they said, philosophical and democratic…" And there is, "In Year of Anti-Muslim Vitriol, Promoting Inclusion"; NYT 1/1/17 S. Maheshwari, an advertisement showing a Christian pastor greeting his friend, a Muslim Imam, as they commiserate about their arthritic knees and lovingly open up a package of knee-pads purchased through Amazon. The Times opines that the ads were "apolitical," a dramatization of two religious in a friendly dialogue. I suspect, however, that gauzy sentimentalities took a back seat to globalization's pursuit of money. The silliest notion is that Google, Facebook, etc. are primarily motivated by ideology and "a vision." No, they are motivated by power, money, and control. Also, in the fullness of time, it became clear that the tech behemoths had little to fear from the Republican establishment. America First was not its top priority.

Unfortunately, the hoped for populist revolution was in part thwarted and the plutocrats have extended their control. The Republican establishment maintains that Mr. Trump was elected because he promised to repeal "Obamacare" and pass "taxreform." No, that's not quite accurate.

He was elected because he hoped to revitalize the forgotten working class and middle class. The Republican foot soldiers for Big Business dug in to head off solutions to the nation's enervating trade imbalance with China, citing scary 1929 scenarios because of short term economic dislocations while ignoring the long term effects of such a massive transfer of wealth to a hostile foreign power. The then President Trump's policy on China took immense courage to enact but he found that Big Business would do everything in its power to reverse course and isolate him. The super-rich were still in the driver's seat. That was indeed what happened in 2020.

For the plutocrats and their politician puppets in Congress, the American people are little more than chattel. The billionaires and corporate America received a gigantic windfall: $1.5 trillion reduction in taxes. Republicans, with a straight face, informed us that only 25% of the public (what's left of the middle class) take deductions on their income tax, so property, state and local taxes deductions can be phased out (how else can the country pay for the billionaire's tax windfall?). Laughably, the Republican establishment pretends outrage because the "rich living in blue states" (the middle class) are getting away with murder by deducting state and local property taxes. Of course, the .01%, making tens of millions to hundreds of millions a year, hardly worry about such trifles. A majority of the public in both parties never felt that slashing corporate taxes was their #1 priority, especially since, prior to "tax reform," the biggest corporations have never been more profitable and already dominate the world stage.

["Tax Cuts Do Raise Pay, for Bosses" NYT 1/28/18 Jim Tankersley]: The Republican tax law has slashed the federal corporate tax rate to 21 percent from 35 percent. It is claimed that this will result in big pay raises for workers. Many economists, however, say that most of these gains will accrue to shareholders and top executives not worker's salaries. Companies will be allowed to repatriate billions if not trillions in untaxed profits stashed overseas by reducing the federal tax load to 15.5 percent on cash held offshore. Apple says it will repatriate most of the $252 billion it holds abroad by making a onetime tax payment of $38billion….a mere fraction of what it would have had to pay under the prior tax structure.

["Big Rewards for Corporations That Moved Money Offshore" NYT 11/30/17, Jesse Drucker] A similar Republican tax law in 2004, the American Jobs Creation Act allowed companies to repatriate foreign profits at a one-time rate of just 5.2 percent. Companies used the money to buy back their stock but didn't expand their American work force. Pfizer, for example, brought home $37 billion and shed 10,000 workers. Hewlett-Packard bought back more than $14 billion while eliminating 14,000 jobs. Thereafter, companies again parked their profits overseas beyond tax authorities and into low or zero tax havens like Bermuda, Ireland and The Island of Jersey (Apple). The stock market is, for the time being, rising parabolically, but 50% of the American public don't have even one dollar in the stock market. On 8/23/18, The New York Times, it was reported that as of 2016, the last year with solid data, the wealth of the median American household was 34% below where it was just before the Great Recession.

Quick to forestall public outrage that could sweep the Republican establishment out of congress (and later did just that), a few giant corporations make a big show of granting bonuses to their employees of a thousand dollars or so (see how the trickle-down theory is already starting to pay off for the little guy!). Of course, bonuses are not pay raises. Neither party is honest. The Democrat candidate was sure that she could win the 2016 election by shrewdly cobbling together the minority vote. She failed. Her party had to wait awhile for enough illegal immigrants to gain voting rights to tip the scales their way. Fabricated issues abound. There was much heat being generated in the so-called left-wing press about Russian meddling in U.S. elections. The average American rightfully yawns at the claim that Russian conniving altered the 2016 election outcome. The Democrat establishment continues to bank on diverting the public from the real issues: appropriate taxation of the billionaires, the despicable gutting of healthcare, the toxic wealth disparity in America, the destruction of the middle class, the impotence of a once vital working class, in short: economic issues. Instead, their so-called "left-wing" media (a tool of multinational corporations) claims that the American people salivate for unrestrained cheap-labor immigration and open borders. The desire to preserve a nation's cultural integrity, both here and in Europe, is deemed "the death of democracy!!" (plus it interferes with the globalization money-agenda). The entrenched establishment of both parties are puppets of the super-rich. The country needs a third party.

"1984" in 2021

President Trump was not re-elected. The billionaires and their allies Communist China did everything possible to discredit him, including relentless propaganda and street mobs, because he attempted in spite of imperfections to put America first. Their goal is to destroy the United States as a nation, destroy Western Culture and destroy individual liberty. Their incentive is money through one-world globalization where they control everything. The political upheaval currently is being described by some as Marxist. Wall Street gave 4x as much money to the new Democrat party than to their old friends, the Republicans. Is Wall Street Marxist? Big Business according to Michael Pillsbury of the Hudson Institute invested 1-3 trillion $ in Communist China (ATT, Apple, Bloomberg, Facebook). Is Big Business Marxist? Facebook's Mark Zuckerberg gave $450,000,000 in the last election to influence the outcome in swing states. The billionaires conceal their motives by pretending to support leftist populist causes. Many Republicans seem the most irate about any suggestion of taxation of the billionaires (that's "redistribution of wealth" !!). If the real enemy are Marxists, not billionaire fascists, you certainly don't want to redistribute the wealth to a bunch of Marxists. The billionaires are not "terrified" by the current trends nor do they "hate business" as one brain-dead Republican guru said.

The problem is fascist wolves dressed up in socialist sheep's clothing. That the Nazis called themselves National Socialists did not make them socialists. Nor was The Union of Socialists Republics other than a dictatorship. A campaign to weaken and humiliate America at home and abroad, thus paving the way for globalization, has a central target: weaken the white working class and middle class. They are the only remaining power block that might resist the plutocrat agenda. Relentless propaganda claims that the #1 problem facing the nation is white racism. While the great majority of black Americans do not participate in these lies, a small minority, including some in Congress, are exploiting this propaganda. They openly encourage looting, arson and violence against whites and Asians while condoning criminals (its justified as reparations for slavery that happened 200 years ago). Remarkably, the white majority is supposed to kneel down before rioting criminals and suffer humiliation including violation of their Civil Rights. Big Media spews relentless propaganda having learned well Hitler's advice: If you repeat a big enough lie often enough, they will come to believe it. Recently, a young man was found innocent of murder by a jury in Wisconsin. For a year, Big Media described him as a white supremacist in spite of the fact that he had no such history and the added fact that the two men he shot were white. Two days later, also in Wisconsin, a black man drove his truck into a Christmas parade, killing 6 whites. His criminal rap sheet was 50 pages long with a long history of anti-white hatred. MSNBC's anchor chose to ignore mentioning him altogether in the tragedy or his obvious anti-white motivation. The Milwaukee D.A. had just released this man on $1000 bail for attempting to run over the mother of his child. Defending the miniscule bail this D.A. intones that releasing criminals like this will no doubt have consequences but the greater good takes precedence. So it is with irresponsible "dirty politicians".

Weakening the power of America is happening militarily as well. America's top general, a worthless sycophant, sees "white rage" as his primary worry. "Diversity" not military preparedness are his burning issues. This same Chairman of the Joint Chiefs of Staff was reported, in a new book by Bob Woodward and Robert Costa of The Washington Post, to have called the top Chinese General and reassured him that he would warn him in advance about any planned American attack, all without President Trump's knowledge. He also labeled Trump supporters Hitlerian "brown shirts", adding: "We're the guys with the guns." This miserable sycophant is quoted as saying "Trump is a fascist to the core." Men are the backbone of any fighting force which should rest on merit not politics. Of course, the armament industry promotes lies for money to prolong unwinnable wars (we were "winning in Vietnam" plus there was "the domino effect" while in Afghanistan "there would be worldwide terrorism if we don't stay engaged for another 20 years in spite of further American blood and more trillions). Granted, the corrupt puppet in the White House mystified the world by pulling out in a rout leaving $85billion in cutting edge military equipment and stranding Americans who now are hostages of the Talaban. After the Talaban suicide bomber killed 13 American soldiers we are told that the Talaban are "business-like and gave their word ($$$)." We learn that a man dressed-up as a woman is the first 4 star "woman" military officer to achieve such an honor. Every cell in his body has the XY male chromosome.

First Amendment rights have been suspended. The billionaires own the news outlets (CNN, NBC etc.). The tech giants (Google, Facebook, etc.) censure any opinions with which they disagree. Former President Trump is denied access to these news organs. Parler and Veritas have been silenced. Noted constitutional scholar Alan Dershowitz, a Democrat, affirmed that we have the right under the First Amendment to freedom of speech, including Communists and Nazis, as long as they do not incite violence.

The ongoing campaign to turn America into a third world cesspool is the top goal of the Biden Administration, thus insuring votes for continued political control and permanent dilution of the white working class who it is assumed are Trump supporters. In a few months hundreds of thousands, soon to be millions, of dirt-poor illegal aliens from around the world are welcomed and ferried all over the U.S. to join the welfare rolls, and win a quick path to citizenship while Americans languish. These illegal aliens are exempt from covid vaccination mandates because they are votes that will hasten the billionaire's agenda of turning America into an obedient satellite that will acquiesce to their one-world economic blueprint. Many of them are criminals and drug traffickers but are deemed exempt from deportation. The Administration plans to offer illegal aliens who were jailed for violating U.S. immigration laws $450,000 per person for pain and suffering, $1,000,000 per family. Americans who died for their country? Gold Star families get a quarter of that. Drug cartels awash young Americans with fentanyl from China leading to over 100,000 American deaths in 2021. The new Democrat party is deeply concerned about gun control because of the huge increase in crime but fights any attempt to enforce the law and advocates defunding the police.

An important destabilizing ploy to destroy America's independence is the strategy of promoting violence. Thus, looting and arson, robbery, home invasion, even murder, are rationalized. Criminals escape being arrested or prosecuted. Instead the politicians call for defunding the police when they themselves should be jailed and prosecuted for encouraging lawlessness. Violent crime has skyrocketed. Criminals should be held accountable for what they do to their victims.

The billionaires cloak themselves in virtue pretending that they are for the little-guy. Major corporations, pretend that they are aghast at America's #1 problem, white racism.

They require their white employees to undergo re-education and admit that they are racists. Thus, in this virtuous endeavor, count Raytheon in (a corporation in the business of killing people). Giant corporations have instituted diversity hiring policies that disenfranchise whites and Asians because they are not black. The Ford Foundation masquerades as a charity. Billionaires stash billions in these so-called charities tax free which in turn fund grants to public and private universities, also tax free. The grant money is geared for anti-American propaganda and decimation of the white working class. The aim is the destruction of American independence and the furtherance of a one-world agenda. At Arizona State University two white students were vehemently vilified by a recipient of a Ford Foundation grant for sitting in a study hall "reserved for multi-cultural students." One student wore an insignia that proclaimed "police lives matter." Advocating black lives matter and police lives matter are equally protected under the Constitution. Big Business is always for the little-guy. That's why they forced Major League Baseball out of Georgia because the state wanted voters to show ID's before casting a ballot. Of course, no mention is made of Big Business's anti-Trump agenda. Corporate America is not beyond betraying America when profits are at stake. The NBA and Hollywood, controlled by billionaires, couldn't care less about what happens to this nation. Enes Kanter Freedom, NBA star, paid a price for calling out Communist China for its human rights abuses. Profits of NBA's owners were jeopardized. Hollywood ditto.

America has one principal adversary on the world stage, that being Communist China. The billionaires, however, have only one priority, money. Schultz of Starbucks states that "China is a friend and an ally." Bloomberg acquiesces to Chinese censorship "because otherwise you are out of the country." Apple readily hands over its apps to China and exploits Chinese sweat shops. Human rights violations against Moslems and Christians aren't even taken seriously. Totalitarian abuses, so what? Bill Gates expressed admiration for the Chinese dictatorship. Peter Schweizer's book "Red Handed" reports that the Biden family earned $31,000,000 from doing business with Communist China, our enemy. The Bush family, Nancy Pelosi and Diane Feinstein made millions as well.

Big Business will adopt these same tactics in regard to Americans. Under President Trump, America became energy independent. To weaken The United States, under the pretext of climate control, President Biden reversed these huge economic gains while exempting China and India from pollution constraints. "Climate control" has become politics for charlatans. 50 million years ago, palm trees grew on Antarctica. "Climate Control" is another way to distract the public from where all the money is going. By the same measure, the armament industry pretended heartfelt concern for women's rights in Afghanistan in order to distract the public from their war profit's agenda. They covered up their motives by the pretext that they could remake a culture thousands of years old. Of course, that was propaganda.

Its time for the armament industry to think up another war. That is not to say that military preparedness and active steps of self defense may no longer be necessary given the world we live in. Had action been taken when Hitler marched into the Ruhr, he could have been toppled. America has been weakened politically and economically, emboldening

Chinese and Russian dictators. Inviting a Russian invasion of the Ukraine by withholding timely military aid to Ukraine and loudly broadcasting Washington's willingness to accept "a small incursion" was a display of incomprehensible weakness on the part of the most powerful nation on earth. Furthermore, one wonders why Germany and Japan lack robust armies or why Japan isn't supposed to develop their own nuclear weapons: China wouldn't like it but they might think twice about starting a war. While the military-industrial complex needs serious oversight, America's military has been weakened by the current administration, emboldening Communist China to aggressively test limits. America's military arsenal and missile systems need modern updating.

Education has been corrupted by the billionaires and Communist Chinese money stolen from the American people. Astronomical tuitions are encouraged by cheap Federal loans to schools and students in contrast to Europe where college is free. The end result was an exponential increase in university administrators and bloated salaries. Half of these parasitic positions could be eliminated. Trade schools are options. Not everybody needs to go to college. Unfortunately, Europe is succumbing as well to the economic one-world agenda of the billionaires.

Under Hitler, the Nazis set fire to the Reichstag, blaming the Communists and Jews. Hitler used this as a pretext to institute a police state. Similar reasoning is at play by the Biden administration in their comical attempt to equate a riot by Trump supporters on Jan.6 to Pearl Harbor and 9/11. Out of many thousands of angry but peaceful pro-Trump demonstrators 200 unarmed individuals broke into the Capital. No appreciable damage was done but a young woman was shot to death by Capital police. The new Democrat party is using the event as a reason to subject working class whites to police state surveillance. Whites who supported former President Trump are equated to Al Qaeda terrorists. President Biden's Attorney General is enlisting the FBI to investigate American parents who criticize school boards for fostering anti-white racist propaganda, pornographic books aimed at impressionable children and gender politics in the routine curriculum. I am not aware of any actual reported violence on the part of parents but Fox News reports that the DOJ's son in law's company, Panorama, has made tens of millions of dollars selling Critical Race Theory (read anti-white indoctrination) course materials to schools fully condoned by School Boards. A small subset of disgruntled homosexual activists who hate the nuclear family have gained control of educational curricula at the expense of the majority who want their children to learn to read and write. In sum, the fascist police state is here.

Brainwashing, mind control and puppetry: the #1 objective of the billionaires is the destruction of individual liberty and human relationships. They control every layer of our culture. In the case of Standard Oil and the robber barons, it took an exceptional person, Teddy Roosevelt, to deal with their lust for power. All references to life experience and human relationships are being deleted from the English language. Official Psychiatry has vilified Freud and psychoanalysis that rightfully brought to light life experience and how it shapes us all. The motive is to obliterate any hint that we can alter our outcome. Big Business wants us to obey the fate they have hard-wired for us. Individuals that value relationships think for themselves and resist enslavement. They are a threat to the dictates of tyrants. Freedom of speech must be suspended unless it yields to mind control. A case in point is the current politics regarding the viral pandemic. Aside from medical efficacy, what is the real reason for requiring two year old children to wear masks, prevent relatives from giving comfort to dying parents, attending church services, or seeing friends? It serves the additional motive of cementing totalitarian control over all of us. We are being groomed to obey from the ground up. Forcing small children to wear masks and concealing the faces of adults with whom they interact will lead to profound emotional illness. Bowlby showed the crucial importance of human relationships for the developing child (Attachment Theory). Psychoanalytic case studies show that autism is a consequence of impaired mother-child interaction. Popular WebMD confirms the benefit of psychoanalysis in autism treatment. In our culture, however, the role of mothers in the origin of mental illness is a taboo and censored. Does that really help the suffering recipients of troubled parenting or the disturbed parent? Bruno Bettelheim removed autistic children from their families that he likened to concentration camps and provided them with total care including psychoanalysis through high school. I can personally verify that the successes he had in his Orthogenic School at the University of Chicago were undeniable. Susan Sherkow,M.D. at Albert Einstein had real successes treating autistic children in four times per week psychoanalysis with the mother present. The approach was to help the child and mother to understand the overwhelming emotions the child had repressed and connect them to life experiences. Psychoanalytic principles are based on free speech. We owe nothing to the gods of mind-control.

Any motive that enriches Big Business is fine, including the chemical castration of children that steals their God-given sexual identity. We are to believe that there is no biological difference between men and women. After all, puppets are puppets. Black is white, white is black. So-called "education" is just another tool for weakening America. On the West Coast, for example, a teacher requires the children to repeat daily "We are living on stolen land." I learn that there are some individuals with a trace of Neanderthal in their genome. France by that logic should be given back to the Neanderthals.

We note also that the destruction of The United States necessitates scrubbing it clean of its history. Employing the tactics of the Red Guard, mobs destroy historical statues they don't like including Christopher Columbus and Abraham Lincoln. Speech must be policed.

Any repetition of claims that there was election fraud in the 2020 campaign and you could be arrested. The Democrat controlled House dictates that the words "assimilation" or "illegal aliens" should be prohibited. Cigna discourages words like "mother," "father," "girlfriend," or "brown bag lunch." Any reference to obvious biologically based differences in ability between the sexes is deemed racist. Both men and women are under attack and to be refashioned as puppets,. Women are no longer mothers but rather "birthing persons." International Pronoun Day is to be celebrated while Communist China has newly developed a supersonic missile cable of deploying a nuclear warhead. A D.C. politician among others informs us that the nuclear family is hardly necessary, even harmful. One official in the teacher's union claims that "Know Thyself" is an old African proverb. Sorry, it originates from the temple of Apollo at Delphi dating from the sixth century B.C.. I know it well. The great god Apollo and his father, Zeus, are at the foundation of Western Culture and, I might add, of psychoanalysis.

Solutions: Tax the majority of billionaires at 90% unless they use their money to create jobs. Ordain a special assessment of assets of those individuals who have amassed over $3billion and return that money to the people. Bill Gates doesn't need to be the greatest farmland owner in America. Prevent Blackstone Group from buying up residential property. Blackstone now has portfolio of over $ 11 trillion, yes trillion. Safeguard single family home ownership. Break-up Big Tech and Big Business monopolies. Billionaires are not the job creators but rather an economically robust citizenry. Protect the Civil Rights of all Americans. Strengthen the military from the incursion of dirty politics. Prosecute those who prohibit First Amendment rights. Double the tariffs on China. Prohibit mainland Chinese students (who now number 300,000) from taking sensitive technology courses in the U.S. Fire teachers who inculcate anti-American propaganda in the classroom. They have a right to express their views but not a right to practice brainwashing on impressionable young minds. Law and order must prevail. Criminals must be arrested and prosecuted. Illegal aliens should be deported and immigrants should be able to assimilate to fundamental Western values as well as enrich the United States economically. America does not have to share the wealth with the rest of the world. Tax the endowments of universities top heavy with worthless expensive administrators. Politicians who purposely promote unconstitutional measures should be impeached and prosecuted.

The ballooning wealth disparity in the U.S. will erode the foundation of our democracy and, if not addressed, America will continue to tread the path that led to the decline and fall of ancient Rome. The Republican establishment points to "bloated entitlements" for the poor and the middle class when the most egregious entitlements have been granted the super-rich. The Republican establishment, given their marching orders from their billionaire donors, to a man, have betrayed the American people and rammed through an unprecedented heist of the nation's wealth that will further enrich the .01%.

The Republican establishment's answer to Obama-care was to choke off needed medical treatment for the poor. The Obama administration itself fomented lies that made it appear that it was going to do wonders for health-care by elevating "quality over volume" (the average doctor was treating people too much and it was eating into the plutocrat's trillions). The wholesale return of "managed-care," welcomed by Mr. Obama and the establishment of both parties, will ensure the rationing if not gutting of medical care, not just for the poor, but for all except the gold-plated politicians and the billionaires. Clinical experience and knowledge of the mind has served to gird me against selling out to dishonest economic forces that hurt those who suffer. The goal should be a cure of mental illness as much as possible to the extent that circumstances allow. Two days a week I treat several of the mentally ill housed in a sheltered care facility, utilizing 1: 1 psychoanalytically oriented individual psychotherapy for the psychiatric hour (unfortunately, daily therapy sessions are not possible). Taking care of a person lost in the shadows of mental illness is the responsibility of a civilized society. Artificial deadlines on the duration of psychotherapy are not compatible with the complex realities of mental illness where significant gradual progress occurs but may require years of treatment. Anyone who experienced what these people experienced in life would have exactly the same problems. Remarkable progress is possible (no longer needing hospitalizations, a glimpse of a better future, a much better hold on reality and yes cures), but forces are underway that will soon put a stop to care of this nature. The #1 priority of corporate America and the government is the reduction of medical costs through the rationing of care. Medicare alone is scheduled for a $500 billion cut. Recently, my patients on Medicare and Medicaid (the poor) have been denied weekly intensive psychotherapy by Medicare's contracted agents who deem this help "medically unnecessary." Detailed progress notes highlighting suicidality, multiple hospitalization the need to work through a terrible childhood are proof enough that these poor people deserve help. What about that the proverb: "There but for the grace of God go I." Further dishonesty is evident in recent fabricated statistics by which the NIMH made 2 million people with schizophrenia disappear (E. Fuller Torrey. MD and Elizabeth Sinclair). The intent, of course, is justification to end long-term treatment of the mentally ill....except for pills. It is also of note that the increase of mass shootings in this country parallels the gutting of disciplined psychiatric treatment. Instead, we get the pronouncements of official psychiatry that it is impossible to predict potential for violence. Impossible? When the history of these perpetrators is replete with their threats to do exactly what they did? "The opioid crisis" is much in the news but the media doesn't connect the dots. Individuals turn to drugs because they are abandoned and no one is listening to them. The "government" (politicians) flushes human relationships and tells us that medical doctors who understand the mind can be replaced with cheap and worthless substitutes like "mindfulness" or shallow 12 session cognitive behavior therapy read off a manual. If such approaches worked we would all be walking gods. Nurse-practitioners have training but only a quarter of the training of physicians. What about "studies show…?" The pseudo-studies have a predetermined bias and that bias is money.

Totalitarians cement their power by controlling education and substituting propaganda for the voice of trained experts. Stalin liquidated the Polish educated class rendering Poland leaderless. Pol Pot murdered a million of his countrymen, anyone who was educated and could think. Perhaps there are similar reverberations currently in aspects of diversity politics that sidelines capably trained,\educated, high achievers. Under the Obama administration prospective candidates for Air Traffic Controller jobs are given a leg up if they did poorly in math and science and were out of work for a long time [reported by Tucker Carlson on Fox News]. Schools have begun to do away with the valedictorian. New York is set to scrap its test for admission to its top high schools (too many hard working Asians score too high). And, of course, "studies show" that highly trained doctors are oftentimes quite unnecessary (except, of course, if you are a politician or a billionaire).

Since free speech is guaranteed by the First Amendment the facts cannot be blacklisted regardless of politics. Yet there is a rolling juggernaut in America, from both the right and the left (if there is really any difference) to suppress the truth.

"1984" in 2024

Former President Trump is again running for President. The alarm bells are going off for the billionaires, fearful that their economic alliance with China will be jeopardized because Trump puts Americans and America first. They will stop at nothing to defeat him. Money and power are at stake. Their organs of propaganda are spewing out lies relentlessly. Their politicized state courts attempted to prevent Trump from being on voting ballots. At present, they aim to jail him through bogus prosecution when their fascist puppet in The White House is breaking US immigration laws every day. They are throwing billions at their man Biden and then V.P. Harris.

However, President Trump was re-elected by mandate. The American people saw through the lies of Big Business smears and propaganda that they had lifted from Joseph Goebbels playbook. Americans realized that Biden-Harris were the real enemies of Democracy. Hollywood and billionaire pop stars were not so virtuous. No one points out the obvious that they knew that President Trump would interfere with the billions they envisioned they would reap from Communist China.

Dehumanization: Censorship

Psychiatric treatment cannot rest upon a foundation of censorship that sacrifices the individual to current politics. In Freud's genius, he realized that nothing valid can come about in the course of psychotherapy unless the patient can fully speak his/her mind. I will investigate the origins of emotional problems as a consequence of interpersonal relationships. We are not hardwired in spite of the "it's genetic" drumbeat of the media and official psychiatry. Plutocrat and government grant money are at the root of the "It's genetic" agenda. An in depth look at the scientific evidence fully supports my statements. Genetic expression, if in play, is responsive to environmental experiences in humans. The giants of literature appeared freer to write about human relationships and the origins of emotional problems than present-day official psychiatry. For example, I have translated relevant passages from "Tod in Venedig" (Death in Venice) by Thomas Mann, Robert Musil, an Austrian novelist, and Billy Budd by Herman Melville, to exemplify various psychological aspects of homosexuality. Homosexuality is a normal part of adolescence but psychological conflicts often underlie its exclusive orientation in adulthood. It cannot be oversimplified, but certainly ancient and fundamental issues of self-assertion and submission are involved. Those who desire a good homosexual relationship should be helped to achieve that. Those who find it a betrayal of their true identity should be helped toward a heterosexual adjustment, to the extent they so desire. It isn't impossible.

The unconscious is the dark matter of the mind. Plato's allegory of the cave, is intuitively psychoanalytic. Bringing to light the origin of repressed childhood conflicts and fears can dispel the shadows of seeming reality, allowing the hidden, real person, to emerge.

The jargon in vogue that pretends to depict a balanced approach to looking at human behavior is, in reality, pseudo-liberal and pseudo-balanced. It is not what this work is all about. No, I will not throw words around like "psychosocial-neuroscience" because such allusions are meaningless. In truth, understanding the mind through a psychoanalytic approach has been eradicated, for economic and especially political reasons. Nor is human behavior to be understood by analyzing the brain, because that knowledge, at this point in time, is extremely primitive and rudimentary. What is clear, is that research shows that brain changes are secondary to environmental experience. That does not mean that I will avoid an in-depth analysis of up-to date brain and genetic research. My dear reader, professional or lay, will find, in a second book, Vol II, an in-depth, detailed elucidation of these issues.

The arts reflect a portrait of a dehumanized society ruled by billionaires

Psychiatry is influenced by the culture in which it is embedded. It is relevant, therefore, to take heed of the arts since they reflect a culture's values. Our culture is controlled by a dehumanizing plutocracy. Contemporary music, the plastic arts, and architecture are devoid of the human face and spirit. The dehumanizing forces that control artistic expression in present day society are the new establishment, a mafia of plutocrats and their designated peons, administrators, and politicians.

As if there wasn't enough fly-by-night ludicrous fragmentation masquerading as creativity, the charlatans that control the art-forums refigure the classics by "updating"(eliminating history) "so that the public can relate the past to our times" (and forget the lessons of the past), usually with some current political message of sufficiently ugly shock value to attract attention or no coherent message at all (I recently saw a production of "Tosca" in which the libretto refers to Napoleon's battle of Marengo but the cast is dressed in WWI costumes). The public, you see, cannot perceive the eternal message of the classics without a lens provided by shallow posturers who can educate them as to how it all fits in with our times. "Our times," however, means indoctrinating the public with current political propaganda that makes the middle class feel guilty for being better off than the down-trodden of third world countries. A current production of Humperdinck's Hansel and Gretel lets us bemoan world hunger. The real message, however, is the morality of globalization, the pitch to eevate the third world and multinational corporate profits at the expense of the West's working and middle classes (the danger to the plutocracy: the scorned middle class might one day resist the apparent inexorable lowering of their standard of living). "The patriarchy" is another code word to justify eliminating the male as a power base (men don't sufficiently realize that they need to obey).The crazy productions at Bayreuth, promoted by Wagner's confused great-granddaughter, are foisted on the German public who fear being called Nazis if they dissent. An American, Yuval Sharon, in charge of a new Bayreuth production of Lohengrin changes the ending of Wagner's opera, anointing the witch Ortrud a heroine while Lohengrin slinks off the stage in defeat. There is nothing wrong with exalting feminist politics (or other politics) but calling such pretentions "art" make it agonizingly clear that under the dead hand of present day culture, artistic creativity is dead.

Again, it's the proven Roman campaign of divide and rule. We will have to hold our breath for another great composer of Wagner's stature to make their appearance anytime soon. And make no mistake, the charlatans and their politician-benefactors play their role churning the homogenization machines: hatred of the family, traditional male-female relationships, and traditional humanistic values. I read of the Shakespeare's Globe current production of "A Midsummer Night's Dream [Wall Street Journal, "All-Too-Modern Nightmare" 5/10/16 S.Ahmari].The theater's new artistic director, Emma Rice, injects contemporary slang and profanity into Shakespeare's dialogue: "Get away from me, you ugly b...h!" "[R]aunchy grinding and nipple tassels" help the audience to grasp the subtleties of sex. Almost every scene includes pop numbers like Beyoncé's "Single Ladies" along with Indian drums and constant sitar strumming and, of course, there must be the obligatory coming-out story as the female Helena becomes the male Helenus as "he" pursues Demetrius. "They have made worms' meat of me" [Romeo and Juliet].

Creativity is dead. But all manner of frantic interlopers hope to attract the attention and money of the plutocrats, who, in turn, hope to unload their garbage onto the next greater fool until the musical chairs stops. It isn't "art" anymore, it's the stock market casino applied to the art market. It isn't about "Truth and Beauty," as Keats idealized, it's about money. Karl Marx warned of the dehumanizing consequences ("die Entmenschlichung") when money becomes the measure of everything and transcends intrinsic humanistic values: "My money makes the coward a hero." Junk isn't junk, it's really wonderful.

Contemporary music is unlistenable, better suited for some distant asteroid. Like antimatter, it exists only as a negative. Music, we are told, had reached a dead-end. Only by turning a positive into a negative could poor music struggle mightily onwards, in spite of the fact that harmony and beauty in the arts seemed to have no trouble persevering for the past three thousand years or so. The talking-heads' music critics, in unison (probably to keep their jobs), opine that the next conductor of a major American orchestra should also be "a composer," that is, a composer of abstract music. This will ensure that failing patron attendance (les grises) will be supplemented by droves of young people flocking to contemporary fare. That may work on the plastic West Coast (temporarily), but New Yorkers are not stupid. Just because some composition is "new," doesn't do it for the most experienced music-goers who, over time, have informed themselves in the music of the spheres. The hypomanic young, many of whose attention span is about a nanosecond's duration, have never been educated in classical music and won't sustain the arts because the classics are no longer part of the educational process. It takes time to see a Rembrandt. Patronage is falling because no really beautiful music is being created. Abstract pings and screeches will not fill auditoriums with human beings. The latter "newly commissioned" works are usually stuck in the middle of a program to discourage patrons from coming late or leaving early and, usually, for good reason, will never be heard again. The human touch may be on the way out anyway. Computer chips are next in line to do away with musicians and their instruments. Popular music is moribund as well. Where are the unforgettable melodies of "Carousel," "Hair," or "Porgy and Bess"? Sadly, Broadway would be dark were it not for revivals. Newly minted musicals boast generic music that one couldn't hum if one tried. "Rap," geared to dumb-down African Americans, can't sing at all but is ballyhooed as the sensational answer to Broadway's death throes.

The restaurant scene mirrors the fragmented manic chaos of contemporary culture as well, with bizarre combinations passing as "creative." Personally, I'll take the French haute-cuisine created meticulously et avec soin (that is if one can find haute-cuisine anymore.) Even in France, the classic sauces have disappeared in favor of vegetable water). Fancy image without substance.

Abstraction has its message but, subjectively, the highest art form presents the whole person. Even in tragedy, the highest art reminds us that we have not been extinguished. Current trends in art have eliminated the face of man. A deadening hand of ugly emptiness has descended on the human spirit and the enlightenment of the renaissance is sorely lacking.

Power, control, and dehumanization

American society is becoming increasingly obsessed with power. The relentless depiction of sadism in movies, television, opera, theatre, and video games is a pure obsessive power distillate. A recent book and movie, all the rage, features a young woman trapped in the sadomasochistic grip of a handsome young billionaire. She is sexually exploited, replete with whips and bondage, and, we are told, sophisticated female theatre-goers are "culturally curious" about this "Zeitgeist moment" [New York Times, 2/16/15 "The movie as a fairytale" Sarah Lyall] because women are thereby celebrating something akin to sexual liberation. True, there is a hint in the movie adaptation that this twisted "romance" has origins in childhood trauma, but that observation escapes the movie critic, as it does our society in general. Cruelty that aims to extinguish the individual doesn't indulge in niceties or conceal its priorities. It is what it appears to be, force reigning supreme over humanistic values. As the later Roman Empire devolved into a dictatorship run by henchmen, the public was increasingly distracted from the real issues, like where all the money was going, by bread and circuses. Sadistic entertainment desensitizes the public and the ongoing celebration of cruelty undermines concern for one's fellow man. Devaluing interpersonal relationships is the prime means by which totalitarian police-states create unthinking obedient puppets. The plutocrats are employing tried and true gladiatorial games to debase and dumb-down the American public all the while accelerating the transfer of wealth to their own hands. I read of a new opera where a boy is sacrificed in a manner especially sadistic. "Not for the squeamish," I read. The audience roared its approval, reverberations of the Colosseum still discernable. Getting down to in vogue minimalism (no need for pretty actors), Then there is current movie fare, a Gallic fright film remade in the United States, replete with close-ups of torture ("horror fans dare horror rookies" to watch it). Force is celebrated. The next Oscar winner will be some digital super-muscular monster smashing its way to domination. There is a church portal in Parma, Italy, that depicts a man eating honey in the tree of life, in Nordic mythology, "Die Welt Esche." But two giant rats are gnawing at the roots of this noble tree and a dragon spews tongues of fire in the direction of this innocent fellow, who continues to enjoy himself as if his pleasures will never end. His dream is not hopeless, however, as the Sun God and Luna, Apollo and Artemis (Selene), speed to his defense. The plutocrats are undermining American culture and our personal dreams for a happy life. The truths embodied in the classics can ensure that the tree of life and our individuality endures. Healing human relationships are the only real solution to problems in living. Falling under the spell of a dehumanizing power-ethic is a detour that dead-ends in spiritual death. Emotional problems are the result of suffering and fears of punishment that starts in childhood. Good experiences later on in life and healing human relationships are the antidote to these wounds. We all have a true identity within us that no alien force can completely extinguish. That true flame within needs encouragement to light our path in life. We may need an ally to accompany us through the darkness. Psychiatry can and should be the public's ally but it has been usurped by Big Business, the Super-Rich (with a few exceptions) who control legislative priorities in America and globally.

What is psychiatry?

By definition, psychiatry is the branch of medicine that treats the emotions. That few psychiatrists are currently trained in the principles of intensive psychotherapy might appear to justify the view that a medical school education is superfluous when it comes to understanding the mind or the origins of psychological symptoms. The essence of medicine, however, is the doctor-patient relationship even more than the application of procedures or medications. In treatment, the mind of another is revealed in the course of a trusted therapeutic alliance. The doctor as healer and friend must also be clinically responsible. A medical education teaches clinical responsibility and discipline.

Understanding the Mind

This work hopes to be of value to professionals, the public, and the individual. It aims to enhance the public's insight into the psychological issues at play in our troubled culture and energize the electorate to change society's priorities so as to better reflect humanistic values (this is not impossible!). I also hope to aid the individual struggling with personal unhappiness, whether or not they need the more focused help of a professional alliance. As for our professionals, my study will hopefully remind them of their true calling and help them to consider all the scientific evidence, including the vast body of scientific data forthcoming from the study of inter-personal relationships. The mind-numbing refrain that "biology and genes" primarily explain mental illness is nothing more than a circular argument motivated by a dehumanizing economic agenda. In-depth research in lower animals, for example, proves that parenting changes the brain and changes it profoundly. Are human beings more regulated by primary brain defects independent of life experience than rats? But that is apparently what official psychiatry and the grant money-hungry cohort expect us to believe. The average person in the street has more common sense regarding the effect of life experience in shaping behavior than the Frankenstein brain-talk "experts."

We are told that we feel overwhelmed by "too much information." The problem, however, is not "too much information" but rather the quality of the information that is allowed a forum. The information overload is selectively skewed by the unbridled capitalist agenda, namely a relentless hurricane of propaganda to convince all of us that our fate is sealed by preordained brain/genetic factors. Individuality and human relationships are anathema to the plutocrats. They want puppets and they want all of the money. In their credo, only the super-rich are to be allowed the luxury of an identity.

What to make, then, of all the seemingly impressive brain data being published? The answer is that no government or drug company grant money is available anymore for the study of human relationships or long term psychotherapy. All current "research" aims to justify cheap therapy (12 sessions or less) to make sure that no personal change is possible and reinforce the dictate that we are mired in our fate along with the corollary that individuality is fantasy. The full scientific picture, however, undeniably shows that the brain is a plastic organ and that it is molded from day one (and earlier) by the environment, of which inter-personal relationships starting with the mother and infant are cosmically paramount. Dr. Jonathan Shedler, a psychologist at the University of Colorado, has extensively researched the studies that claim that cheap cognitive behavior therapy works. He shows how baseless these claims are and how the findings are manipulated [see Chapter 12].

Why this book is being written

While in the course of my clinical experience (and echoing Charles Darwin's tournure de phrase), I have been much struck with certain facts that have come to light in my treatment of patients regarding the origin of their symptoms and the path to emotional healing, It occurred to me that light could be shed on this question by presenting and reflecting upon relevant facts and observations in as objective a manner as possible, realizing that psychiatry, if not medicine itself, is part science, part art. As for the art component, it should not be dismissed since science is not the only road toward understanding and not all truths, as complex as they are, can be translated into physical properties without losing their essence. Let me say, in personal terms, if you have ever experienced the tragedy of losing someone close to you, you will understand why this book has been written. Living in the dark ages, as we do, it will no doubt elicit gnashing of teeth to bring to light the whitewashed details, namely, that the most disturbing manifestations of human behavior (serious mental illness, suicide, murder) are byproducts of disturbed parenting and dehumanized cultures.... and the gathering storm starts in impressionable childhood. The New York Times [6/7/18 "Defying Prevention Efforts, Suicide Rates Are Rising Across the Nation" Benedict Carey] reporting on suicide, notes a 25% increase in suicides in every state from 1996 to 2016. It adds: "Treatment for chronic depression and anxiety – often the precursors to suicide – has never been more available." In reality, however, nothing could be further from the truth. Treatment limited to pills will not solve these problems. The need for intensive psychodynamic oriented psychotherapy in the hands of an adequately trained therapist is a necessary even if inconvenient truth. Trauma is instilled in childhood and festers both consciously and unconsciously. The mind is like an iceberg, where the greater part of its reality is below the surface. A healing therapeutic human relationship is essential. Nothing will be gained by whitewashing one's parenting. Looking at brain scans and looking for culpable genes is futile. Our dehumanized culture suppresses both adequate support and the truth. If hospitalization is required, it cannot be truncated to save money for vampire billionaires. Expensive? Yes. But unbound productivity could be unleashed if people really believed that the state cared about them. Skimming through the official newspaper of the American Psychiatric Association, one notes a complete absence of any mention of the need for long-term treatment, especially if it concerns intensive psychotherapy. Page after page touches upon every politically correct hot topic especially if it involves emergencies or the politically fashionable. Headlines report breakthroughs as: "Children who have been routinely beaten have emotional problems as adults!!!" Rome is burning but official psychiatry fiddles.

Nor can a psychiatrist understand another's emotional conflicts without having undergone rigorous training that by necessity must include a personal psychoanalysis to avoid, as much as possible, the blurring and mixing up of the therapist's personal emotional problems with those of the person he is treating. By "psychoanalysis," I mean a method of treatment for understanding and healing conscious and unconscious psychological roadblocks that interfere with personal happiness. The smartest person in the world is rendered stupid when held hostage to the irrational tyranny of unresolved emotional conflicts. The goal of therapy, through understanding and support, must aim to free the person seeking help from conflicts and patterns that are self-destructive. The ultimate goal should be the realization of an individual's inner potential.

The mind's empire comprises domains and principalities

The facts which clarify the origin of emotional conflicts and symptoms and their connection to the process of healing is my focus. In our society, however, distortions regarding these issues requires an understanding of more than one aspect of the puzzle in order to clarify the whole. In America, political pressures, economically motivated, have distorted psychiatry. Ethics have gone by the wayside and treatment has been correspondingly decimated. Understanding the emotions will therefore also require an analysis of the cultural milieu in which we find ourselves, a careful weighing of the motivation of organizations, cultural values, and ruling politics of the times. Political agendas have unfortunately been well documented historically to take precedence over the search for the truth and, often, those who persisted in the noble endeavor of fact-finding, have been punished by those at the helms of power.

Since, in recent years, little has been published in psychiatric circles that has not consciously or unconsciously been unduly influenced by our culture's current power oriented value system, and since those at the helms of power also control the means for dissemination of information, it is important to publish a work whose priority is the enlightenment of the individual, regardless of current political dictates. Undoubtedly it is smart politics to avoid punishment by offering obeisance to the brainwashing machine of the plutocracy and the politicians they control, but healing cannot rest on a foundation of lies where the individual's best interests are secondary to "the greater good" (Big Brother-speak for the interests of the powerful). The fanatics of the organized right and left, as committed as they are to the principal of thought control, will not look favorably on this work but then neither did they find much to their liking in George Orwell's "1984" or "Animal Farm." A society of individuals is healthier than a colony of marionettes.

Current politics says that emotional problems are inborn. Treatment presentations (supported by current research on the brain) will show, however, that environmental experience rules. Recurrent patterns of thought and behavior that emerge in the course of intensive treatment reveal connections that clarify causation and subsequent coping mechanisms and adaptations. In a second book some histories will be presented in detail, others as vignettes. Psychotherapeutic studies can reveal the origin of emotional problems with great clarity. Our times overlook the fact that what a person says and how he or she behaves has psychological meaning. The powers that be no longer listen to the individual. An iron curtain has descended over the mind. "The Era of the Brain" has become "the Era of Brainwashing."

But understanding the origin of symptoms is only half the story. The power of a healing human relationship within a therapeutic alliance can lead to resolution of deep emotional problems. Depression, panic, schizophrenia, the spectrum of homosexuality, etc. are addressed without the "Heils" to politically correct propaganda.

Schizophrenia:

For example, those suffering from schizophrenia are capable of remarkable recoveries. One such case is that of an "incurable schizophrenic" who was treated five times a week in psychotherapy (with medication) over a period of years. That patient achieved a complete and enduring recovery in every aspect of his being, for all intents and purposes, a cure. There other "remarkable" outcomes. Of course, the ignorant, using circular reasoning, state that schizophrenia and many other emotional problems are, by definition, incurable: "If the schizophrenic is cured, he or she wasn't really schizophrenic." There are, however, many well known cases that contradict that dogma, John Nash, who won the Nobel Prize in economics, being one such example. In contrast to the current attitude that schizophrenia is incurable and hopeless, recovery and reclaiming a normal life pattern for those suffering from this illness is not a rarity. "Treatment resistant" schizophrenics is not the problem. It is treatment-resistant-therapists who retreat from developing the long-term intensive treatment relationship that the person suffering from this difficult illness usually requires. That is the problem. The focus on primary brain defects rationalizes the denial of funding for treatment of serious emotional illness: "It's an inborn brain problem, so why waste money on 'unproven' intensive long-term treatment of hopeless cases?" In general, the remaking of medical treatment by instituting bureaucratic criteria of "Quality" care and "value based care" to replace "volume," as well as the promotion of "integrated care" as opposed to intensive personal care is a cover-up to camouflage cheaper watered down treatment and a two-tiered system of medical care, one for the public and the other for the rich. I recently heard that Walgreen's drugstore chain will start offering mental health counseling (there is money to be made). And it isn't only psychiatry that is being undermined. "Studies show" that we really don't need trained doctors that much. Nurse-practitioners are even better (and much cheaper).

The Spectrum of Homosexuality:

Homosexuality is a complex topic. Gay-activist journalists of The New York Times limit information for public consumption to the opinions of other gays in the sciences. The latter suggest that, for male children, the mother develops hypothetical antibodies to the male fetus or something else biological is at play. Evidence for the latter, we are told, is a male child's increasing risk of becoming homosexual the more older male siblings he has. No such antibodies, however, have ever been found. On the other hand, a mother who was resentful of a favored brother in childhood may tolerate the first born son but, not the second or third. The mother has the power to change the sexual orientation of the child and the child complies out of fear of abandonment. We are told that homosexuality is inborn and cannot be changed. There is not the slightest evidence, however, that it is genetic, hormonal or inborn. It is a normal part of adolescence, but, when it persists as the dominant pattern in adulthood, it can be shown to originate in a particular family environment in which the child had no choice but to adapt homosexually. Contrary to taboo dictates and political correctness, yes, the mother has the power to change sexual orientation (for males, the "momma's boy"). To give one example, a small boy whose self-assertiveness has been relentlessly suppressed by the mother has a great risk of growing up a masochistically oriented homosexual, particularly if a resentful mother has done everything she could to drive a psychological wedge between father and son, thus preventing male identification from taking place. The homosexually oriented who have no interest in changing their sexual orientation should be helped to have a good and caring homosexual relationship. A good homosexual relationship is better than no relationship. Enduring homosexual relationships are not a rarity. Those who feel that their homosexual patterns are a distortion of their true identity should be allowed to resolve their conflicts heterosexually, to the extent they so desire. The latter is not "religious conversion therapy" but arises in the course of psychodynamic psychotherapy just as other realizations emerge when a patient's thoughts are freed from censorship. It is false that homosexuality is fixed. That adolescents resolve these conflicts is common place A true same-sex friendship can abort homosexual impulses that originate in self-doubts and depression. Homosexual "coming out" is celebrated, considered politically correct and "happens all the time," but heterosexual "coming out" for a homosexual is never acknowledged or given credence. This, of course, is politics and bias. The official condemnation of psychotherapy on the part of the politicians that control the professional organizations is inexcusable politics.

Homosexuality was not so long ago viewed by the state as a crime and homosexuals were persecuted. Now, however, anyone presenting facts that show that homosexuality is anything other than "perfectly normal" is muzzled, refused a forum, and, in spite of the Constitution and the First Amendment, likewise threatened with persecution and prosecution. We read in The New York Times (6/26/15 "Conversion Therapy"; no author given) that courts and politicians aim to outlaw all psychotherapy for children and adolescents who struggle to overcome the anguish of unwanted homosexual conflicts, even if the child doesn't want to be homosexual (and most don't). Crazy "therapies" by charlatans are quoted as blanket justification for suppressing the First Amendment. By contrast, The New York Times [8/22/15 and 8/23/15 editorials] champions free speech for topless women who expose their painted breasts and thongs in Times Square and demand "tips" while their male handlers stand guard, even devoting their frontpage and a long editorial to the issue. The nomenclature "prostitutes" and "pimps" would seem to fit. The Times pretends it is at the forefront of visionary and liberal causes as long as it doesn't irritate its plutocrat benefactors unduly.

Science is turned on its head by preposterous court opinions [NYT 7/22/28 "Who Should Be Allowed To Compete As a Women?" Roger Pelke] that distort biologic facts through the lens of politics. We are supposed to believe that "sex is part of a spectrum, not a this or that definition..."and "...sex in humans is not simply binary.... Nature is not neat." Sexual expression is certainly on a spectrum but true physical sexual anomalies, like hermaphroditism or Klinefelter's syndrome, that occur as rare outliers, hardly constitutes a gradual spectrum. Someone declaring themselves the sex opposite to their birth sex does not alter the fact that every cell in their body retains either the XX or XY chromosome, with very rare exceptions. Both males and females secrete testosterone and estrogens. Somewhat elevated testosterone in women does not make them male or change their chromosomal make-up. The plutocrats aim to homogenize individuality and redefine reality. Getting rid of the family and the Father as an authority creates the rudderless society they welcome.

An article in the New York Times, "How Changeable Is Gender?"8/23/15, by Richard A. Friedman, M.D., Director of the Psychopharmacology Clinic at Weill Cornel, ends up a high-wire balancing act between scientific fact and political correctness. He is cognizant of "the inescapable biology at the heart of gender identity" but adds that "recent neuroscience research suggests that gender identity may exist on a spectrum and that gender dysphoria fits well within the range of human biological variation." He refers to an investigator who claims to have found brain differences that "may" point to a neural basis for the transgender experience. Those who want to change their body, he continues, is a very rare phenomenon, about 5 per 100,000. He refers to Dr. Richard Green's study of gender dysphoric boys and Madeleine S.C. Wallein's research, as well as others, who found that in young children upwards of 80% no longer wanted to change their gender after ten year follow-ups. Nevertheless, some groups, he notes, recommend pharmacologically delaying puberty in children until age 16 and then proceeding with gender reassignment unless there is reason not to. Dr. Friedman finds that agenda misguided in view of the fluidity of childhood perceptions. On the politically correct side, he states, like a law of physics: "In fact attempts to change a person's sexual orientation, through so-called reparative therapy have been debunked as quackery and rightly condemned by the psychiatric profession as potentially harmful." He admits that one can be straight or gay "or anything in between but variability in behavior shouldn't be confused with malleability….sure you can change your sexual behavior, but your inner sexual fantasies endure."

Comment: The above writer maintains that there is an insurmountable wall between childhood sexual identity fluidity and the ability of adolescents or adults to "really" change sexual orientation. He acknowledges that sexual behavior can change but not "inner" sexual fantasies, whatever that is supposed to mean. How is he so sure? Since his training is in psychopharmacology, what does he know about psychodynamics? Has he ever treated a patient in intensive psychotherapy or come to understand the fluid potential of a grown-up and the power of positive human relationships in effecting change, even of longstanding behavioral patterns? Why are occasional homosexual "inner fantasies" the determining factor if someone has direct heterosexual experience? Moreover, I have male patients in my practice whose sole conscious erotic awareness is exclusively homosexual yet periodically have dreams of sexual excitement and erections when experiencing, in sleep, friendly non-threatening women. Consciously intervening homosexual fantasies are usually related to self-doubts that have their origin in childhood fears of parental punishment. His silence regarding the dysfunctional family's imprint on behavior and his talk of nuanced brain changes without alerting the reader to the fact that the brain responds to environmental experience highlights the fact that he is uncomfortable with fundamental psychology. He states that "I was surprised to discover how many professional colleagues in this area either warned me to be careful about what I wrote or were reluctant to talk with me on the record for fear of reprisal from the transgender community." Political correctness is motivated by fear. Should science be sacrificed to politics? Although there are no guarantees, there is overwhelming data to show that homosexual to heterosexual change is possible. Homosexuality is not a sin but, it is a clinical fact that many individuals struggle with a truly unwanted homosexual behavior pattern that dead-ends in depression, even suicide. He states that the "psychiatric profession" considers psychotherapy for homosexual conflicts "quackery" but the majority of rank and file clinical psychiatrists never ascribed to these official policy statements which were political in nature and a consequence of activist threats. Those that run organizations are, above all, politicians. The cold hard facts evidenced by the Karolinska Institute exposes the nonsense that mutilating surgery cures psychological conflicts.

Charles M. Blow, columnist for the New York Times and champion of minority rights, wrote a remarkably courageous op-ed entitled "Sexual Attraction and Fluidity" [9/7/15]. He refers to the market research firm YouGov that, in 2015, asked British adults to plot themselves on a sexuality scale created by Alfred Kinsey in the 1940s, with zero being exclusively heterosexual and 6 being exclusively homosexual. For 18-24 year-olds, 43 percent place themselves somewhere in between. Only 46 percent say they are completely heterosexual and 6 percent as completely homosexual. YouGov released the data for the United States and found that 29 percent put themselves somewhere in the category of bisexuality. The survey was meant to measure the "the possibility of homosexual feelings or experiences." It showed that well beyond adolescence, and even into older adulthood, the awareness of homosexual feelings is a fluid awareness. Mr. Blow rightfully points out that resistance to this fact "comes from straight and gay people alike."

Highlighted in the very same paper [9/7/15 "Ousted as Gay Aging Veterans Battling Again for Honorable Discharge" Dave Philipps] and reminiscent of Hitler's use of the S.S., the U.S. military, in the 1950s and 60s, embarked on a campaign to purge homosexuals from the service, some 100,000 individuals between World War II and 2011.The records of good soldiers were smeared with dishonorable discharges. They were barred from veteran's benefits and government jobs. Several such cases were reported among which was that of a 21-year-old who was labeled a "Class II homosexual." He was rated excellent in reviews but, while on the street, was propositioned by a young man and caught in a military sting. Later, he married, had children, including 12 grandchildren.

Comment: Nazi laws against homosexuality are, of course, wrong. But there is an additional issue here, that being the report of a young man who gave up a homosexual orientation for a heterosexual orientation, in spite of this papers repeated canon that homosexuality is "inborn" and cannot be changed.

One has quite possibly noticed the pessimistic, negative pall being cast over hope for positive changes of any kind in our present day society. These pervasive feelings of hopelessness are directly linked to the campaign to instill the conviction that we are all genetically determined. Reading the newspapers and listening to the media, the only group who can self-energize and blossom is our youth, but only youth in an abstract sense. Any particular young person in real life is hopeless too. Thus, we are led to believe that older men shouldn't be fathers, women will be victimized by motherhood, there is no money for Medicare or Social Security, upward mobility for the impoverished is dim and so on. But the public and professionals need to know that depression, panic, fear and despair are the product of real life experiences and are not immutable even though the path toward emotional freedom may not always be smooth going. There are no guarantees in life, but human beings have remarkable positive potential for growth. Sometimes, to varying degrees, a trusted ally may be necessary. Powerful hidden forces of the mind can free the true self from a time-warp's prison. Steven Pinker, a cognitive psychologist at Harvard, recently addressed the issue of optimism in his book: "Enlightenment Now: the case for reason, science, humanism, and progress." All the aforementioned (reason etc.) light the way for the human spirit but, above all, is humanism, the sine qua non of civilization, true civilization, which has yet to make its appearance on the world stage. Surely we need to be armed with realistic optimism as we make our way in a difficult world, and I have presented case studies of real people that bear witness to the positive potential within us all, including those who have been written off by society. Yet the truths that would fortify us will not be furthered by glossing over the looming threats that exist. Perhaps Mr.Pinker is not a sophist and is sincere in his endeavor. Perhaps he is just guilty of oversight. Granted, there is evidence of progress: we have antibiotics now, most don't live in extreme poverty in America (but far too many still do), one need not undergo surgery without anesthesia, Social Security is a magnificent achievement etc. On the other hand, one cannot ignore recent history when upwards of 100 million people were extinguished in World War II etc.. With justification, he casts a harsh light on the economic conditions of the1950's, but a 2014 Credit Suisse Global Wealth Report does not paint an encouraging picture for Americans: the average networth, per adult, was $301,000, putting Americans fourth in the world. That statistic is skewed, however, owing to the top-heavy effect of US millionaires and billionaires. 42% of the world's millionaires and 49% of those with a net worth greater than $50 million were Americans. The median net worth of adult Americans was only $45,000 (half have less, half have more), ranking the US 19th on the world stage, behind Japan, Canada, and much of Western Europe. The median American household income in 2012 was $ 51,017. In 1999, it was $56,080 (owing to the destruction of unions, shifting jobs overseas etc.). In the 1950's, inflation was a sliver of what it is now: apples 10 cents/pound, gasoline 25cents a gallon, a big house $20,000 and both spouses didn't have to work to make ends meet.

Turning to present day, insight into the relentless march toward puppetry and the elimination of personal identity is nowhere to be found in his book. Was the good docteur Pangloss Mr. Pinker's inspiration? "Enlightenment Now" is a far cry from The Enlightenment. It is politically safe whitewash of the plutocracy and of its inroads into American culture. The good docteur Pangloss states the case for Pinker well: "Car, dit t'il, tout ceci est ce qu'il y de mieux…car il est impossible que les choses ne soient pas où ells sont, car tout est de bien." [Voltaire] (everything is for the best because it is impossible for it to be otherwise). Mr. Pinker also wrote: "The Blank Slate: The Modern Denial of Human Nature." This supposed "brilliant" and objective book opines that human nature is the product of biologic evolution. He states that parents have next to nothing to do with their children's emotional outcome because our attitudes and behavior are determined by genes. Thus, we are not born "blank slates" but are a creation of preordained genetic factors with perhaps the added influence of peers. He states "that every study" of identical twins proves his point (sorry, not quite: see an in depth discussion of the facts as detailed by the geneticist Richard

Lewontin and others in my book on psychotherapy. One example he presents as proof is a pair of identical twins, "raised apart," who meet someday and are identical down to the tiniest details: Both were wearing navy blue shirts with epaulets, both flush the toilet the same way, both like to sneeze in elevators to see people jump etc. (the college students whom he addressed were also plied with glib jokes to entertain them). One cannot underestimate the appetite of the publishing industry for shallow feel-good books. Armchair philosophy as pontificated by the evolutionary biologists cannot be taken seriously. Maintaining, as he does, that there are no studies that verify the role of parenting in their child's outcome is an incredible falsehood and my case studies, for example, show otherwise. I would add that the brain is not "just a computer" because computers do not have emotions. Roman writers, even after The Republic, and under dictators, seemed freer to speak the truth than in our society. Mr. Pinker is confusing humans with worms. Human beings are blank slates. It is worms who are not. By the way, is maintaining that we are all genetically programmed really optimism? One has been led to believe that hard, scientific research offers indisputable proof for genetic causation of emotional problems and inborn brain dysfunction. Quite the opposite is true, however, as my second book shows in an extensive review of current research and scientific literature.

Of course, there are strong headwinds that would oppose a study that confronts directly those that control our society. Power brokers prefer brainwashing to enlightenment (60% of Americans do not believe in evolution, less than any other major country except Turkey according to the journal Science).Their news organs endlessly market recycled "one liners," and diversionary pseudo-news. My esteemed reader has surely noticed how ingrained the art of lying has become in our society and at the highest levels, including the office of the presidency, Wall Street, journalistic lying, false advertising (brainwashing), and yes, scientific investigation, manipulated as it is by corporate money. The "information" aimed at the public is outrageously distorted, filtered, and controlled by the plutocrat-media.

These two books will attempt to present a more complete picture of relevant issues than is usually the case, a factual accounting requiring in-depth details. In those sections that are somewhat technical, the reader will find that the truth concerning the origin of emotional problems is morally and scientifically the exact opposite of what he or she has been led to believe.

Do genes cause emotional problems? The environment? Can we still ask such questions? The public is, I'm sure, acquainted with the current view that human behavior is genetically determined and that emotional problems are the result of genetic variation or faulty genes. It goes something like this: "If they haven't found the gene or combination of genes that explain it all, they are on the verge of finding it, them." Official psychiatry and the media tell us that we live in the "Era of the Brain" and that, therefore, makes psychiatry more scientific. The old psychoanalytic approach that focused on the mind has never been verified we are told and, furthermore, was disproved, long-ago disproved, leading to the current attitude: "We will not even listen to you." Anxiety, panic, depression, obsession compulsion, schizophrenia, the spectrum of homosexuality (Freud noted that everyone has a potential for homosexuality), drug and alcohol addictions, attention deficit disorder, criminality, even "curiosity seeking," are all due to genetic variation we are told. Looking objectively at the mother – child/parent-child relationship is currently deemed unethical if not immoral and parents should "breathe a sigh of relief" that they can no longer be held responsible for their child's problems. A thinking person is likely to raise the question, however, if only genes are to be held accountable, why are there laws that make people responsible? Are laws just not yet in sync with psychiatric science? But if parents aren't responsible, then people in general are not responsible, nor is the state, or corporate America, or the billionaires who hold the reins of power. Our culture denies the significance of parenting and, in particular, that of the powerful mother-child symbiotic bond. Hardly a revolutionary or subversive concept, the importance of the mother-child relationship has been subjected to scientific research for quite some time now. We know it by the familiar name, "attachment theory." Of course, insight and introspection are in the cross-hairs of an increasingly efficient brainwashing machine that aims for a colony of humanoids who will have neither a past nor a future. It is our memories, however, á la recherche du temps perdu, that make us human.

Of course, all human behavior must somehow be explainable ultimately through genes but the success of the human species resides in its ability to adapt to disparate environmental conditions. That is, after all, fact. It is the flexibility of the brain in response to environmental stimuli that allowed for human ascendancy over other animals and, of course, the genes allow for this potential for adaptation and variability. There may possibly be a predetermined genetic proclivity for certain emotional problems but, in the vast majority of cases, the final determining factor, is not genetic, it is environmental, and foremost among environmental factors is the mother – child relationship. For humans, there is strong evidence that the psychological environment has the power to turn genes on and off, the so-called "epigenetic phenomenon." Of course, the facts don't sway everybody. We hear over and over again, from investigators who are beholden to corporate and government grant money. Lay people are brainwashed by one-liners from the media, that "it's genetic." Perhaps humans given to mindless repetition can learn something from the African Grey Parrot, a remarkably intelligent bird that actually has the ability to listen to the other party and respond logically.

Polygenic propaganda of the puppet-masters

Unable to find the gene or genes which, independent of environmental experience, initiate and dictate human behavior, the organicists are now apt to use the term "polygenic."

Thus, we are led to believe, hundreds, even thousands of genes are the innate brain factors that cause variations, big and small, in human behavior. A psychologist writing in The New York Times [7/28/18 "Why progressives should embrace genetics in education" K. P. Harden] states that a study in the journal "Nature Genetics" analyzed the genes of 1.1million people of European ancestry and found "thousands of genetic DNA variants that are correlated with educational attainment." These results are then given a single number and a "polygenic score." 10% with a low score didn't complete college while 55% with a high score did, "as big a disparity as the difference between rich and poor students in America." She claims that genes shape "nearly every aspect of our lives." She attributes opposition to this kind of research "left-wing thinking" and states that the "reality of genetic differences between people is a necessary step for us to ensure a more just society." For some reason, genetic variants only minimally predicted educational outcomes for African-Americans, which in itself raises questions.

Comment:

The assertions of the psychologist are next to worthless. One "study," without replication from other research, will join the junk heap of false positives that characterizes such claims. That she cobbles together such complexities with scarcely a disclaimer or qualification is rather inexcusable from the standpoint of science. These issues will be thoroughly reviewed in my second book but may it suffice in this overview to refer to the following:

[Nature, 8/9/2014] Hugh Fletcher (The Queen's University of Belfast): "That mental health is subject to chaos theory. None of these alleles are necessary or sufficient.

Dr. Kevin Mitchell, a geneticist at Trinity College Dublin, 2014 Apr 04: "Regrettably, the use of the term polygenic implies the causal involvement of multiple genetic variants in affected individuals...Using it to refer to the implication in the etiology of a disorder of many different genes across the population bastardizes the term and renders it ambiguous at best and actively misleading at worst". The finding is an excess of rare disruptive mutations.....across a sample of cases compared to a sample of controls. While genetic heterogeneity across the sample is acknowledged, this "does not imply that disease is caused by multiple variants per individual."

A recent journal article highlights the efforts of investigators to demonstrate statistically significant proof of genetic combinations that will substantiate the assumption of genetic causation of schizophrenia [Am J Psychiatry; Sarah Bergen et al.; "Joint Contributions of Rare Copy Number Variants and Common SNPs to Risk for Schizophrenia" January 2019] The investigators acknowledge that research has failed to prove assumptions that schizophrenia is primarily caused by genetic variations involving either SNPs or Rare Copy Number Variants independently. What about combining the contribution of both variations? Results shed little additional light on this issue after investigating over 40,000 cases. It was stated, however, that certain rare CNPs supposedly do have a possible link to this illness but only 1.4%-2.5% of individuals with schizophrenia carry one of them. Risk for schizophrenia conferred by these CNVs is not deterministic, and many carriers do not develop schizophrenia. The article states that it is not known whether the additional factors affecting disease liability are environmental….

Laura C. Lathatzzeroni, PhD, Stanford University, points out the risk of finding false statistical significance when statistical measures are applied to very complex data [JAMA Psychiatry; "Evaluating the Evidence of Replication for Genetic Associations With Schizophrenia" January 2014, Vol.71, No.1 p.94]. She critiques another's (KA Aberg et al.) attempt to replicate their findings (see the article for details). Conducting her own simulation, she demonstrated the potential for large deviations from the plausible, but potentially false, sign test assumption. She states that this study illustrates a troubling statistical trend toward more complicated analyses comprising multiple filters, steps, and heuristic algorithms joined together, applied to large complex data sets ascertained from multiple sources. The statistical significance can be impossible to evaluate. She adds that permutation tests and computer based methods can maintain validity by simpler study design and adhering to clearly understood performance properties.

[Am J Psychiatry; R. Border et al. "No Support for Historical Candidate Gene or Candidate Gene-by-Interaction Hypotheses for Major Depression Across Multiple Large Samples"; May 2019] In a well-powered study, the researchers demonstrated that an analysis of prior studies of 18 candidate genes and their link to depressive phenotypes showed that the prior statistical conclusions were in error and the genetic underpinnings of common complex traits such as depression appear to be far more complicated than originally hoped. Large collaborative efforts have not supported the existence of common genetic variants with large effects on depression liability. The presumed candidate genes were no more liable to be associated with depression than genes chosen at random. This study showed that the purported statistical links were really false positives.

Our fundamental core is the emotional and psychological product of our human relationships with others, not the Frankenstein model of primitive brain-talk. At the present state of knowledge, the accumulating body of facts gleaned from the study of brain functioning does not explain complex human behavior and such knowledge remains at a rudimentary, primitive level. At the level of brain-knowledge, even consciousness itself eludes understanding let alone such complex behaviors as panic, the spectrum of homosexuality, depression or schizophrenia. Neuroscientists cannot explain "thinking." Brain changes may reflect emotional distress but such phenomena are not necessarily explanatory in and of themselves. Most emotional problems are not simple phenomena. They are complex learned maneuvers in adaptation to a particular and pathologic childhood environment.

Some, without reading this work, will dismiss it out of hand. For them, adhering to the reigning politics of the times creates an illusion of security.

Therefore, no issues exist. Of note [The New York Times, D.T. Luhrmann; "Redefining Mental Illness"; 1/18/2015] is the fact that the British Psychological Association recently affirmed ("Understanding Psychosis and Schizophrenia") that hearing voices and feeling paranoid are often a reaction to environmental trauma and that it is "vital" for those suffering from these distressing symptoms to be given an opportunity to "talk in detail about their experiences and to make sense of what has happened to them."

An analysis of present-day American culture reveals profound trends of dehumanization. Psychiatry has, as a consequence, been politicized and become a tool for the plutocrats. "The Era of the Brain" sounds praiseworthy on the surface (who could be against scientific study of the brain?) were it not for the fact that references to the mind and the human being to whom the brain belongs are being systematically deleted from the English language. "The Era of the Brain" has proven to be a wolf in sheep's clothing. Exclusively focusing on the brain at the expense of the mind serves a political end: dehumanization of the people, "The Era of Brainwashing." The plutocrats aim to create the equivalent of a homogenized humanoid insect colony where only they control the money. All people are equal as human beings and clearly no race is superior to another, but the plutocrat controlled media instructs the public that they have no right to preserve the culture they personally value and with which they identify. The dictate that all cultures are equal serves the globalization agenda and plutocrat profits. A recent film sheds a tear for giant antlike aliens whose attempted invasion of the earth was repelled. Undeterred, the aliens ready an invasion fleet anew but are vanquished by an earthling preemptive counterattack led by an adolescent who commands super-technological know-how. Our fabricated hero is heartbroken, however, that the alien hordes were wiped out with the exception of one remaining queen and her eggs (in other words don't blame the mother). He feels certain that the giant ants and humans could come to be friends and co-habit the earth. The humans, however, racists that they are, have intemperately rejected this accommodation so our hero turns his back on the human race and off he flits with the egg to populate some receptive (and unsuspecting) planetary domain. The message: just accept change. The super-rich have already prepared a niche for you in the colony.

A prerequisite for a brainwashed compliant public always necessitates thought control and dehumanization of the individual. Perhaps not in so many words but in their actions, if the powers that be can convincingly brainwash the public into believing that the mind and human relationships are irrelevant they have effectively voided an individual's personal history and identity. We become as mindless cogs to be exploited by the real culprits, the stewards of unbridled capitalism, the billionaires (with a few exceptions), whose only agenda is to complete the unfinished transfer of wealth into their own hands. Money is power. Of course, there are the billionaire philanthropists who sooth their egos with gifts here and there, perhaps charitable sums of a billion or so, but they still have trillions left over. And how did they get those trillions? Thinking people who realize that they have a mind of their own are a potential threat to the plutocracy. A thinking public might start to wonder, for example, where all the money is going. As a consequence, who knows whether or not a forthcoming angry ripple might turn into a tidal wave of retribution. As for official psychiatry, it has unfortunately been hijacked and corrupted by the money of corporate power brokers. It has been lured down a path that promotes the interests of those who seek to eliminate the thinking individual and the personal accountability we owe our fellow human beings.

Take, for example, the statements of Joshua R. Sanes, then director of the Center for Brain Science at Harvard as he addressed law students at Fordham School of Law [The New York Times; 9/18/13,"The Day When Neurons Go On Trial", Jim Dwyer]. Dr. Sanes, commenting on "the legal implications of unlocking the mysteries of the brain" states: "Fifteen years from now, somebody is going to say it's the 489th neuron from the back of your ear that made you do it, along with a mutant gene. That's going to be hard to dismiss. You guys have got a lot of work to do." Such statements are as absurd as they sound and have no scientific basis even if they have clear political implications. The brain is a plastic organ that is shaped by experience. Criminal behavior is a consequence of culture and parenting. It is the consequence of a mind and a person who has been exploited and psychologically damaged, not brain disease. But one might ask, how could a director for "Brain Science" at Harvard be so wrong? Easy, when one takes into account the fact that universities and the government have been corrupted by pharmaceutical and big business grant money. Money talks and "science" listens.

Official psychiatry's spokespersons have lobotomized the individual and amputated the brain from the mind. The entire culture, and, with it, psychiatry, have undergone a dehumanizing transformation, eine Verwandlung, as Kafka would say. If, according to the self-appointed brain experts, little energy need be expended on trying to understand how human relationships affect us, why are the arts so preoccupied with the impact that others have on our lives? If the human bond is so minor, why the fervid preoccupation of poets, composers and painters with our relationships one to another? Tragedy, love, success, failure, hatred, and fashion, would have no meaning if we lived alone, in a vacuum, without others. Yet, the currently quoted "experts" in neuroscience-talk, those who command the billions of dollars of grant money, continue to describe some fanciful species that inhabits another planet rather than the reality of human beings living on the planet Earth. In "Blazing Trails in Brain Science" [NYT 2/4/14 B. Carey], a reporter interviews Dr. Thomas R. Insel, the director of the National Institute of mental Health. The reporter, steeped in learning, states that in the 1970's psychiatry was "ruled by a cabal of Freudian theorists and lacked a scientific infrastructure."

Dr. Insel admits that his primary goal is biological. He states: "The future of psychiatry is clinical neuroscience, based on a much deeper understanding of the brain."....a path he is not likely to wander from no matter who disapproves, adds the reporter. Dr. Insel, of course, need have no fear of disapproval from the pharmaceutical industry or the government, controlled as it is by the billionaires. Yet, Dr. Insel admits that decades of research on the mechanisms of drugs has taught scientists nothing about the causes of mental illness and mentions, for example, serotonin, the target of antidepressants. "We've had this huge...a 250% increase in the use of antipsychotics without any change in the morbidity or mortality in people with mental disorders; it hasn't budged."

Dr.Insel, of course, has not spent a lot of time treating patients in intensive psychotherapy. It is doubtful that he has spent ten years in a personal psychoanalysis to find out more about himself. Were he to do so, he might question his current priorities. Be that as it may, as a scientist, it is inexcusable that he ignores incontrovertible research that proves that the brain in human beings, as opposed to song birds and worms, changes in response to how we are impacted by interpersonal relationships., the environment. Well intentioned former President Obama unveiled "the next great American project": a $100 million initiative to probe the mysteries of the human brain. "We can't afford to miss these opportunities while the rest of the world races ahead," The background for this project can be traced to Paul Allen, a co-founder of Microsoft who had set up a brain institute in Seattle and Fred Kavil, a technology and real estate billionaire who established a brain institute at Yale. It all sounds inspiring except for the fact that knowledge of environmental/interpersonal experiences as they affect the human being and its brain is light years ahead of brain knowledge, even if this knowledge, for economic reasons (read the control of money), is silenced. Furthermore, current brain research proves that it is the environment that rules.

In "All Circuits Are Busy" [NYT 5/27/14 James Gorman], Dr. H. Sebastian Seung, a neuroscientist at Princeton with a Ph.D. in physics from Harvard etc. discusses the connectome, the wiring diagram of the brain, as seen at the level of the electron microscope. For a human, that would be 85 billion brain cells, each with up to 10,000 connections, equal to a trillion gigabytes. The article describes Dr. Seung as a realist who states: "We've failed to answer simple questions. People want to know 'what is consciousness?' And they think that neuroscience is up to answering that. They want us to figure out schizophrenia and we can't even figure out why this neuron responds to one direction and not the other." He left physics because it seemed that string theory would be impossible to test. "Little did he know, he said, that neuroscience would be the same."

Promising that magical solutions to emotional problems lie just on the genetic horizon

For decades, the hunt for the gene, and then, later, the genes, that cause schizophrenia and other disorders has come up empty-handed in spite of the outlay of billions and ongoing billions in grant money funneled into what is turning out to be a wild goose chase. Hundreds, perhaps thousands, of claims made for important discoveries have not held up under scientific scrutiny. The claimed results could not be replicated nor could the assumptions based on circular reasoning be substantiated. The facts have not slowed the tempo, however, for ever more expensive "research" launchings. Recently, a billionaire, has earmarked $650 million for academic research to ferret out these theoretically causative genes. A study in the journal "Nature" (7/24/14 "Biological insights from 108 schizophrenia associated…" S.Ripke et al.) involving 36,989 cases of those suffering from schizophrenic illness and 113,075 healthy controls claimed to have found 108 genetic "risk loci" linked to schizophrenia of which 83 of these genetic variants are newly identified. The genes involve dopamine, the immune system, smoking, proteins, neuronal transmission and other as yet unknown functions. Over 40 different investigators from different facilities as part of the Psychiatric Genomics Consortium contributed to the samplings. The genetic variants in question are, individually, all of "small effect" (no blockbusters here), but the claim is made that in combination they are fundamentally involved in schizophrenic illness. A psychiatric newspaper says that the study sheds incontrovertible evidence for the genetic causation of schizophrenia. Curiosity regarding all this prompted me to contact the authors of the "Nature" study as well as a very prominent expert in the field of genetics. What is not highlighted in the news accounts but is nevertheless buried in the data is the fact that the 113,075 healthy controls, including people like you and me, also exhibit these very same risk loci and the percentage difference between cases and healthy control, is small, somewhere on the order of one or two percent. The reason for the huge sampling numbers is a consequence of the fact that without such vast samplings, and the laws of statistics, no statistical significance would be forthcoming. I asked the researchers in question why the controls didn't manifest schizophrenic illness, sharing as they do the same risk loci. Essentially their response was "No easy answer here." In other words, they don't know. But they did note that "clearly some kind of environmental risks are also impacting." This study and others like it including correspondence with the above researchers will be detailed in another book.

Sadly, a gifted comedian and actor, Robin Williams, recently committed suicide after a lifelong struggle with depression. As with many comedians who are laughing on the outside but crying on the inside, there is, at the root, depression. News commentators interviewed someone from a "brain institute" for their insights on the matter. One is left wondering, however, what planet the brain "experts" inhabit and what alien species they are talking about. It certainly couldn't have anything to do with people when they fully ignore a human being's life experience yet claim to be scientists of the planet earth.

Reading some telling details about Robin William's life and childhood, one is struck with the following: His early childhood was a lonely one, growing up in a forty room farmhouse with wealthy parents, both of whom worked, while he was attended to by maids. Much of his time was spent isolated, playing with his 2000 soldiers. He described himself as a quiet, shy, child whose first imitation was of his grandmother's voice to his mother and making her laugh. He revealed that his upbringing left him with an acute fear of abandonment and a condition he described as a "love me syndrome." He told jokes to his mother to make her laugh. At the Academy Award's ceremony, he thanked his father (with a slight twist) for giving him the confidence to go into acting. No mention was made of the mother.

What can one conclude? One suspects that his whole role as a comedian was a manifestation of his wounded attempt to emotionally connect with a remote mother, "to make her laugh." Jim Carrey, also a gifted comedian, states that a sick mother is behind the comedian's depression: "my own mother was sick."

Even commonsense would tend to indicate that parenting and culture play the dominant role in shaping human behavior. How else can one explain the capricious diversity of mankind and his myriad vicissitudes of behavior from one culture to another? Class differences, for example, are clearly the result of economic imbalances (poor blacks and whites behave differently from privileged blacks and whites). Role expectations in Japan hardly resemble Western standards and appear to be, as they are here, inculcated. How medieval Europe conceptualized the meaning of life was molded by the Church and remains incomprehensible to present-day Americans. Even the most unschooled observer, if they are honest, must admit that the high prevalence of alcoholism, crime, mental and physical illness in the American inner city is the result of poverty, illiteracy and inadequate medical care.

Of course, there are investigators who claim that genetic factors explain such cultural phenomena, which only proves, that prejudice and underlying political agendas are impervious to the facts.

Take, for example, those who claim that adoption studies of separated identical twins show that the heritabilty of I.Q. is 85%, the premise being that if identical twins with identical genes show high correlation of I.Q. even though one twin was adopted out to an unrelated family, there must be a strong genetic basis for the correlation. In reality, however, a detailed analysis of the background data reveals that the "unrelated families" are, for the most part, anything but unrelated. Or, it is claimed that heredity explains why whites of European origin have on average higher I.Q's than blacks of African origin. If that were true, one would expect that blacks who have a greater percentage of European genes would have higher I.Q.'s. That is not, however, the case. that the latest genetic and animal research roundly fails to confirm the intemperate claims that genes are the primary cause of emotional problems. An analysis of the scientific evidence involving genes, brain-environment interaction, animal research, brain plasticity studies, epidemiological data, statistical bias, and up-to date genetic research (including "de novo" gene claims), will show that the environment rules. It is human relationships that underlie mental health and mental illness.

Even the psychiatric news organ's habitually shallow presentation of the facts are posting articles that acknowledge the effect of environmental experience on the biology of the brain [Psychiatric News "Early Life Trauma of Brain Changes Biology"; July 19, 2019].

Technology and increased mobility have accelerated changes in behavior that in the past required centuries to evolve. To attribute these phenomena to unproven genetic mutations seems highly improbable. On the other hand, social forces, particularly economic factors, do explain these transformations quite well.

Part I

Psychiatry and Culture

1

The Role of Economic Factors, Unbridled Profit Motive and the Ultimate Dehumanization of the Person: Historical Perspective

The following investigation details the behavior of plutocratic unbridled capitalism in the marketplace and its influence on culture. While one may wonder about this investigation's relevance to psychiatry, bear in mind that psychiatry is profoundly influenced by economic forces and, since the super-rich control the dissemination of information, a review of these forces is more than relevant, lest we forget.

It has been said of our times that, curiously, they have failed to produce the great figures of prior ages, giants who extended the world's horizons and radically altered our perception of reality. The computer (and beyond the computer) is heralded, but rather than liberating man, it seems increasingly to be serving those who would manipulate him (ferreting out his private proclivities, spying on his whereabouts, usurping his free time, eliminating individuality). Furthermore, faster and faster computing, while a remarkable achievement, does not necessarily expand the landscape of reality. But, at another time, owing to a unique confluence of forces toward the end of the 19th century, discoveries by Einstein, Darwin, Mendel, Freud and Marx revealed heretofore hidden perspectives and forever altered our perception of the world.

Since the destruction of psychoanalytically oriented intensive treatment can be attributed to political and economic factors, one would be remiss in our review of seminal contributions to the understanding of the human condition if one did not make reference to Karl Marx, unpopular though he may be in the United States. Of course, mentioning Marx in our discourse will undoubtedly lead to accusations of "class warfare", socialism, communism and the like. Needless to say, the "free enterprise system" claim seems increasingly suspect and hypocritical for what in reality has become criminally unbridled monopolies. Moreover, the current dilemma facing psychiatry cannot be understood without realizing the extent to which economic factors influence every aspect of culture, including medicine and scientific research. A historical background follows. Later, we will continue our expedition into the realm of the mind.

Marx and the undeniable historical influence of economic factors on society

Since one may not fully agree with all of Karl Marx's analyses regarding human motivation, Marx, while not the first to recognize the influence of economic factors on society was certainly one who examined the real problems of people caught up in a particular social dilemma and related them to political and economic realities. He states in his "Vorwort zur Kritik der politischer Oekonomie" (1859) (my translation): "...my investigation resulted in the following findings, that the system of laws and the structure of the state can neither be understood by itself alone nor by the so-called general evolvement of the human spirit, but is much more rooted in the material living conditions whose totality Hegel, following the lead of the English and French of the 18th century, conceptualizes as the "bourgeois society" and that the anatomy of the "bourgeois society" can be clarified by the study of the politics of economics." "People, enter into particular necessary relations quite independent of their own will when it comes to that which they produce for society, and which corresponds to their particular level of material productive capacity. The totality of these relationships related to production creates the economic structure of the society, the real basis upon which the juridical and political superstructure is built and which determines the corresponding social consciousness. The modes of production of a person's material life determines the social, political and spiritual life processes. It is not man's consciousness that determines his being, but rather the reverse, his social being that determines his consciousness."..... "In considering [social] upheavals, one must constantly distinguish between the material, truly scientific contributing factors to upheavals in the economic conditions of production and the juridical, political, religious, artistic or philosophic, in short the ideological forms by which men become conscious of these conflicts and deal with them." "Just as one cannot judge an individual entirely by what that individual thinks he is, so one cannot judge an era of social upheaval by what society consciously says it is, but rather it must be understood much more from the existing contradictions in material living conditions, and the existing conflict between the social forces of production (the workers etc.) and the relationships related to production (the bosses etc.)."

[The original text]: "Meine Untersuchung muendete in dem Ergebnis,dass Rechtsverhältnisse wie Staatsformen weder aus sich selbst zu begreifen sind, noch aus der sogenannten allgemeinen Entwicklung des menschlichen Geistes, sondern vielmehr in den materiellen Lebensverhältnissen wurzeln, deren Gesamptheit Hegel, nach dem Vorgang der Englander und Franzosen des 18.Jahrhunderts,unter dem Namen 'buergerliche

Gesellschaft' zusammenfasst,dass aber die Anatomie der buergerlichen Gesellschaft in der politschen Oekonomie zu suchen sei......In der gesellschaftlichen Producktion ihres Lebens gehen die Menschen bestimmte, notwendige, von ihrem Willen unabhängige Verhältnisse ein,Produktionsverhältnisse,die einer bestimmten Entwicklungsstufe ihrer materiellen Productivkräfte entsprechen. Die Gesamtheit dieser Produktionsverhältnisse bildet die Oekonomischen Struktur der Gesellschaft,die reale Basis,worauf sich ein juristischer und politscher Ueberbau erhebt, und welcher bestimmte gesellschaftliche Bewusstseinsformen entsprechen. Die Produktionsweise des materiellen Lebens bedingt den sozialen,politischen und geistigen Lebensprozess ueberhaupt.Es ist nicht das Bewusstsein der Menschen,das ihr Sein, sondern umgekehrt ihr gesellschaftliches Sein, das ihr Bewusstsein bestimmt.... In der Betrachtung solcher Umwälzungen muss man stets unterscheiden zwischen der materiellen naturwissenschaftlich treu zu konstatierenden Umwälzungen der oekonomischen Produktionsbedingungen und den juristischen, politischen, religioesen, kuenstlerischen oder philosophischen, kurz ideologischen Formen, worin sich die Menschen dieses Konflikts bewusst werden und ihn ausfechten. Sowenig man das, was ein Individuum ist, nach dem beurteilt, was es sich duenkt, ebensowenig kann man eine solche Umwälzungsepoche aus ihrem Bewusstsein beurteilen, sondern muss vielmehr dies Bewusstsein aus den Widerspruechen des materiellen Lebens, aus dem vorhandenen Konflikt zwischen gesellschaftlichen Produktivkräften und Produktionsverhältnisse erklären].

In a word, Marx brought to light in unflinching fashion the overweening power that economic realities have in influencing if not distorting every facet of society-and that includes science, the arts, medicine and psychiatry. Bringing forth these important insights into the nature of economic realities as Marx investigated them, acknowledges a historical basis. Denying observations which have verified again and again over thousands of years the role of money and economic power in shaping the manifestations of societal structure and man's consciousness, denies reality and aims to suppress dissent. Freedom to think without censorship and to search for the truth, are the necessary conditions without which no person can experience his reality as an individual. Denying historical facts is to deny time itself, the fourth dimension of reality. Of course, one might not agree with all of Karl Marx's postulates, but his ground breaking research into the effect on man's consciousness of economic realities cannot be denied. Nor was he merely motivated by pre-existing political prejudices as the research was based on hard facts. Much of the data was supplied in meticulous detail by Engels in firsthand observations of the plight of British laborers.

Marx also laid bare the dehumanization of the individual when money and power become the only value, replacing all others. In his "Entmenschlichung durch das Geld" (Karl Marx, "Nationaloekonomie und Philosophie," Pariser Manuskript-1844), he states and I translate: "When money becomes the reigning and self-proclaimed measure of worth and falsely succeeds in representing and substituting for all other things, so is the world falsely transformed and along with it all natural and human qualities." "He who can buy bravery, that one is considered "brave," even if he is a coward. When money becomes the measure not just of one specific quality or thing, as related to human capacity, but rather substitutes as a measure of the whole human and natural objective world, so it becomes from the standpoint of its owner, a replacement and substitute for every existing quality, even contradictory qualities and objects; it brings about the brothering of impossibilities, it forces contradictions to kiss. If you stipulate that man and his relationship to the world indeed reflects the "human", then you can only compare love to love, exchange trust against trust. If you want to enjoy art, you must become educated in art; if you want to exercise influence over other men, you must be effectively energetic and demanding of other men. For every aspect of your relationship to Nature that corresponds to the objective of your will, there must be a true expression of your real life as an individual. When you love, without being able to call forth love in return, that is when your love does not produce a return of your love, when you as a loving person by your expression of love do not make yourself beloved, then your love is impotent, a misfortune."

[Original text: "...Da das Geld, als der existierende und sich bestätigende Begriff des Wertes, alle Dinge verwechselt, vertauscht, so ist die allgemeine Verwechslung und Vertauschung aller Dinge, also die verkehrte Welt, die Verwechslung und Vertauschung aller natuerlichen und menschlichen Qualitäten." "Wer die Tapferkeit kaufen kann, der ist tapfer, wenn er auch feig ist.Da das Geld nicht gegen ein bestimmte Qualität, gegen ein bestimmtes Ding, menschliche Wesenskräfte, sondern gegen die ganze menschliche und natuerliche gegenständliche Welt sich austauscht, so tauscht es also – vom Standpunkt seines Besitzers angesehen – jede Eigenschaft gegen jede – auch ihr widersprechende Eigenschaft und Gegenstände aus; es ist die Verbruederung der Unmoeglichkeiten, es zwingt das sich Widersprechende zum Kuss. Setzte den Menschen als Menschen und sein Verhältnis zur Welt als ein menschliches voraus, so kannst du Liebe nur gegen Liebe austauschen, Vertrauen nur gegen Vertrauen etc.Wenn du die Kunst geniessen willst, musst du ein kuenstlerisch gebildeter Mensch sein; wenn du Einfluss auf andere Menschen ausueben willst, musst du ein wirklich anregend und foerdernd auf andere Menschen wirkender Mensch sein. Jedes deiner Verhältnisse zum Menschen und zu der Natur – muss eine bestimmte, dem Gegenstand deines Willens entsprechende Äusserung deines wirklichen individuellen Lebens sein. Wenn du liebst, ohne Gegenliebe hervorzurufen, d.h. wenn dein Lieben als Liebe nicht die Gegenliebe produziert, wenn du durch eine Lebenäusserung als liebender Mensch dich nicht zum geliebten Menschen machst, so ist deine Liebe ohnmächtich, ein Unglueck."

Marx apprises us of the unnatural condition in which money becomes the measure of everything. The individual is dehumanized and his natural essence is subrogated. There is nothing inherently evil about capitalism (or socialism for that matter) unless an oligarchy controls so much of the wealth and productivity of a nation that the silent majority are reduced to the status of puppets. Free enterprise is different from unbridled monopolistic capitalism. In pursuit of wealth accumulation, the means of production, communication, entertainment as well as the judicial and legislative organs of the state are bought up by ever more powerful corporate monopolies. Congressmen are purchased and laws passed that wink at and validate corporate crime but annihilate some luckless "three-time loser" in California with life imprisonment for stealing the equivalent of a loaf of bread. As I will show, official psychiatry has succumbed to this corruption. Big Business has supplanted humanistic values with a money oriented ethic and turned psychiatry on its head.

perspective on Marx:

Tempering some of Marx's views in accordance with what has been learned from the study of human behavior: whereas his conclusions regarding the potential influence of economic factors on all aspects of society is undeniable, one would not conclude that economic realities on a societal level are the soul determinant of individual consciousness, though economics certainly contributes to shaping conscious perceptions. The culture can brainwash individuals who then comply out of fear. It is also true that desperation for food and shelter understandably takes precedence over "the finer things of life" and, on a societal level, is the engine for revolutions. Our essential human consciousness is, however, innate and intrinsic to us as human beings even though corrupting life experiences may distort us. Is not Marx also upholding the basic truth that we all have an intrinsic sense of what is fair or unfair in human relationships?

The need for positive human relationships is also intrinsic. One turns to money and power in response to rejected love, as we see in Wagner's Das Rheingold" The last cell phone call from those doomed on the 911 flight was 'I love you", not how much money do I have?"

2

The Psychology of Unbridled Capitalism: Its Sociopathic Roots

"In these days friends are won through flattery. Truth breeds hatred"
Veritas odium parit
Terence, playwright of the Roman Republic

Throughout history, it has more often been the case then not, that a small faction of society gains monopolistic control over the production of capital. To secure, broaden and maintain that end, preventing competitive economic inroads by the majority in the society who would then limit, reduce, or even supplant the ruling class is a prerequisite. Expansion of political power then becomes the means to achieve this end. A necessary stratagem mandates the dumbing down of the electorate (if there is one). Ply them with immediate gratification of the baser variety, especially if profit is involved, thus killing two birds with one stone, distract them with unwarranted fears from some fictitious "enemy," or just distract them by any means possible from the real issues like where all the money is going. Above all, prevent the emergence of a competing intelligent opposition. This is best accomplished by eliminating thinking at all levels through corruption of the educational process. Maintain the status quo and stifle dissent that could potentially threaten those who have all the money. Change could lead to revolution. The "Era of the Brain" is a manifestation of an underlying agenda that is promoting a policy of thought control ("everything is in-born"). We are not to be the captains of our destiny.

Marx in "Das Kapital, The General Law of Capitalist Accumulation" highlights these time-tested principles as put forth by a candid Bernard de Mandeville at the beginning of the 18th-century: "It would be easier, where property is well secured, to live without money than without poor; for who would do the work?... as they (the poor), ought to be kept from starving, so they should receive nothing worth saving. If here and there one of the lowest class, by uncommon industry and pinching his belly, lifts himself above the condition he was brought up in, nobody ought to hinder him;... but it is the interest of all rich nations that the greatest part of the poor should almost never be idle and yet continually spend what they get… those that get their living by their daily labor… have nothing to stir them up to be serviceable but their wants, which it is prudence to relieve but folly to cure. The only thing, then, that can render the laboring man industrious is a moderate amount of money, for as too little will, according as his temper is, either dispirit or make him desperate, so too much will make him insolent and lazy… from what has been said it is manifest that, in a free nation, where slaves are not allowed of, the surest wealth consists in a multitude of laborious poor; for besides that, they are the never failing nursery of fleets and armies…. To make the society happy and people easier under the meanest circumstances, it is requisite that great numbers of them should be ignorant as well as poor; knowledge both enlarges and multiplies our desires, and the fewer things a man wishes for, the more easily his necessities may be supplied."

Mon. de Mandeville states with enviable clarity his principles for controlling and exploiting the "lower" classes. Would that today's "liberal media" dared as much to uphold the rights of the common man (but, then again, the "liberal" press are owned by big business too). If Monsieur de Mandeville's value system sounds familiar, it is because these very same principles of exploitation are as much in force today as 300 years ago. True, there is still a middle-class, but it is in the plutocracy's cross-hairs. Republics, and democracies, in time, succumb to empires as oligarchies gain control and personal freedoms succumb. Greece and Rome are cases in point.

3

Psychiatry is influenced by the Culture in which it is Embedded Who Controls Present Day American Culture?

"The right to tell people what they do not want to hear"

– George Orwell

One might ask: What does a detailed accounting of unbridled capitalism's effect on American culture have to do with psychiatry? In a word, the current impoverishment and destruction of inter-personal psychiatry in this specific society is a byproduct of economic and, especially, political forces. Many psychiatrists command lofty incomes. They opt out of Medicare and charge high fees for dispensing pills for a few minutes contact with a patient. They are ignorant of the mind and psychodynamics and have ceded psychotherapy to others, many of whom have little or no training. In this approach, long term healing relationships with patients becomes impossible, insuring the status quo and aborting the patient's chance of realizing their healthy inner potential. Totalitarian political processes (totalitarianism is the logical endpoint of unbridled capitalism) consolidate power through a program of thought control. A politically ignorant and culturally impoverished public, leaderless, poses little threat to a powerful oligarchy. The eradication of psychoanalytic exploration of the mind, memory, and the life experiences that made us unique individuals, our personal history, is one of the necessary prerequisites for mind control and the creation of mindless puppets (Hitler and Stalin certainly thought so).The goal of the plutocracy is power and the control of money. The following is a detailed historical review of the evidence that highlights the psychology of unbridled capitalism as revealed by its consistent behavior patterns. Of course, there are those who will say: "everybody knows all that anyway." If the reader is fully aware "anyway" and seeing it in print is redundant, then spring immediately to the rest of the book. Yet, people may indeed know lots of things but, unless they take to the streets, who listens to them? Everybody subjected to the tyranny of the

Bourbons, Nazis, and Soviets must have known "all that anyway" but fear of the powerful stifles open dissent.

The know-it-alls who guided the Titanic knew all about the tips of icebergs too.

How powerful is the plutocracy? A Historical Review of Selfenrichment "No money for Medicare" "No money for mental health"

The circles of the very rich, the media they control (including the so-called "liberal newspapers") and their political representatives claim that there is no money available for social benefits. France and Germany are ridiculed for squandering capital and stifling economic growth because they provide too many benefits for the average person. Available data, however, disputes these claims. It is instructive to take a factual look at the history of compensation, chronologically, of corporate executives:

Nicolas D. Kristof, columnist for the New York Times, reported that the average CEO of a major corporation (2004) received $10.8 million a year, almost 20 times as much as in 1981. But in 2017, the median pay for the 200 highest-paid chief executives was $ 17.5 million and they received an average raise of 14% compared to 5% in 2015.

[The Wall Street Journal April 12, 2004]: Pay is usually determined by a compensation board appointed by the CEO himself and composed of other CEO s (often friends) who sit on one another's boards, determining each other's salaries. [By contrast, under German law, half of the company's board seats must be filled by employee representatives.]

[The New York Times, March 17, 2004 "$111,000 per Day" Patrick McGeehan]: In 2003, the chief executive of Citigroup earned $30 million for just nine months work amounting to $111,000 per day. In addition, he sold shares of stock back to the company for $262.4 million, as well as $23 million from exercising options. Keep in mind that in 2002, Citigroup also agreed to pay a $400 million fine (a paltry sum compared to current punitive standards) as part of an industry-wide settlement to end regulatory investigations and conflicts of interest among stock analysts.

[Forbes, May 10'2004 "Executive Compensation" Forbes Staff] for 2003 (including cash, stock and options) for the following CEOs are as follows: Merrill Lynch $28 million, Wells Fargo $71,396,854 (in 2001 it was $114,367,721), Metlife $26,298,454 (in 2002 it was $33,799,343), Occidental Petroleum $29,470,293, MBNA $46,285,747, Morgan Stanley Dean Witter $15,097,889, SBC $28,894,652, Metropolitan Life Insurance $11,273,771, Schering-Plough $ 9,500,436, Sprint $27,157,374, Aetna $16,860,141, Altria Group$ 23,936,679, AT&T $18,301,630, Apple Computer $74,750,001, Bear Stearns $ 39,533,712, Cardinal health $ 13,383,468, Colgate-Palmolive $148,000,000, United Technologies $70.5 million, Lehman Brothers $67.7 million, Cendant $ 60 million, NVR $58.1 million. Wall Street paid out $15.8 billion in bonuses in 2003....and much more later.

[The Wall Street Journal, December 28, 2004 "Fannie Details Its Payout Plan for Ousted CEO" by John D. Mckinnon]: In December 2004, the CEO of Fannie Mae Corp. was ousted because of accounting irregularities but is eligible for monthly pen-sion payments of $114,393 for life. He is also owed $8.7 million deferred compensation.

Additional benefits include 1.6 million shares of stock, plus options for 368,800 shares that he becomes eligible for upon retirement. He also has life insurance benefits of $5 million until age 60 with the benefit of $2.5 million afterwards.

[Wall Street Journal August 17, 2004, "Conseco Gives CEO Rich Severance" by Joseph Hallinan]: Executive compensations have risen even when the value of the company's stock collapsed. Conseco Inc.., the insurance company, announced that its chief executive was leaving and taking with him a severance package worth $13.5 million in cash and stock. In 2003, Conseco emerged from bankruptcy court protection. The cost of he executive severance package amounted to 6% of what the company had expected to earn in 2004. [Tne New York Times, 4/25/2004, "Broadcom's Defense: Options Plan Works" Gretchen Morgenson, columnist for the New York Times, reports that the compensation board of Broadcom Corp. proposed a stock option plan that would enrich its executives and retain the express right to re-price options in the event the stock does not go up (Broadcom lost $1 billion in 2003). The Wall Street Journal [April 8, 1999 "Companies move to reprice stock options" Alix Stuart] noted: "Many businesses are re-pricing worthless executive stock options – a reprieve beyond the reach of ordinary shareholders."

[The Wall Street Journal April 8, 1999, "The Bosses Pay" compiled by William Mercer] compensation records indicate that these figures are not the exception but rather the rule in recent years. Here are some company's CEO's total compensation packages for1998: Walt Disney Co.: $576.6 million (up from$318 million in1995), while Disney's stock plummeted, America Online:$159.2 million, General Electric: $83.6 million, CocaCola: $57.3 million, Bristol-Myers Squibb: $56.3 million, Morgan Stanley Dean Witter: $53.4 million, Colgate-Palmolive: $52.7 million etc.: "These days, CEOs are assured of getting rich however the company does."

The Wall Street Journal continued: "Even staid utilities are playing the game": Cinergy Corp. gave its CEO a grant of 535,400 options." A spokesman for the utility states that 'with the jumbo award, the board is saying we want to retain you as CEO.'" Even though the utility links a portion of the annual bonus to a per share earnings goal which the company missed in 1998, Cinergy doled out the money anyhow (The CEO's bonus swelled to $619,200). The board pay panel wrote in its proxy statement report: "Employees should be rewarded for their commitment, dedication and achievements facing the company and the industry in this era of change."

Then there is a CEO of Eastman Kodak & Co. whose contract included a five-year 8.2 million-dollar loan from Kodak with which to buy company stock. Kodak waved interest payments, then forgave the principal over a period of five years. [As of 2011, Kodak was in bankruptcy].

The Wall Street Journal further reported: "Many CEOs serve on compensation boards to determine their own salaries." A chairman and CEO of Innovex Inc. and head of its compensation committee stated that he "generally leaves the room, coming back only after the panel's outside board members 'decide what I should be making. I was looking out for shareholders.'" He also, according to the Journal, "helped make compensation decisions for his wife." As one executive quoted in this Wall Street Journal article stated: "I don't want to know what anything costs. Once you're well-to-do, price doesn't really make any difference. That's part of the freedom."

[Forbes magazine, May 20, 1996 (Sherwin Rosen now deceased)]: Forbes magazine, a propaganda vehicle for big business, asked the question: "Is it fair for people to make so much money? Economics is not about fairness, it is about productivity." They quoted University of Chicago economics professor Sherwin Rosen: "It's not fair for Michael Jordan to be such a damn good basket-ball player, either, let's cap his salary!" [Are these CEOs, however, so "damn good" or, in many cases, just unethical political manipulators?" Sports figures and movie stars at least generate the money they earn.]

Nicholas D. Kristof in his New York Times column states: "There is a huge supply of would-be CEO's and negligible demand from companies for new ones, so their price should be cheap – if boards would use their leverage. When Jack Welch retired, General Electric held a contest among three underlings to succeed him. Each was desperate to get the job. If GE had applied its usual tough bargaining, it could have signed up Jeffrey Immelt on a 15 year contract for a mere $750,000 a year in salary, plus reasonable incentives for long-term success." In response to the claim: "If you don't pay the chief executive an obscene sum, you lose him," Mr. Kristof notes: "except for a turnaround experts, CEOs have few transferable skills and are in little demand elsewhere. The average 63-year-old head of a plastics company has almost zero chance of finding a better job elsewhere. One study found that of 77 cases when a major company had to find a new boss, only twice was this because the CEO had left for another corporate job."

The quest to determine whether money is available in America and where it is going

The New York Times [October 13, 1996, "Special Tax Breaks Enrich Savings of Many In the Ranks of Management" Christopher Drew et al] highlights the issue of special tax breaks, "deferred compensation" for corporate executives. These deferred pay plans work like this: "Rather than take all their pay and pay taxes on it, executives let the company hold on to some. The company invests the money and executives don't pay taxes on any of it until they take the money years later." Unlike the minuscule allowances of IRAs for millions of Americans, this deal has "special benefits": "there are no government limits on how much can be put away and many top executives have put away millions. A lot of companies guarantee then high interest rates on the money and throw in a matching contribution." The late CEO of Coca-Cola accumulated $936.4 million of company stock by virtue of this practice. Companies do not even have to disclose the amount deferred to the government, even on the executives W-2 tax form. Nor are stockholders privy to this information. A case in point is that of the head of the New York Stock Exchange, an administrative bureaucratic position, who received $140 million in accrued pension and salary (awarded by his friendly compensation board) but felt he was due $200 million. Big business owned media expressed their dismay at his critics – after all, he worked 36 years at one job! (Of course, so did millions of average Americans who have little to show for their loyal service).

Additional examples: [The New York Times January 9, 2005 "Mayday Payday Hit the Silk Timothy Obrien]: Bank of America plans to bestow on its soon to retire chief executive a promised 16.36 million-dollar cash payment, $8.67 million in incentives payments for work done over the past 13 months and $3.1million a year for life. "If he dies before his wife, she will receive $2.3 million a year, also for life. The bank also guarantees him $50,000 a year in consulting fees, and 120 hours of free flight time a year on the company's jet, an office and a secretary. "All of this is on top of the $38.4 million in company stock that he has accrued over his 38 year career." "And now that other forms of compensation are simpler for investors and shareholders to scrutinize, critics are concerned that chief executives may be quietly bundling potential riches in outsized retirement plans." When Bank of America Corp. was acquired by NationsBank in 1998, it's then chief executive who was 50 at the time, was rewarded with a new retirement package that included annual pension payments equal to 95% of his 1997 salary and bonus at Bank of America, making him eligible to receive annual payments of $4.98 million from his retirement until his death. If he died before his wife, she would receive $3.7 million annually until her own death. Prior to the bank merger, his pension was worth $810,153 a year. Six months after the merger was announced, he resigned from Bank of America and began receiving benefits.

[The New York Times February 9, 2005 "Hewlett Packard's chief forced out" Gary Rivlin rt al]: yesterday, the Board of Hewlett Packard ousted its CEO, a person known for flashy self-promotion. Although she was fired, she will walk away with $21.1 million in a severance package as well as millions more in stock and stock options. How long had she labored at the company?: About five years. She was "shot down" according to the plutocrat's television commentators.

In contrast to the astronomical windfalls of corporate CEOs, their employees receive short shrift indeed. [The New York Times February 9, 2005 "Retirement Turning Into a Brief Rest Stop As Pensions and Benefits Dwindle." Eduardo Porter et aj]. "As companies have whittled away at benefit packages, they have pushed their retirees back to work." Corporations apparently have the right to "realign benefits" as was the case at AT&T that, in 1996, replaced its defined benefit pension plan with a defined contribution system, thereby in some cases slashing benefits by half. "Downsizing" and globalization, forcing employees to work overtime without overtime pay, firing higher earning older workers, hiring part-time employees who are not entitled to any benefits whatsoever, and slashing health care benefits are the current trends. Curiously, it is consistently reported that American companies are "flush with cash." [As of 2018, nary a day goes by when we do not hear about burgeoning corporate profits].

[New York Times April 9, 1998 author not listed]: "getting kicked out of jobs is lucrative as well for the superrich." The past CEO of Apple Computer obtained a 6.7 million-dollar severance package. He asserts: "Without such downside protection, you would not get good people to take difficult jobs." Colombia/HCA Healthcare Corp. gave its chairman $10 million after ousting him amid a Medicare fraud investigation. This included a fiveyear consulting contract costing $950,000 a year, $50,000 more than he earned in annual salary. Circus Circus Enterprises refunded two million dollars to its resigned CEO to reimburse him for stock options which had become worthless. "That's why they are called CEO's" asserted Circus Circus's president. [When a CEO leaves] they have more negotiating room than people in the ranks."

American Medical News, August 23, 2004 observed "but what's getting some regulators and physicians even more upset these days are the enormous sums insurance chieftains are being paid not to work." Top executives have benefited from golden parachutes guaranteeing bonuses and benefits should their company ever be acquired by another. California insurance commissioner John Garamendi cited a potential 600 million dollars in golden parachutes to Well Point Health Network's executives as a reason to refuse approving the California firm's 16 billion-dollar merger with Indianapolis-based Anthem Inc. (other state and federal regulators had approved the merger). United Healthcare's 4.7 billion-dollar purchase of Oxford Health Plans would be accompanied by a 37 million-dollar cash and stock's option bonus to Oxford CEO's. This merger was contested by the medical society of New Jersey. When Aetna Insurance in 1996 bought out US Healthcare, the latter's chairman stayed on as an advisor for $2 million a year plus benefits. Aetna immediately supplemented that with a $10 million merger bonus and an extra $1 million a year to sign a non-compete agreement as well as an I.O.U. for another $10 million when he left the company completely. In addition, he got a gift of a 25 million-dollar airplane and was paid up to $2 million a year to operate it. So it is that the beleaguered healthcare industry has little money for adequate healthcare benefits.

Incomes of the super-rich, [Wall Street Journal = WSJ; The New York Times = NYT]

[WSJ] [Kristof, NYT 11/7/06] C.E.O. Barry Diller, 2005 take home pay $ 469 million. [WSJ, 9/8/2006] Typical winnings of managers when their company is sold to private equity firm in a $5 billion buyout: $ 150 million (or 3%) cash and $350 million additional equity.

[WSJ, 12/6/2006 "Lehman's 186 million haul" Randall Smith"12] CEO of Lehman Brothers set to receive $186 million in stock over 10 years by changing terms of stock grants dating back a decade (the company no longer exists).

[WSJ, 12/15/2006 "Street chiefs in for big payday" Susanna Craig et al] The paychecks: John Mack of Morgan Stanley $ 41 million; Lloyd Blankfine of Goldman Sachs > $50 million, CEO of Bear Stearns "possibly" $40-50 million (this investment bank subsequently failed in the "credit crisis") etc.

[WSJ, 12/15/06] "Manhattan real-estate is humming"; "projected $36 billion in bonuses will be doled out this year by the 5 top investment banks in New York"; representative property purchases (mansions, condos): $ 53 million, $40 million, $30 million etc.

[NYT, 12/17/2006 "Goldman Sachs profits at a record" John Holusha] Goldman Sachs showers "$16.5 billion in compensation" to its employees including as much as $100 million to some of its traders.

[NYT 12/22/2006 "Ex-Pfizer CEO to leave $180 million richer" Associated Press] "The former chief executive of Pfizer, Hank McKinnel, who was forced into early retirement in part because of investor anger about his rich retirement benefits, will get every penny of it and perhaps more…" (more than $180 million).

[WSJ 12/27/2006 "Bosses pay: How stock options became part of the problem" Maek Maremont et al] Executive stock-options profits from 1992-2005: Dr. William McGuire, United Health Group $2,121,000,000; L.Ellison, Oracle $1,524,000,000; S. Weill, Citigroup $ 979,000; M.Eisner, Disney $919,000,000; S. Hemsley, United Health Group $853,000,000; R. Fairbanks, Capital One Financial $781,000,000; as well as 19 other individual CEOs who averaged around $500,000,000 each.

[WSJ 1/4/2007 "Nardellis departure may spur renovation of a different kind" Michael Connolly] Being "forced out" was also lucrative, the exit package: R. Nardelli, Home Depot $210,000,000 including $20,000,000 in cash; T.Freston, Viacom 59,000,000; P. Purcell, Morgan Stanley $62,000,000; C.Fiorina, Hewlett Packard $21,000,000; M. Ovitz, Walt Disney $140,000,000; J.Barad, Mattel $50,000,000.

[WSJ] Stanley O'Neal, pay package of $48,000,000 in 2006 as well as $37 million, $34 million, $30 million, $23 million for four Vice-Presidents.

[WSJ 2/21/2007 "Fannie wont pay $44 million in bonuses…" James Hagerty et al] Fannie Mae, the quasi federal mortgage institution, won't pay $44.4 million in bonuses because of fraudulent earnings growth linked to a $6.3 billion accounting scandal. The 2006 CEO received $14.4 million in compensation. In 2008, Fannie Mae and Freddie Mac were near default, threatening to topple America's financial house of cards.

[WSJ 2/24-25/2007 "The golden touch of Stanford's president" John Hechinger et al] John Hennessy, president of Stanford University, in November, 2006 made $1 million, including $75,000 from Cisco Systems on whose board he sits, plus $133,000 in Cisco stock, $452,000 from selling stock in Atheros Communications Inc., where he is cofounder and chairman, and a $384,000 profit from Goggle Inc. stock options. He sits on Google's board. In the past five years he has collected fees, options etc. totaling $43 million. "...about a third of presidents at four year universities served on at least one board. Ruth Simmons, president of Brown University, sits on the board of Goldman Sachs Group, Pfizer Inc. and Texas Instruments. "In 2005, she took in about $732,000 from those posts in cash and stock awards ....". She has a current paper profit in Texas Instrument options of $160,000. Brown paid her $685,000. Princeton President Shirley Tilghman joined Mr. Hennessy on Goggle's board and received a stock grant of $ 1.9 million and options with a paper profit of $1.8 million. The schools say that "the presidents recuse themselves from any matters involving the companies." Mr. Hennessy was and is involved in various venture capital funds and start-up technology companies with other Stanford faculty which have been extremely lucrative. Stanford itself has profited handsomely because some of the technology, that in turn spawned private companies. Google licenses its Internet search technology from Stanford where Google's co-founders were doctorate students. "Stanford's library is one of a handful that has participated in Google's project to digitalize books so the public can search the texts." Google is being sued for copyright law and Mr. Hennessy's holdings in Google have come under criticism. Princeton also participates in Google's enterprise and their president also sits on Google's board. Google made a contribution of $2 million to a division of Stanford's law school that believes copyright law should be liberalized.

[CNN News 4/6/2007] Ford Motor co. paid Alan Mulally $28.2 million in his first four months on the job. Ford had losses of $13 billion.

[Microsoft Bing 202 salary] J. Dimon, CEO of J.P.Morgan was paid $27 million. Net worth $2 billion.

[WSJ, 4/7/2007 "Occidental's $416.3 million pay package..." Russell Gold] R. Irani CEO of Occidental Petroleum received a pay package of $426.2 million. Former Exxon Mobil Corp. CEO received $69.7 million. He also got a lump sum payment of $98.4 million because he was retiring.

[WSJ 4/27/2007 "A pension to retire for..." Dionne Searcey] "Big Pension Packages":

R. Handler, Jefferies Group $201.8 Million; E. Whitacre, ATT $158.5 million; J.Kindler, Pfizer $156.4 million; R. Ulrich, Target $134.8 million; R. Irani, Occidental Petroleum $124 million; R Davis, U.S. Bancorp $111.4 million; J. Mulva, ConocoPhillips $101.3

million; K. Lewis, Bank of America $83 million; etc. [WSJ 2007] R. Tillerson, CEO of ExxonMobil received $22.4 million in 2006, not including $102,587 for personal use of company aircraft etc.

[NYT 11/7/2007] The communist party police state of China has no problem embracing the extremes of unbridled capitalism which has "put China near top of billionaire rankings" while per capita income in China is less than $ 1000 a year. Other news sources report that if the poor in China don't pay upfront, they cannot obtain admission to hospitals. Their schooling also comes to an end if they cannot afford the taxes. Young laborers are herded into sweat shops to make t-shirts for Walmart etc.

[NYT 11/18/2007] "Creative Loans, Creative Compensation": Hundreds of billions of losses spread through the economy as result of the corrupt Wall Street subprime loan debacle. Yet, even when their companies went bankrupt and shareholders lost all their money, many executives still made off with millions (see article for details by G. Morgenson.)

Bloomberg News, 11/15/2007, reports that subprime CEO's exit pay averaged $66 million.

[NYT 11/23/2007 "Banks gone wild"] Paul Krugman, commenting on the current financial crisis and the staggering sums the Wall Street titans managed to lose, states: "And they were encouraged to make socially destructive decisions by a system of executive compensation that should have been reformed after the Enron and WorldCom scandals, but wasn't." Millions of homeowners lured into crooked mortgage loans have been wiped out and none of the greedy executives have been forced to give back their huge paychecks. [NYT 12/6/2007] "Conflicts in Consulting on Executive Pay" G. Morgenson] A congressional committee's analysis showed that 179 of the largest 250 companies disclosed hiring at least one of 6 firms to advise them on executive pay. 63% of those companies paid the same firm to provide other services to the company, thus creating a conflict of interest. [NYT 12/22/2007 "Nightmare before Christmas"] Bob Herbert reports that Bloomberg News tells us that the top Wall Street securities firms will be handing out $38 billion in bonuses, the highest total ever.

[WSJ 12/22/2007] CEO of Goldman Sachs, L. Blankfein received $69 million in compensation in 2007 (just prior to a government $ 10 billion bailout of Goldman Sachs). "Goldman's $69 million man" by Kate Kelly.

[NYT 3/7/2008 "Executive pay on the hill" Deal Book] Countrywide Financial's CEO A. Mozillo received total compensation of $250 million from 1998 through 2007 and an additional $456 million from stock sales. The company subsequently lost almost all its value.

[WSJ 3/7/2008] "KB Toll Brothers award bonuses amid gloom" M.Corkery. Mr. Toll:

$17 million bonus in 2006 plus a $1.3 million salary and stock options valued at $7.1 million. The company says "he should be compensated for preparing … for a housing market recovery." The company's stock lost most of its value. A similar scenario played out for KB homes CEO. Washington Mutual recently set compensation targets for top executives that will shield their money from the fallout of the mortgage meltdown.

[NYT 3/13/2008]"Blackstone's golden one…" by Deal Book. S. Schwarzman, CEO of Blackstone Group was paid $350 million in 2007, on top of the $4.77 billion he received when his stake in the firm was converted into stock in an initial public offering.

[NYT 3/14/2008] "V.Pandit's payout from Citigroup…" Eric Dash. 4 Pandit receives $216 million, the price tag for becoming Citigroup's new chief.

[NYT 3/16/2008] According to Show boats Int., there were 916 yachts measuring 80 feet or longer under construction, four times the number in 1997. The CEO of Oracle Systems ship is 454 feet in length, outshining Paul Allen's of Microsoft which is only 417 feet.

[WSJ 4/12/2008]"CBSs Moonves receives a 29% pay raise" by M. Marr. L. Moonves, CEO of CBS Corp. received a 29% pay raise in 2007, a package worth $36.8 million. [NYT 4/16/2008] "Housing Bill Includes Big Tax Breaks for Businesses." By Stephen Labaton et al. "Automakers, airlines and home builders are to get aid." (at least $ 25 billion through 2010 "but potentially much more"). "Automakers Are Among Industries Asking for Help in Congress." "…how the credit crisis, while rattling the housing and financial markets, has created beneficiaries in the power corridors of congress."

[NYT 4/6/2008] "A brighter spotlight" by Claudia Deutsch. John A. Thain, Merrill Lynch's newly hired CEO was coaxed aboard with a $83.8.million bonus. See article for the parade of multimillion dollar CEO pay packages. (A more detailed list is tallied in The WSJ 4/14/2000).

[CNBC 4/10/2008] Freeport McMoran's CEO's pay doubled to $74 million.

[CNBC 5/1/2008] The head of Goldman Sachs "earned" $74 million or $314,894 perday. [WSJ 8/11/2008] "A trader lands $300 million to stay put at Fortress" by Peter Lattman.

Fortress Investment Group, a hedge fund has lost two-thirds of its market value from its peak value "amid brutal markets…."

In 2008, a trader for Citigroup is slated to receive compensation for 2008 topping $125 million. The failed bank is about to be nationalized, its share price about one dollar. In 2008, huge corporate payouts posthumously to heirs: B. Roberts, CEO Comcast $

298.1 million; E. Isenberg, CEO Nabors Industries $288 million etc.

[WSJ 6/13-14/2009] "A payday for Barclays Diamond" by Sara Schaeffer Mu. More than 400 top executives of Barclay's PLC will pocket $630.3 million from the sale of the bank's money-management arm to BlackRock Inc. as the world's financial situation faces a monetary precipice reminiscent of the 1930's. B.Diamond of Barclay's (who will get $36.5 million) and BlackRock chairman L. Fink are shown smiling ear to ear.

[WSJ 4/28/2009] "Chesapeake holders denounce executive pay" by Ben Casselman. Chesapeake Energy corp. directors paid the chief executive A. McClendon $112 million in 2008 "even as the company's stock tumbled."

[WSJ 4/29/2009] V. Pandit, C.E.O. of Citigroup argues for U.S. approval for retention reward bonuses "designed to perk up demoralized employees." One such energy trader made $100 million in 2008. The bank's stock sunk to a low of around a dollar a share.

[NYT 6/4/17] "Dissecting Marissa Mayer's $900,000 a week salary" by Vindu Goel. Marissa Mayer C.E.O. of Yahoo received nearly $240,000,000 during her five year tenure. [NYT 4/6/2008] Ben Stein writes: "In the Boardroom, Every Back Gets Scratched."

He explains why executives of American corporations are paid far more than their counterparts at comparable companies in Europe or Japan. Stockholders may legally own the company "but they have almost no say in how their employees, the executives, are paid." It is the board, the compensation committee that determines pay. Those board members are appointed by the C.E.O. himself. As a board member you get good pay for just sitting in on meetings. You get insurance, a pension, stock options, use of the private jet. "The compensation committee knows that its hiring and rehiring are dependent on Mr. Big's being happy. So it crafts a package that will keep him happy and throws in a few goodies for the directors." "You have to make sure you stay on the inside." "The amazing fact is that as the economy goes through challenges, as the stockholders fume and workers fume, the executives can basically set their own pay."

[NYT 3/23/2008] Ben Stein writes about the financial debacle facing the economy, the subprime mortgage crisis, the hedge funds that are running amuck, destroying the retirement hopes of millions: "...there are laws against schemes and artifices to defraud. The current Securities and Exchange Commission basically ignores them." "...we have basically turned over the securities markets to the Crips and the Bloods. It's time to reclaim them for semi-decent people."

[NYT 4/9/2008] "For many a boom that wasn't" by D. Leonhardt. In 2007 in what looks to have been the end of the most recent expansion the median family made about $60,500. At the end of the previous expansion in 2000,the median American family made about $61,000 (in inflation adjusted terms). "This has never happened before."

[NYT 11/20/2007] "In Thanksgiving Speech, Bush Urges Americans to Give Back."

An announcer for CNBC financial news network (NBC) feigns dismay at the criticism of these payouts and asks if it doesn't represent "war on the wealthy." At the time, some Democrats timidly suggested a 4% surcharge on those earning more than $500,000 per year. In alliance with the Republicans, any tax increase on the super-rich was later scuttled by Mr. Obama. Grave concern for the "middle class" was the expressed excuse.

A history of how the ultra-rich escape taxation

A 75% – 90% tax rate on income of more than three million a year is justifiable. In Frank Sinatra's era a 90%+ graduated tax rate was the norm but today's militant plutocracy and its propaganda machines rage on uncontrollably if anyone proposes taxing them equitably, this at a time when "official" unemployment overlooks real unemployment as individuals drop out of the work force and unemployment among African-Americans is devastating. In the 2008 financial crisis, millions lost their homes and life savings owing to crooked Wall Street practices. The arrogance of those who find it natural that a plutocracy should have more rights than the economically disenfranchised rests on a double standard, namely, that it is O.K. to harm the defenseless if you have more money than they do. Illogical as it may be that some people in this country have billions while others have nothing, it is justified as, "well, that's capitalism." The divine right of kings attitude is alive and well. As Louis XIV said: "l état c'est moi." (I am the state).

A detailed look at the propaganda regarding Medicare and Social Security will be found in Chapter 14: "No Money for Medicare" – "Health costs out of Control!" (Did you know that the recent income for one year for the 400 richest Americans averaged $385 million apiece and was taxed at less than 17%?).

Overall, the compensation of CEOs in the United States compared to that of their employees is unconscionably high and at a far higher multiple than their equivalents in Europe or Asia.

A pattern evolves that absolves giant corporations of paying taxes

Let's also take a look at the tax structure. [New York Times September 23, 2004 Robert S. McIntyre]: A study released in September 2004 showed that America's largest and most profitable company's paid less in corporate income taxes the prior three years even as they increased profits. Robert S. McIntyre, the lead author of the study, wrote: "The fact that America's companies were allowed to report less than half of their actual U.S. profits to the I.R.S., while ordinary wage earners have to report every penny of their earnings, has to undermine public respect for the tax system." Tax breaks enacted in 2002 and 2003 prompted the decline in corporate payments. 28 corporations paid no taxes from 2001 to 2003 despite having profits in the period of nearly $45 billion. Pretax corporate profits rose 26% from 2001 to 2003 but corporate tax payments fell 21%. Meanwhile, capital investment by corporations dropped 12% in 2002 and 3% in 2003. "Corporate taxes as a share of the national economy are at their lowest sustained levels since World War II the study said, and financed only 6%of government expenses in the last two fiscal years."

[Wall Street Journal, April 13, 2004 Justin Layhart]: "One reason U.S. corporate tax rates have fallen, according to Lehman's Mr. Willens, is that more earnings are being generated in countries with lower tax rates. General Electric Co. paid 21.7% in income tax on earnings in 2003, down from 28.3% in 2001. This was due, the company said in its 2003 annual report, to the increasing share of earnings from lower taxed international operations." [New

York Times September 13, 2004]: A study conducted by Martin A. Sullivan, a Treasury Department economist, shows that "many companies try to lower their taxes by setting up foreign subsidiaries and using internal lending so profits are taken primarily in tax havens and costs are incurred in high tax countries." In 1991, only a small part of profit was taken from tax havens. Currently, however, 58% of offshore profits are now taken in tax havens. "The sharp rise in profits taken in tax havens like Bermuda had no relationship to economic activity there. American companies took $25.2 billion in profits in Bermuda in 2002, yet total revenues there were only $34.3 billion." Congress, "through laws and treaties that favor the use of tax havens, is shifting the burden of taxes from multinational companies to individuals and purely domestic companies." Mr. Sullivan states: "...the torrent of profits now taken in tax havens may indicate that future job growth by American firms will shift offshore." "Congress also permits perpetual deferral of taxes on profits earned offshore-but only if they are not returned to the United States." [no wonder American Big Business is frantically expanding into Asia where the many billions they reap are tax free. Consider also that, aside from the taxation question, their investments enrich Asia, not America]. Recently, the New York Times reported that Congress passed scores of special interest tax rates, including $30 billion in tax reductions on foreign corporate profits and dozens of tax breaks for timber companies, oil and gas drillers, movie studios, wine distributors and manufacturers of bows and arrows. Some tax analysts say that the bills would ultimately cost several hundred billion dollars. Yet, the facts don't deter the plutocratic media from indignantly demanding that corporate taxes be slashed.

[NYT, "What Apple Pays in Taxes, and Doesn't", 5/4/12]. Responding to a Times front page 4/29/12 article of "How Apple Sidesteps Billions in Taxes," Robert McIntyre, Director, Citizens for Tax Justice, states that in its annual report, September 2011, Apple parked $54 billion offshore (since grown, as of 2018, to $252 billion). These billions in foreign tax havens are not taxed by any government. This money originates from profits born in the U.S. "Congressional scorekeepers estimate that ending the offshore corporate tax exemption would increase overall federal revenues by about $600 billion over the next decade" (and appreciably more as of 2018).

[Reuters, "Pfizer Proposes a Marriage and a Move to Britain,..."; 4/29/14, Ben Hirschler]. Pfizer, a behemoth American drug company founded in Brooklyn in 1849, offered to buy British rival AstraZeneca for $99 billion (the offer has since been rescinded due to hefty opposition). The overture was motivated by Pfizer's desire to renounce its U.S. citizenship and incorporate in Britain to take advantage of lower corporate tax rates there. The deal would allow it to follow dozens of other large American companies that have already incorporated abroad in such countries as Ireland and the Netherlands. 50 American companies engaged in mergers that allowed them to incorporate in other countries in the past two years. Pfizer had $49 billion stashed away abroad (to avoid U.S. taxes) that it could have gotten its hands on.

President Obama rightfully proposed in his 2015 budget to ban such mergers. Another option is to turn the drug companies into public utilities.

[NYT, Floyd Norris; "Switching Names To Save On Taxes"; 4/14/14] Caterpillar found a simple way to duck billions of dollars in U.S. taxes on parts made in America but shipped overseas. In 1999 it simply took the parent name off invoices and substituted a Swiss subsidiary. Although the manufactured parts never came near Switzerland, the company negotiated a deal with Switzerland to tax its invoices at far below the normal Swiss tax rate, somewhere between 4 to 6 %. "Under current corporate tax law, it is easy for multinational companies to park profits in subsidiaries based in low-tax countries." As Caterpillar testified before a Senate hearing, only Senator Levin seemed troubled by the company's ethics: "The revenue lost to those strategies increases the tax burden on working families, and it reduces our ability to make investments in education and training, research and development, trade promotion, intellectual property protection, infrastructure, national security and more – investments on which Caterpillar and other companies depend for their success." As for the corporate tax rate of 35%, "virtually.

No multinational company pays anything near that amount."

The ultra-rich relieved of tax burdens, a recent history

Edmund Andrews, reporting in the New York Times, August 12, 2004,"Bush's remark touches off new debate..." Fully one third of President Bush's tax cuts in the prior three years had gone to people with the top one percent of income, who had earned on average $1.2 million annually, according to a report by the nonpartisan Congressional Budget Office. "The report calculated that households with incomes in that top 1% were receiving an average tax cut of $78,460 this year, while households in the middle 20% of earnings – about $57,000 a year-were getting an average cut of only $1090." According to the Congressional Budget Office, two thirds of the benefits from the tax cuts of 2001 and 2003 went to households with an average income of $ 203,740. Those in the bottom fifth of earnings received an average tax cut of only $250. Richard Yancey, author of "Confessions of a Tax Collector: One Man's Tour of Duty Inside the I.R.S. writes: "An astounding 63% of United States corporations paid no federal income tax at all in 2000." "The I.R.S. goes where the money is owed and the money is owed by the little guy. When the service was reorganized in the late 1990's, it moved collection personnel to the small business/ self-employed division; the other compliance division, which handles medium and large businesses, has no collection employees at all. Squeezed between a complex tax code that favors big business and an agency that marshals the entirety of its resources against him, the little guy doesn't stand a chance."

In 2018, the Republican's "tax reform" giveaway to the billionaires outdid the Bush windfall by $1.5 trillion.

4

How the Economic Pie is Divided Between Rich, Poor and Middle-Class: A History (Remember, Costs for Healthcare must be Slashed !)

Back in 1995, John Cassidy writing in the New Yorker [Oct. 16,1995] pointed out that in September 1979, the median middle-class income was $25,896 in inflation-adjusted dollars. In September 1995 it was $24,700. In contrast, during the same time frame, the richest 5% of American families earned $137,482. By 1993 it had risen to $177,518 and in the top 1% between 1977 and 1989, income rose from $323,942 to $576,553, a gain of 78%. living standards have fallen for the majority of Americans, while a small minority have enjoyed a bonanza. Between 1979 and 1995, the median male worker saw an 11.5% drop in annual earnings to $ 27,716, while high school graduates and high school dropouts saw earnings fall by 14.7% and 22.5% respectively, forcing women into the workforce. Mr. Cassidy went on to state that 20 years ago, the typical CEO of a large American company earned about 40 times more than a typical worker. Now[1995] he earns 190 times as much In 2003, William J. McDonough, the former head of the Federal Reserve Bank of New York who later ran the Public Company Accounting Oversight Board, testified that the average Fortune 500 CEO in 2003, made 530 times more than the average person who worked for him or her in 1980. The demise of trade unions, part of the Reagan "legacy," and the high tide of unskilled immigrants, legal and otherwise, from countries that place zero value on educating the masses, adds to the woes but provides the conglomerates with cheap slave labor.

In 2008, the compensation ratio of the top 100 CEOs compared to the average worker was 1,071 to one [Les Leopold, author of "Why Are We Afraid to Tax the Super-Rich?" www huffingtonpost.com, 4/15/2010].

[The New York Review of Books, July 18, 2002]: In 2002, Jeff Madrick reviewed "Wealth and Democracy: A Political History of the American Rich" by Kevin Phillips Here are some of the statistics: 1) more than 40% of total income in America now goes to the highest 10% of earners; 2) the wealthiest 1% of households owned more than 40% of all assets, including homes and financial investments-higher than in any year since 1929; 3) the compensation of top executives rose five times faster than did profits between 1990 and 1998. 4) corporate CEO's made 419 times the hourly wages of production worker. Even in 1988, they made only 93 times as much. Mr. Madrick also highlights the fact that the richest families in the 1950s and 1960s could not really compare to the fortunes of Rockefeller and Carnegie during the Gilded Age. This changed by the late 1980s. President Reagan enacted a major tax cut for high income Americans, making the top individual and family fortunes of 1992 two or three times the size of their 1982 counterparts. The gap between the rich and everyone else was at levels unseen since the 1920s and 1930s. By 2002, family incomes were only modestly higher after inflation than in the 1980s, but even this improvement required both spouses to work many more hours than in the past.

Have things improved? [NYT 9/11/13] "Top 10% Took Home Half Of U.S. Income in 2012." And according to Fortune the average C.E.O. made 271 times their employees in 2017.

[NYT, 2/8/12] "The Zuckerberg Tax" David S. Miller, a tax lawyer, writes about the chicanery of allowing multibillionaires to hold onto billions of dollar's worth of their company's shares and never pay taxes on those holdings even though the stock may explode upwards in value over time. The spouse then inherits that money after the executive's death. If the beneficiary sells those shares, they are only taxed on the increase in value of the stocks that might accrue after the executive's death. Executives, like Lawrence J. Ellison, C.E.O. of Oracle, can also borrow against their tremendous wealth. Mr. Ellison reportedly borrowed more than a billion dollars against his Oracle shares and bought one of the most expensive yachts in the world. President Obama proposed a minimum 30 % tax rate on the millionaires. But, as Mr. Miller points out, that so-called "Buffett rule" would only represent a trivial amount of additional taxes for Mr. Buffett. Mr. Miller proposes instead taxing any gain in a stock's value on a market to market basis at the end of each year but the taxation would be limited only to the top one-tenth of 1 percent of those who pay taxes....the super–rich.

In contrast to the windfall tax cuts for the wealthiest 1% of Americans, the ranks of the poor and those without health insurance grew in 2003 for the third straight year, the government reported. The national poverty rate rose to 12.5% in 2003, from 12.1% in 2002.

Forbes magazine annually lists the 400 richest Americans, whose net worth ranges from the hundreds of millions of dollars to the billions upon billions.

Ian Ayres and Aaron S. Edlin of Yale and University of California Law Schools [NYT 12/19/11; "Don't Tax the Rich. Tax Inequality Itself"] state that when Reagan took office the ratio of the income of the richest 1% to the median household income was 12.5. In

2006 the ratio rose 36 times greater than the median income family income. If inequality continues to grow at the current rate, the ratio will be 80 times the median.

Additional data:

[WSJ 7/23/2008 by Jesse Drucker] "In a new sign of increasing inequality in the U.S., the richest 1% of Americans in 2006 garnered the highest share of the nation's gross income for two decades, and possibly the highest since 1929, according to Internal Revenue Service data. Meanwhile, the average tax rate of the wealthiest 1% fell to its lowest level in at least 18 years."

While Americans are getting poorer, The Republicans in congress are battling to slash estate taxes for the top 0.1% of the people, a $200-300 billion giveaway over 10 years.

[NYT 3/11/2008] Bob Herbert: "It is disgraceful that in a nation as wealthy as the United States, nearly a third of the people are poor or near poor."

[NYT 12/15/2007] "Report Says the Rich Are Getting Richer Faster, Much Faster." By David Cay Johnston. From 2003-2005, for the bottom 20%, incomes were up $200; for the top 1%, a rise of $465,700. The top 1%, the total tax rate dropped 1.8%, from 2003-2005, while their average income tax rate declined to 19.4%, because of tax cuts.

[WSJ 3/19/2007] "What's Wrong With Billionaires?" A. Brooks writes that Larry Ellison, founder of Oracle Systems, would need to spend $30 million per week, or $183,000 per hour, just to avoid INCREASING his wealth. The writer finds nothing wrong with this. It's a case of what's good for Larry Ellison is good for the country. (in August, 2008 it was reported that his salary might increase by 38%).

[NYT 11/19/2006] "A New Class War: The Haves Vs. The Have Mores": While the % change in average real household income between 1990 and 2004 was an increase of 2 % for the bottom 90% of American households, it was 57% for the top 1%; and shot up to 85% for the top 0.1%; and up to 112% for the top .01%." The richest are getting richer almost twice as fast as the rich. (by Eric Konigsberg).

[WSJ 7/25/2008] The Wall Street Journal editorial board bemoans the increase in the federal minimum wage by 70 cents to $6.55 per hour and blames "left-wingers": "Bad Law, Worse Timing."

Both political parties aim to lower corporate tax rates. [NYT 8/18/2008] "Pity the poor corporations" by Paul Krugman. notes that U.S. corporate tax rates are among the highest in the industrial world but the taxes that U.S. corporations actually pay are among the lowest. Two-thirds of American companies pay no corporate income tax (CEO salaries etc. are deductible). A paradox. (by 2018 corporate tax rates were reduced to 21 percent).

[NYT 8/29/2008] Carmakers have upped their demands for a federal bailout to a "deserving $50 billion" by Nick Bunkley (remember the Hummer etc.?).

[CNBC 9/17/2008] A financial news network reports that AIG (American International

Group), the largest insurance conglomerate in the world collapsed today, the greatest financial debacle for a single company in the history of The United States, and was taken over by the U.S. government at a cost to the taxpayers of $85 billion (it was "too big to fail"). Shareholders in the company lost everything but the C.E.O. who had been on the job for a grand total of three months was given a severance package of more than $7 million.

[NYT 9/18/2008] Nicholas D. Kristof writes that Richard Fuld, the C.E.O. of now bankrupt Lehman Brothers, took home nearly half-a-billion dollars in total compensation between 1993 and 2007. In 2007 he was paid about $45 million or "$17,000 an hour to obliterate a firm." "Do we truly believe that C.E.O.'s like Mr. Fuld are more deserving of tax dollars than sick children?" "E. Stanley O'Neal, the former chief of Merrill Lynch, retired last year after driving the firm over a cliff, and he walked away with $161million." [WSJ 2/18/09 "Goldman Officer quits; Got $67.5 Million 07" by Susanne Craig. [WSJ 2/12/09 by M. de la Merced et al.] "Merrill Lynch & Co. 'secretly' moved up the date it awarded bonuses for 2008 and richly rewarded its executives despite billions of dollars in losses, giving bonuses of $1million or more apiece to nearly 700 employees…", $3.6 billion altogether.

[WSJ 3/21/09] "Wagoner's $21 million at the exit" by P. Dovrack. Rick Wagoner, ousted as CEO of General Motors for helping to destroy the company will exit with $21 million.

[NYT 6/7/12] The average executive pay for the top 200 chief executives in 2011 was $19,801,485.

[Barrons 1/2/12] Alan Abelson reports that former Hewlett – Packard CEO, Leo Apotheker reaped more than $25 million in severance and benefits after 11 months on the job during which the stock fell 40 %. IBM's departing CEO Samuel Palmisano is eligible for $170 million by waiting past 60 to retire. Nabors Industries is paying CEO Eugene Isenberg $100 million severance as he bids fond farewell to the company.

[NYT 6/1712] "CEO pay is rising despite the din" Nathanial Popper. The new CEO of Apple Computer, Timothy D. Cook, is to be compensated $378 million for a year's work. His photo shows him grinning ear to ear.

[NYT 6/17/12] David Simon of Simon Property: $137 million. Nathanial Popper [NYT 6/1713] Lawrence J. Ellison of Oracle: $77.6 million. Nathanial Popper [NYT 11/2/13 by Deal Book] "David Tepper giving Carnegie Mellon…" In 2009, in the depths of the "Great Recession," David Tepper, founder of Appaloosa Management, earned an estimated $4 billion. James Simons of Renaissance Technologies, made $2.5 billion.

[NYT 3/5/14 "Apollo global chief earned $ 546.3 million..." William Alden.] In 2013: Leon D. Black, chief of Apollo Global Management made $546.3million; the three founders the Carlyle Group including David M. Rubenstein together earned $749 million; Henry R. Kravis of Kohlberg Kravis Roberts made more than $160 million; Stephen A. Schwarzman, head of the Blackstone Group took home $452.7 million.

[NYT 4/13/14] "Still number one and doing what he wants" David Streitfeld Larry Ellison of Oracle Systems: $78.4 million.

[NYT 4/13/14] "Oligarchy in the 21 century" National Review, Mathiew Coninetti Robert A. Iger of Walt Disney $34.3 million.

[nbcnews 4/30/14] "One of nations top paid CEOs..." Entrepreneur, Geoff Weiss Cheniere Energy CEO Charif Souki $142 million in 2013.

[Motley Fool 5/27/18] "Snap hits all-time low months after CEO..." by Natalie Walters. Evan Spiegel, CEO of Snap received a stock award worth $636.6. million. Yahoo finanee Matt Weinberger, 5/27/18] "Dropbox CEO Drew Houston made $110 million..." Drew Houseton, CEO of Dropbox was awarded about $110 million.

[NYT "The Rich Get Richer", 3/26/12] Steven Rattner, a longtime Wall Street executive, states: "New statistics show an evermore startling divergence between the fortunes of the wealthy and everybody else and the desperate need to address this wrenching problem." In 2010, 93% of the additional income created in America that year compared to 2009 – $288 billion – went to the top 1% of taxpayers, those with at least $352,000 income. But the super-rich got rich faster than the merely rich. "In 2010, 37 percent of these additional earnings went to just the top 0.01 percent, a teaspoon–size collection of about 15,000 households with average incomes of $23.8 million." The bottom 99% received an $80 increase in pay per person in 2010.

In 2018, The Republicans in congress enacted gigantic tax cuts benefiting the ultrarich. It will be paid for by draconian cuts in Medicare and eviscerating programs that help lift up the disenfranchised at the social bottom.

[NYT "U.S. Families, Net Worth Falls To 1990's Levels", 6/12/12] by B. Appelbaum. [NYT "Two French Economists Say the Richest Ought to Pay More Than the Buffet Rule", 4/17/12 Annie Lowrey]: The work of Piketty and Saez and supported by Peter Diamond, a Nobel laureate at M.I.T., concludes "the United States is getting accustomed to a completely crazy level of inequality...People say that reducing inequality is radical. I think that tolerating this level of inequality is radical."

[NYT 5/30/14] "Thomas Piketty responds to criticism of his data" Neal Irwin. Thomas Piketty, a professor at the Paris School of Economics and author of the bestselling book: "Capital in the 21st Century," was challenged by The Financial Times that accused him of arbitrary manipulation of financial data and dismissed his conclusions that, over decades, there has been growing wealth inequality in Britain, and, on a broader scale, soaring inequality globally. In a response of 4,400 words, Mr.Piketty, answered these accusations point for point and suggested that The F.T. journalists refer to his reasoned conclusions supported by the facts. According to the data selected by The F.T., Mr.Piketty notes that Britain would come out more egalitarian than Sweden has ever been: "This does not look particularly plausible."

The sophist-foot-soldiers of the plutocrat-media maintain with a straight face that burgeoning income inequality between the classes is just so much leftist propaganda. Although I am a psychiatrist, not an economist, the economic data related to our culture, which I have detailed, cannot be dismissed so easily.

[NYT 2/11/14; Annie Lowrey reports "Even Among the Richest of the Rich, Fortunes Diverge"] The fortunes of the 1% and the 0.1%, or the 0.01% or the 0.001% have diverged even more than the economic fortunes of the 99% and the 1%. The richer you are, the more you have pulled away. Data from the Paris School of Economics together with the University of California, Berkeley, found that the average household in the bottom 90% of the income distribution earned about $30,997. For the top 1% the figure is $1,264,065 (41 times greater) and for the top 0.1%, $6,373,782 (206 times greater). In 1990, the same multiples were 21 and 87 and in 1980, 14 and 47. The Economic Policy Institute found that compensation for chief executives swelled about 725% in real terms from 1978 to 2011, far outpacing corporate earnings. At the same time worker compensation grew just 5.7%. The ratio of chief executive compensation to worker compensation has grown from 18 to 1 in 1965, to 209 to 1 in 2011.

[NYT 12/30/15, N.Scheiber and P.Cohen, "By Molding Tax System, Wealthiest Save Billions – Hiring an Army of Lobbyists and Lawyers to Exploit Loopholes and Steer Laws"] An extensive exposé reveals the exploitation of esoteric tax loopholes that enables the super-rich, through the courts and private negotiations with the IRS, to set-up a private tax system unavailable to the public, fueling the greatest wealth disparity in America in a hundred years. Twenty years ago the 400 hundred highest-earning taxpayers paid 27% of their income in taxes. In 2012 that figure dropped to 17% and they took home on average $336 million. The ultra-rich plutocrats insure the allegiance of presidential candidates and politicians being the greatest benefactors and contributors to their election campaigns. They also finance conservative groups that attack any effort to raise taxes on the wealthy. Through convoluted partnerships, opaque family trusts and foreign shell corporations, the billionaires convert one type of income into another type taxed at a lower tax rate. For example, hedge fund magnate, Daniel S.Loeb, Louis Bacon and Steven A. Cohen have earned billions of dollars while saving millions in taxes by routing the money to Bermuda and back. Another strategy is to place income in a special charitable trust, generating a deduction that offsets the income tax. The trust then purchases a private placement life insurance policy, which invests the money on a tax-free basis. Once the trust pays out a certain percentage each year, the heirs can inherit the rest tax free. The bottom line: the exact opposite of a progressive income tax system. The Republicans, to a man (or woman), are fighting to reduce taxes on the plutocrats further, some aiming for a 10% tax rate, and elimination of the inheritance tax completely (the "Club for Growth")

The national poverty rate

[The New York Times August 26, 2004] "More Americans living in poverty". In contrast to the windfall tax cuts for the wealthiest 1% of Americans, the ranks of the poor and those without health insurance grew in 2003for the third straight year, the government reported. The national poverty rate rose to 12.5%in 2003, from 12.1% in 2002. (by B.Knowlton)

[The New York Times, 1/26/2015] "The shrinking American middle class" A shrinking middle-class is documented: the percentage of households with income between $25,000 and $75,000 had dropped from 51.9% in 1980 to 44.9% in 2003. Since 2000 middle class income has alarmingly fallen. By A. Parlapiano et al.

[NYT editorial 4/13/14 "Recovery for Whom?"] 16% of those in their mid-20s to mid-30s were in poverty in 2012.Only 38% of those who were on their own were homeowners compared with 46% from this age group who were on their own in 2000

[NYT editorial 6/8/14] There is a current shortage of 7 million jobs. In 1970, 13.9% of people between the ages of 18 to 24 were in poverty. In 1990, 15.9% were poor; in 2012, the last year of available data, 20.4% were poor. Young people living alone or with roommates or spouses boasted a median household income of $30,604, nearly $4,600 less than in 1970, adjusted for inflation.

[NYT "The Typical Household Now Worth A Third Less" 6/27/14, V.Bajaj] Such a household's net worth was $87,992 in 2005. Ten years later it was $56,335.

[NYT Eduardo Porter "A Proposal To Help Falls Short"; 7/15/15] In the four decades long effort to ostensibly help American business compete globally, the laws that supported the middle class "were crushed." "More than 30% of men in their prime are either unemployed or earn less than what's needed to keep a family of four out of poverty…" The Economic Policy Institute states that wages in the middle of the distribution have only increased 6 percent since 1979.

The marginalization of the white working class

The destruction of the unions and rising income inequality between the ultra-rich and the white working class is creating a new underclass of poor. The specter of wrenching poverty that has shackled African-Americans is spreading to white working class Americans. Nicholas D. Kristoff [NYT, "The Decline Of White Workers," 2/9/12], writes that "…A chunk of working-class America risks being calcified into an underclass, marked by drugs, despair, family decline, high incarceration rates and a diminishing role of jobs and education as escalators of upward mobility." 80% of Mr. Kristof's high school cohort either dropped out or didn't pursue college because a solid living could be made in the steel mills etc. as their parents had done. Those jobs either disappeared or were taken by immigrants [I assume no small percentage were illegal immigrants who were favored as cheap labor once the unions were crushed]. He isn't afraid to blame the collapse of the traditional family, torn apart by poverty, as an essential factor in the rapidly increasing crime rate and drug abuse among unskilled white workers. "Among white American women with only a high school education, 44 percent of births are out of wedlock, up from 6 percent in 1970,... (according to Charles Murray's book, "Coming Apart"). [Mr. Murray apparently blames "liberals" rather than the real source of the problem].

In eliminating the white blue collar power block, the plutocracy succeeds in rendering impotent the last remaining organized opposition to its agenda of globalization. Now the whites will join the blacks and illegal Hispanics as cheap labor cogs for the plutocracy, if they can even get a job (the jobless rate for blacks is over twice that for whites). Of course, there will be a few disingenuous grand gestures. Mr. Obama, as reported in an April 2013 issue of the New York Times has given away hundreds of millions to African-American claimants who say they were unfairly denied farmland loans. The minimum payout is $50,000 per person for starters. No proof is necessary as long as they are African-Americans and make the claim. Whole families fabricated these stories including school children. Rushing to grab a chunk of the give-away, Hispanics and women are also to be included, no proof necessary. The cost to the taxpayers: over four billion dollars projected. Who said bread and circuses was ancient history?

The bailout of the Wall Street titans who hatched an unprecedented financial crisis and caused the "great recession" has been the top priority of the Federal Reserve and both political parties. Social programs are blamed for the nations escalating debt, not the trillions wasted on wars (for the profits of the armament and oil companies) or the astronomical incomes of the plutocracy who pay 15% income tax (It's "investment income") while the people pay 35%. Wall Street executives of failed firms were showered with billions in "compensation". The stockholders of these crippled companies are not so lucky. Their retirement nest egg vanished.

Former President Bush had his own idea of "fairness." He is of the belief that the transfer of wealth to the superrich is still a work in progress. He proposed a "flat tax" to "simplify the tax code" (income tax deductions would be eliminated – after all, billionaires have no need of mortgage deductions). In addition, the estate tax would be abolished and, ultimately, taxes on dividends and savings completely eliminated. Supposedly, according to Republican theorists, the middle-class and poor would benefit because the superrich could then invest in new factories with their ballooning riches. Government would be downsized because the increased taxes on the backs of the middle-class would not be enough to offset the loss of tax money from the rich. This doesn't trouble the Republican-establishment theorists (and their fellow-traveler – Democrats) because social programs for the poor and the middle-class could be cut to the bone, thus making up for the lost revenue. Budget proposals by the President Bush included slashing social programs, Medicaid, vital environmental, education and housing programs, programs for the working poor people, including childcare assistance and food stamps, community development, and health care. Programs benefiting low income citizens.... are destined to bear close to half of the cuts even though they accounted for less than 10% of spending increases during the first Bush term." As of this writing, in 2018, the Republicans succeeded in ramming through a $1.5 trillion tax relief for the super-rich. The plutocrat juggernaut is advancing.

The Republican establishment finger wags excitedly to head off any talk of repealing the tax cut giveaway to the superrich and, at the time, were successful. This is not the Republican Party of trust-buster Teddy Roosevelt.

There is no Money?

In sum, what can we conclude from the above statistics? The facts show that there is indeed sufficient money available for social programs and health care. This issue will be addressed further in chapter 14. As for the fabricated hysteria that the Social Security system is in a state of crisis, some sources estimate that if the tax cuts for the top 1% were rolled back, the resultant revenue stream would finance Social Security for the next 75 years. The nation's wealth is being siphoned off by a plutocracy, one resembling increasingly the oligarchies of imperial ancient Rome and France under the Bourbons and Louis XIV. There are only sprinkles of articles in The New York Times and The Wall Street Journal in this regard when there should be relentless headlines. Core values of American life are at stake and the American public, distracted by corporate propaganda, is broadly comatose.

With the destruction of the unions a fact, a vision of a "sweatshop" culture is already perceptible on the horizon. The plutocrats compare American workers unfavorably to the Chinese who are housed in nearby dormitories by Chinese technology conglomerates, ready at a moment's notice to work 12 hour shifts, and eager to labor for their masters in exchange for a bowl of rice. Now that's efficiency! Meanwhile, the plutocracy, through its control of entertainment and the media, manipulates a bread and circus agenda to divert the middle-class and poor from the truth. Television soap operas depict the superrich carrying on in multimillion dollar mansions with living rooms the size of football fields. Those who can't find a job or who are scraping along financially are lulled into fantasizing that, this being the land of opportunity, they too, with a little luck, could someday achieve great riches (someone has to win the lottery, why not them?). The latest statistics, however, belie this myth. European class structure has recently been shown to exhibit greater upward mobility than here in America (more on this later). Corporate marketing tells the public they are losers unless they rack up mountains of debt in conspicuous consumption. Pathetically, providing free advertising for the fashion industry by exhibiting their logos distinguishes one as "having made it." To be seen in public fully absorbed with the latest must-have technology (it will be obsolete next week) proves one is important (is anybody noticing?). Human relationships are out and score cards are in... but none but the superrich ever really score. The 2008 worldwide financial upheaval is but further proof of unbridled capitalism's ruthless quest for wild profits and its lethal consequences. The arrogant plutocrats are racing to rescue their ill-gotten billions (and succeeding) while the public is thrown to the wolves: Pension plan wiped out? So what.

The greatest threat to American society lies within. The Roman Empire declined because it succumbed to inner dehumanizing forces and history is repeating itself. The American family is disintegrating. Both spouses are forced to work whether they want to or not. Children are neglected, dismissed as "ADD" or "ADHD" and raised on pills because "researchers" (drug industry's lackeys) proclaim that these are the findings of modern science, if the couple can even afford to have children.

5

The Ethics of Unbridled Capitalism: Its Goals And Ultimate Consequences. Is the Public Fully Aware of the Extent to which America has been Hijacked?

The sociopathic pattern of individuals and business entities who can operate without moral or legal constraints, governed solely by their own self-interest and profit, is historically well documented. Power tends to corrupt and absolute power corrupts absolutely, stated Baron Acton. "The Jungle" published at his own expense in 1906 by Upton Sinclair exposed the conditions in the Stockyards and meatpacking industry: "Rats were a nuisance and the packers would put poisoned bread out for them, they would die and then the rats, bread, and meat would go into the hoppers together."; "The History of the Standard Oil Co," by Ida M. Tarbell published in 1904, detailed the rise of a business monopoly that prospered through unscrupulous gangster tactics; "The Shame of the Cities," by Joseph Lincoln Steffens, published in 1906 uncovered abundant evidence of the corruption of politicians by businessmen seeking special privileges.

Turning from the Gilded Age of the Robber Barons to our own times, is there widespread evidence of unethical business practices? A review of recent history:

The backdating of options scandal

[Wall Street Journal 11/11/05] "Authorities probe improper backdating of options" Mark Maremont. One finds that staid and solid mutual funds (Bank of America, Bank One, Janus Funds etc.) were cited by New York's attorney general to have colluded with a hedge fund to allow buying and selling of their mutual funds at the 4 p.m. New York closing price but actually several hours afterwards, thus taking advantage of earning reports and breaking news after the bell. The price? A cut of the criminal profits. The ordinary citizen, of course, could not exercise transactions until the close of business the following day. "First, Canary conducted late trading with Bank of America by faxing before 4 p.m. a series of proposed trades which would later be either canceled or confirmed with a pre-close time stamp, but then was given a trade processing system with direct access to the securities unit mutual funds clearing system."

The backdating of options was a common place scheme on the part of the corporate mafia. For example, [WSJ 2/16/2007], "Probe of backdating options moves to faster track" by James Bandler et al. "On Jan. 4, 2002, the chief financial officer of Broadcom Corp, tapped out an email about stock options to his chief executive and others.' I VERY strongly recommend that these options be priced as of December 24,' he wrote. They were, and that was fortunate for recipients. Broadcom's share price rose 23% between the two dates. The pretense that the options had been granted on the earlier date made them extra valuable." A former general counsel of Monster Worldwide Inc. pleaded guilty to securities fraud in federal court and the founder of Take-Two Interactive Software pleaded guilty to a backdating scheme.

[WSJ 1/20/2007] "Executives get bonuses as companies reprice options" by Charles Forelle. The backdating scandal caused dozens of companies to fire top executives, take charges totaling billions of dollars. But now a number of companies are making special payments to compensate officers who weren't involved in options wrongdoing but saw their profit reduced when their options were adjusted to reflect the actual dated issued. At least 140 companies are being investigated by federal authorities.

[WSJ 12/30/2006] "Jobs helped pick favorable dates for option grants" by Nick Wingfield et al. Apple's CEO helped pick 'favorable' dates for option grants but ex-executives were to blame according to the company.

[WSJ 12/12/2006] "Backdating done to avoid paying more income tax" The Mercury News, the Associated Press. "New evidence suggests that corporate executives may have found another way to manipulate their stock options, this time to cheat on their income taxes."

[WSJ 2/7/2007] "SEC alleges fraud at DRS unit" Charles Forelle et al. "Federal regulators charged two former executives of Engineered Support Systems Inc. with a long running scheme to backdate stock options at the defense contractor, saying the pair improperly increased their own pay and that of other top officials by a total of $20 million."

The unending parade of greed

[WSJ 3/2/2007]"SEC charges 14 in Wall Street insider trading ring" no author given. Discussing the millions illegally earned through insider trading: "... how easy it can be to get and trade on market-moving information before its public disclosure."[

[WSJ 12/20/2011] "Inside Capitol, Investor Access Yields Rich Tips": Brody Mullins et al. On Dec. 8, 2009, a group of hedge funds were let in on the Senate's brokered proposed health care law, hours before a public announcement. "They belong to a select group who pay for early, firsthand reports on Capitol Hill".... and it's all legal. For example, Senator Dodd signaled to the hedge funds that a proposed provision wouldn't be included, a position favorable to Visa and MasterCard. Among the hedge funds attending, Conatus capital Management, then increased its holdings in VISA by 50 %. Visa's share price rose from $81 at the end of January to a high about $96 in April (see the article for details of other such examples).(And how many of the public know that members of congress cannot be prosecuted for acting upon and financially profiting from their access to insider information?) [WSJ 1/27/2007] "In call to deregulate business…" Greg Ip et al. "Prominent figures in the U.S. are warning that the nation's financial markets have been handicapped by post Enron regulatory overreach." Former Treasury Secretary Paulson made the problem "a signature political issue." The dean of Columbia's business school says that increasing costs to U.S. companies "threatens investment and growth." (The U.S. faced a financial precipice as a result of unregulated investment banker's unethical excesses in the housing industry).

[NYT 6/20/2008] "2 face Fraud Charges in Bear Stearns Debacle." Louise Story. In the spring of 2007 as the mortgage market disintegrated, two Bear Stearns executives shared their growing fears via e-mails: "I'm fearful of these markets," one wrote. The other said later, "Believe or not – I've been able to convince people to add more money."

[The Wall Street Journal Europe October 3, 2003, author not available]: Here are a few of the more than two dozen corporate scandals that "rocked Wall Street, shattered reputations and cost investors billions of dollars in recent years": 1) Arthur Andersen LLP, "the once august accounting firm"-accused of shredding documents in an attempt to obstruct an SEC investigation into the collapse of Enron, an important client; 2) Citigroup Inc. agreed to pay $400 million to settle government charges that it issued fraudulent research reports and engaged in IPO spinning. Their stock analysts allegedly issued overly rosy recommendations to win investment banking business; 3) Enron Corp., a symbol of corporate fraud that reported annual revenue of $100 billion, employed 26,000 people but collapsed after it created off the books partnerships with names like "Raptor" and used aggressive accounting to hide massive debt and inflate the bottom line, enriching top executives in the process. One executive is in prison, another pleaded guilty to money laundering and wire fraud; 4) Global Crossing Ltd-the SEC issued rules essentially saying that global Crossing acted improperly in booking revenue. The company fell apart under $12 billion in debt; 5) HealthSouth Corp., "…prosecutors allege some of its top executives orchestrated a massive accounting fraud, now exceeding $3 billion, to boost earnings." 15 former executives have agreed to plead guilty. 6) Imclone Systems Inc.executives guilty of insider trading;

7) Merrill Lynch & Co.agreed to pay $200 million for issuing fraudulent research reports plus $80 million to settle civil allegations that it aided Enron's fraud 8) WorldCom Inc.-"the biggest accounting scam ever". "Several top executives helped deep-fry the books

to the tune of $11 billion to hide costs and inflate profit and revenue over several years." It's former CEO was ousted over the issue of $408 million in personal loans he owed the company; 9) Tyco International Ltd. – New York prosecutors found that it's former chief executive and its chief financial officer stole more than $170 million from the conglomerate and illegally reaped $430 million from stock sales and used questionable accounting to hide their actions. Tyco has admitted to finding more than $2 billion of erroneous accounting. The Tyco chief executive was charged with stealing $1 million from Tyco funds for a Sardinia party for his wife. Included in the weeklong festivities were an ice sculpture of Michelangelo's David urinating vodka and a life-size female shaped birthday cake with exploding nipples. 70 some guests were greeted by chariots, gladiators and male models dressed in skimpy bathing suits. His New York apartment was decorated with company funds including a $6,000 shower curtain. The executive was later convicted and sent to jail; 10) Goldman Sachs agreed to pay $9 million in damages to The Federal Trade Commission for failing to stop insider trading in bonds.

[WSJ 1/17/2008] Justin Sheck, Steven Stecklow, Network computing "Brocade Ex-CEO Gets 21 Months in Prison" and ordered to pay a $15 million fine for backdating. [NYT 5/15/17] "To spur small business. first free the banks" op-ed by Hal S. Scott, a Harvard Law professor warned against excessive federal and state regulation of the capital markets. [How could Wall-Streeters make money if they are regulated?]

High frequency trading

There is more than one way to skin the public. The Wall Street titans have discovered high frequency trading techniques that, according to CNBC financial network [2/27/12], now account for over 70% of daily stock market trades. Massive banks of super computers now sniff out trading opportunities in a fraction of a second. Millions of in and out trades are performed per second and markets are moved, often wildly.

[WSJ 2/7/14 "Speed Traders Get an Edge"] by Scott Patterson. Traders have been paying to gain direct access to market-moving news releases from Business Wire, the Philadelphia Federal Reserve, and from Marketwired. Privy to instantaneous incoming data from news wires, light years ahead of "news" that finally reaches the poor public, the giant banking houses take advantage of manipulations and reap billions of dollars in shady profits per year. Meanwhile, the public must make do with their idle savings at zero interest, that is, unless they care to risk swimming with sharks. No value is created by any of this.

Why No Outrage?

[WSJ 7/19/2008] "Through history, outrageous financial behavior has been met with outrage. But today Wall Street's damaging recklessness has been met with near – silence, from a too-tolerant populace, argues economist James Grant."

Part of the answer to Mr. Grant's important question can be explained by the propaganda tactics of the corporate controlled media. Where are the headlines that could serve to awaken a comatose public? Even when the corporate media cannot sidestep the evidence, as in the case of the corrupt practices and psychopathic self-interest of those that ran the insurance mega-giant A.I.G., any proposal to tax astronomical executive incomes is met with vociferous propaganda ("it would be the end of America"). There are, of course, historical parallels: the repressed masses under the Bourbons being a case in point.

Sudhir Venkatesh, a sociologist at Columbia, also wonders about the American public in "Feeling Too Down to Rise Up" [NYT, 3/29/09]. He points out that Americans today are less likely to rebel and that may not be such a positive sign. "We are hearing a lot about "populist rage" but so far no riots have broken out in front of the Treasury Department or the A.I.G. headquarters....In fact the only mass disturbance to make news lately was at an 'America's Next Top Model Audition.'" Dr. Venkatesh does not attribute this phenomenon to greater love for one another or the public's capacity for patience but rather to the individual's increasing social alienation: "But these days, technology separates us and makes more of our communication indirect, impersonal and emotionally flat. With headsets on and our hands busily texting, we are less aware of one another's behavior in the public space ...cell-phones...personal entertainment devices ...self-involved bloggers, readers of niche news,... Effective rebellions require that we sing in unison." He points out that if "American anger remains corralled on the internet, into e-mail messages to congress and in sporadic small group protests, it is unlikely that the Obama administration will do much to assuage the anger of taxpayers." I would add that reducing human relationships to the virtual world of the internet and the meaning of existence to the latest technology furthers unbridled capitalism's agenda. Emotional isolation with Big Brother as the only reference point insures a brain washed bread and circus puppet. Puppets don't rebel. There were some stirrings, however. Young people created a ruckus in the "Occupy Wall Street" movement. They are mostly ignored if not vilified by the establishment press and quickly pushed out of the news. It was dutifully reported that they were not bathing regularly.

Nobel laureate Joseph E. Stiglitz's book "The Price of Inequality" rejects the apologists for unbridled capitalism who feign apathy that the monstrous economic inequalities foisted upon the American public are impervious to any cure owing to the inexorable forces of globilization, world-wide competition etc.. He rightfully holds responsible the moneyed interests that sway politics and shape policies that favor the affluent at the expense of the public. A flailing middle class and a burgeoning poor cannot revitalize productivity or economic well-being.

The plutocracy is above the law: recent history

The hope was, of course, that the Obama administration would correct these social inequalities. That, however, was not to be the case. The plutocrats wield too much power. The campaign promise of taxing the super-rich was shelved "temporarily," the excuse being that the American financial system was teetering on the brink of a 1930's style Depression. There was feckless talk of increasing taxes on those earning $200,000 a year, as if that were a bold step toward a solution. No mention is made of the real solution whereby tax revenues could be redistributed to the vast majority of Americans, the only resource capable of energizing the economy.

Increasing the tax rate slightly on those earning over $200,000 yearly, as was, at the time, proposed, is a joke. The inequality lies with those earning tens of millions and hundreds of millions a year while the poor and middle class (what's left of the middle class) see their life savings wiped out by plutocrat thieves. It is the latter who defrauded Americans of billions upon billions of dollars, if not trillions. One example is the A.I.G scandal that was the consequence of a gambling venture on the order of a gigantic ponzi scheme. The American taxpayer was billed for a $170 billion bailout of A.I.G, a sum which may still be insufficient to resolve the giant insurance company's future debt obligations, even though we are now told that all is well. The fact that A.I.G. was insolvent did not prevent the directors of the company from taking the taxpayer's bailout money to bestow $165 million (later $218 million) in "bonuses" to the very same executives at A.I.G. who were responsible for bringing the company to financial ruin [WSJ, 3/18/09]. More than 70 A.I.G executives grabbed $1million or more each (one got $6.4million and five, more than $4 million – although some of this money was supposedly returned after a public outcry.

The then Democratic administration was "outraged" that this had come to pass but felt little could be done to get the money back (dynamic sounding toothless rhetoric is used to imagine "clawing back" the money somehow). Others were also "outraged." Add to this the fact that $40 billion of taxpayer's money was given to just 10 financial institutions who had been A.I.G.'s counterparties. They were compensated at 100 cents on the dollar [NYT 3/18/09]. "Dissecting the AIG bonus contract" by Deal Book. Curiously, one would have thought that such a potentiality was a risk before A.I.G received taxpayer bailout money. Incredibly, the government-appointed chairman of A.I.G (a Bush appointee) had the gall to write the Treasury Secretary: "We cannot attract and retain the best and the brightest talent to lead and staff the A.I.G businesses-which are now being operated principally on behalf of American taxpayers – if employees believe their compensation is subject to continued and arbitrary adjustment by the U.S. Treasury." Lawyers for the plutocrats solemnly warned of constitutional issues if these bonus contracts were to be cancelled.

Lawrence Cunningham, a professor at George Washington University Law School, deflates these arguments [NYT, 3/18/09], as he pointed out that given the company's then current disastrous financial straits, there was ample legal precedent for voiding these contracts. Some honest members of congress offered that the "outrageous" bonuses of this and other companies that have received taxpayer bailout money could be taxed at a 90% rate.

That proposal failed owing to the opposition of Mr. Obama and the Senate stooges for Big Business. We also learned that President Obama's treasury secretary specifically approved a clause in the bailout provision that excluded executive bonuses from scrutiny.

Resourceful corporate America has found a way to get around the "outrage" over astronomical bonuses. Bank of America will increase salaries by 70% instead.

6

How the Plutocracy Masters Propaganda

The proposed (and now failed) taxation of A.I.G. executive bonuses unleashed a carefully engineered media blitz that pretended disgusted bewilderment at the unseemly behavior on the part of those that want to do something about unbridled capitalism's politics of entitlement. Rhetoric like "punitive," "unfair," "hysteria," "unconstitutional," was spinning its way through all news outlets. A journalist [NYT, 3/21/09 "The problem with flogging AIG" James Nocera. "Why Flogging A.I.G. Isn't Solving the Underlying Problem"] maintained that just because A.I.G.'s "shenanigans" caused worldwide problems doesn't mean that the taxpayers should get back the bonus money. He shook his head at one person's e-mail who hoped that the executives in question "should be executed with piano wire." Getting the bonus money back "is beside the point," he stated. He was more concerned about "death threats," and "ignoring far more troubling problems surrounding the A.I.G. rescue" (to my knowledge, no executive has yet been guillotined!). He quoted a banking consultant that accused Congress of "economic arson." "Taking away their bonuses-after they've already put the money in their bank accounts – hardly seems like the right way to motivate them." The journalist mentioned a "bigger issue that has barely been touched by Congress," namely the bailout of A.I.G. counterparties. One can't be too impressed by the pretense of concern for "far bigger issues," however. After all, the journalist realized that it wouldn't sound right to favor corrupt executives raking in millions willy-nilly. His angry defense of executive pay should show a little pretended concern for the public too.

Jamie Dimon, chief executive of J.P. Morgan Chase bemoans "the constant vilification of corporate America."! In a 2012 dinner at a private mansion hosted by J.P.Morgan for prominent plutocrats, Mr. Dimon, used the occasion to ridicule Paul Volcker and Richard Fisher, Federal Reserve Bank of Dallas President, calling them "infantile" for advocating the "Volcker Rule," part of the Dodd-Frank Act, which would bar banks from gambling with government insured bank deposits along with other measures designed to prevent another worldwide banking crisis through the manipulation of arcane index and credit derivatives. None too long thereafter, this bank's trader in London gambled on massive positions in indexes related to corporate defaults which proved a disaster (around $6 billion in losses), the very same reckless activities that initiated the 2008 debacle [NYT, Gretchen

Morganson,"JPMorgan's Ghost of Dinner Parties Past," 5/12/12]. Mr. Dimon was personally vilified with compensation of $23 million in 2011 [WSJ, 4/5/12 "Dimon has top banker pay"].

Vikram Pandit, chief executive of Citigroup [NYT, 3/2/09] wrote his employees about "the work we have all done to try to stabilize the financial system…would be significantly set back if we lose our talented people because Congress imposes a special tax on financial service employees" (it would be impossible for them to pay it back, he adds).

One letter to the editor of The New York Times (all the letters that day supported the A.I.G. bonuses), likens the bill to tax bonuses to the country's great shame in interning Japanese-Americans during World War II and the Salem witch trials.

All the top bankers met with President Obama. They aped grim faces as if they had been read the riot act (for television). Rest assured they won't have to give up any of their hard earned billions. Notice that the usual palaver goes something like this: We can't do anything about what happened so they get to keep all their billions, but we have to find out how to fix the system so that it won't happen again (if you can believe that).

The New York Times informed us that since June 2007 the net worth of U.S. households fell at least $12.9 trillion (subsequently magically reversed by the current stock market's levitation). Current bank bonuses are on schedule to eclipse 2007 figures and reach all-time highs. Let them eat cake.

The sad fate of a 90% tax on AIG thievery: The plutocrat/ politician evil axis

Here are the facts: The tax would only have affected those who earned $250,000 or more a year base salary. It applied only to bonus money awarded after Jan.1, 2009 (Merrill Lynch paid out $2.5 billion in bonuses in December 2008, earlier than usual, and those bonuses would not have been subject to the 90% rate). It involved companies that received government (taxpayer) bailout money, taxpayer money that would have enriched those very same individuals who exploited the moral vacuum created by lax governmental oversight. It is claimed that taxing these individuals risks losing their exceptional talents. Con-artistry is a respected talent in some circles.

Practical solutions to the exploitative entitlements of the super-rich do exist

There are remedies available when "talent" flees to foreign shores to evade taxes levied against them including mutually beneficial agreements with foreign governments, confiscation of assets, and restrictions of commerce with those entities that shelter such individuals or companies, and controlling access to U.S. markets. A 75% to 90% tax rate on any income over two or three million a year is just. It can hardly be justified that some accumulate billions while the majority languish in the maw of poverty. A civilized society acknowledges that we do not all start out on a level playing field. No one needs more than a hundred million dollars. Consider levying a special assessment of 50 % on all assets over $100 million. The money could be used to fund education and health care. The ultra-rich would still have many trillions left over. How rational is it to allow an oligarchy of superrich to augment their strangle hold on America's wealth by dismantling opportunities for the great majority? If the super affluent were called upon to sell two or three of their superfluous villas or gargantuan yachts to meet the country's dire social needs, reality and humanity would be well served and the "lower classes" would have real money to spend to revive the economy. Utopia is not built on a foundation of oppressive greed.

Some object to the giveaways to Wall Street

Joseph Stiglitz, Nobel Prize winning economist at Columbia [NYT 3/25/09] "Too big too fail or too big too save" states that the bank rescue plan is "very badly flawed" and offers "perverse incentives" that amounts to "robbery of the American people." He adds "... the banks win, investors win, and taxpayers lose." "Under the plan by Treasury Secretary Timothy Geithner, the government would provide 92% of the money to buy the asset but would stand to receive only 50% of any gains, while absorbing almost all of the losses. Some partnership! Assume that some investor is willing to pay $150 for a bank asset. The private investor puts up $12, and the government supplies the rest – $12 in equity plus $126 in the form of a guaranteed loan. If, in time, the true value of the asset is zero, the private partner loses the $12, and the government loses $138. "Paying fair market values for the assets will not work. Only by overpaying for the assets will the banks be adequately recapitalized. But overpaying for the assets simply shifts the losses to the government....when taxpayers lose big time." "So what is the appeal of a proposal like this? Perhaps it's the kind of Rube Goldberg device that Wall Street loves – clever, complex and nontransparent, allowing huge transfers of wealth to the financial markets."

Paul Krugman, Nobel Prize winning economist and columnist for The New York Times [NYT, 3/23/09 "Financial policy despair"] notes the increasing perception that Mr. Obama and his circle's ties to Wall Street are clouding their vision: "... the Geithner scheme would offer a one-way bet: if asset values go up, the investors profit, but if they go down, the investors can walk away from their debt" (and taxpayers are on the hook).

The executives at private equity firms and hedge funds, however, voice anxiety concerning the uproar over millions of bonus payments. If they win big buying up bank assets, will they be taxed big? Some executives have told the administration (and gotten reassurances from the Obama administration) that they will participate only if they are no compensation limits.

A good example of outrageous if not shady collusion between politicians and Wall

Street is highlighted by William D. Cohan [NYT, "Big Profits, Big Questions," 4/15/09]. Mr. Cohan details the partnership between Goldman Sachs, the bank, and the Presidency of the United States. Robert Rubin, Goldman's former chairman, joined the Clinton administration in 1993 as Treasury secretary. Then, "Henry Paulson, who followed Mr. Rubin to the top at both Goldman and Treasury, played in the decision to shutter Bear Stearns, to force Lehman Brothers to file for bankruptcy and to insist that Bank of America buy Merrill Lynch at an inflated price.." How convenient for Goldman Sachs who saw its competitors vanish from the landscape as it posted an unexpected $1.8 billion profit in the first quarter of 2009. Mr. Cohan points out that A.I.G. was Goldman's "great masterpiece of self-interest." Mr. Paulson refused to save Lehman Brother's for a mere $45 billion but rescued A.I.G. for $170 billion and counting. Why? Goldman and others might have gone under since they insured many of their adventures through the insurer. [According to The New York Times, 3/18/09, Goldman received 100 cents on the dollar for their gamble, $ 8.1 billion. Mr. Cohan quotes $ 13 billion]. Mr. Paulson also appointed Edward Liddy, a former Goldman Sachs board member, as A.I.G.'s chief executive. Mr. Liddy, it is revealed, still owns millions of dollars in Goldman holdings.

The reader will not be surprised to learn that the bank conglomerates reported astounding profits in the first quarter of 2009, after crippling prior losses. Taxpayer money works wonders, especially when combined with accounting manipulations, like the elimination of market to market accounting rules. After losing hundreds of billions, the biggest Wall Street firms can once again payout stratospheric levels of average compensation, spending about the same amount on employees in 2009 as they did before the financial crisis: Goldman Sachs average 2005 pay $377,000, 2009 $ 569,000; J P Morgan $293,000 in 2005, $510,000 in 2009 etc..

How Wall Street controls the Presidency: Recent history

President Obama had a campaign slogan that got him elected: "Change you can believe in." Unfortunately, the slogan proved to be toothless and a mandate was squandered. Action, not "compromise," is the only measure that can right robber baron wrongs. In the case of Mr. Obama, he went out of his way to reassure the billionaires that he is on their side: "As a general proposition, you don't want to be passing laws that are just targeting a handful of individuals....And as a general proposition, I think you certainly don't want to use the tax code ...to punish people." [WSJ 3/24/09]. One could point out that stealing is a crime and that the plutocrats have been getting away with theft for decades. President Obama called for a "more robust supervisory regime" but the plutocracy will always be several steps, if not light years, ahead of any bureaucratic agency (composed for the most part of the foot soldiers of the super –rich anyway), especially when they know that "you certainly don't want to use the tax code ...to punish people." Clearly, the only way to cure this fiscal corruption is to tax the super-rich, thereby substantially reducing the incentive to steal from the public. In 2016 the Republican establishment, definitively sealed the public's fate with an enormous tax swindle courtesy of big business that will be paid for by gutting medical care for everyone but the politicians and the .01% and ensuring that the incomes of the 95% will continue to falter.

The justice system crushes the little guy and winks at the powerful

Paul Krugman [NYT 1/16/09] "Forgive and forget?" quoted Mr. Obama's answer to the question of whether or not he would seek an investigation of possible crimes by the Bush administration: "I don't believe anybody is above the law, but we need to look forward as opposed to looking backwards." (does that apply to you and me and the law too?). So torture, illegal wiretapping and, in Iraq, handing out billions of dollars in no-bid contracts to politically connected companies is just so much spilled milk. A WSJ news release, 4/16/09: "CIA memo released; immunity for harsh tactics" S. Gorman et al. "Attorney General Eric Holder says the government won't prosecute CIA officials who used waterboarding and other harsh interrogation tactics [like murder?] on terror suspects." The army sergeant who murdered Iraqi insurgents after their capture wasn't so lucky – life imprisonment. Not even the fact that he witnessed the torture and murder of his own men by Iraqi insurgents was viewed as extenuating circumstances. Of course, the little guy doesn't have friends in high places.

Any hint of a third political party will undoubtedly incur the wrath or ridicule of the plutocrat's media arm. Nevertheless, an energized populist ground-swell is preferable to a revolution terrifyingly updated for the 21st century. But let us pursue our investigation of unbridled capitalism's tactics.

7

A History of Killing Americans for Profit: The Leopard Never Changes its Spots

The Tobacco Industry

In addition to fraud, unbridled capitalism is not averse to killing people for the sake of profits. The Journal of the American Medical Association (10/7/98 vol. 280,no. 13; R.Hurt, Channing etc.) analyzed The Brown and Williamson tobacco papers published in 1995 following a Minnesota suit against the tobacco industry. On December 15, 1953, tobacco executives met secretly to develop a response to data linking cigarettes to lung cancer. Then came the published: "A Frank Statement of Cigarette Smokers". "We will never produce and market a product shown to be the cause of any serious ailment." "We accept an interest in people's health as a basic responsibility paramount to every other consideration in our business." However, in-house secret documents state: "There is only one problem, confidence, and how to establish it.... and most important how to free millions of Americans from the guilty fear that is going to arise deep in their biological depths every time they light a cigarette... so that the public will believe [our] assertion of their own interest in Public Health." Research directors interviewed in early 1954 commented: "It's fortunate for us that cigarettes are a habit they can't break" and "boy, wouldn't it be wonderful if our company was the first to produce a cancer free cigarette. What we could do to the competition."

The industry's deliberate manipulation of nicotine levels to ensure continued smoker addiction is shown in a 1980 Lorillard document: "To determine the minimum level of nicotine that will allow continued smoking. We hypothesize that below some very low nicotine level, diminished physiological satisfaction cannot be compensated for by psychological satisfaction," and, in 1982, "The simple answer would seem to be to offer the smoker a product with comparatively high nicotine delivery so that with a minimum of effort he could take the dose of nicotine suitable to his immediate needs." 1972: "[if we] move toward reduction or elimination of nicotine from our products, then we shall eventually liquidate our business." A 1984 cigarette industry's research and development memo stated: "Irrespective of the ethics involved we should develop alternative designs (that do not invite obvious criticisms) which will allow the smoker to obtain significantly enhanced deliveries should he so wish another area of importance is the exploitation of physical and chemical means to increase nicotine transfer, i.e. to increase the effective utilization of nicotine transfer and to improve our ability to control the level of nicotine in smoke." These goals were accomplished with a biotechnology company and genetically engineered tobacco plants to manipulate nicotine levels and by recognition of the consequences of P.H. regulation and ammoniation in tar to increase nicotine delivery. A retired senior scientist at Philip Morris writes in a memo: "If important letters or documents have to be sent, please send to home. I will act on them and destroy."

The Wall Street Journal [April 28, 1998] "Tobacco industry documents" author not given. reports, Re: secondhand smoke dangers, internal tobacco memos state: "Reynolds cannot ignore this issue and stay in the tobacco business." In 1996 cigarette companies conducted a campaign in Europe to debunk the health risks of secondhand smoke with advertisements like this: "Life is full of risks," declares one headline above with a picture of three cookies. "But they're not all equal." One remembers as well the penis faced Joe Camel's appeal to vulnerable adolescent males.

Historically, the leopard never changes its spots: [Wall Street Journal, September 16 1996] "Tobacco launches magazine for regular guys" by S. Goll. Phillip Morris launches the magazine "Unlimited": "action, adventure, good times." A sample cover promises lush color photography and articles about rock climbing ("let's rock"), the country's best pool halls etc. It's destined for 2 million young men between 21and 29 and experiments with new ways to pitch cigarettes to young adults. The publisher says the magazine is aimed at "regular guys who have broad interests." Readers can redeem "Marlboro Miles" when they turn in empty cigarette packages.

The History of American Automotive Industry Ethics

Also of interest is the General Motors Corp. and its handling of vehicle gas tank explosions. In 1995, [Investor's Business Daily, September 12, 1995] G.M. settled a lawsuit with a man whose 22-year-old son was killed when a side mounted gas tank exploded. "Fifty similar suits against General Motors are pending over its C/K model pickups." "The automaker also has avoided a government attempt to force General Motors to recall the trucks". [New York Times, July 10, 1999]:"4.9 billion verdict in fuel tank case" by Andrew Pollack. "In what is believed to be the largest personal injury lawsuit, the General Motors Corp. was ordered to pay $4.9 billion to six people severely burned when the fuel tank of their 1979 Chevrolet Malibu exploded after a rear end collision." There were 30-60 other lawsuits involving fuel tank fires of the Malibu and other A body cars by General Motors. In a 1999 verdict, evidence showed that G.M. lobbied in the early 1970s against tougher standards for protecting fuel systems in crashes.. "Central to the case was a 1973 value analysis written by… an Oldsmobile engineer….. who calculated that fuel tank fires after accidents were costing the company $2.40 per vehicle. Assuming a value of $200,000 per fatality, a safer design would have cost GM $8.59 per vehicle, but the company, said the plaintiff's attorney, decided it would be cheaper to settle any lawsuits that arose. In the past, GM succeeded in keeping the memo secret. Another memo in 1974 made similar cost analyses of deaths and a January 1, 1973 memo said: "cost/ safety benefit is to be evaluated before releasing components for performance that exceeds federal requirements for fuel system integrity."

[NYT 3/14/14 "303 Deaths Seen in G.M. Cars With Failed Air Bags" by Danielle Ivory et al.]

"As lawmakers press General Motors and regulators over their decade-long failure to correct a defective ignition switch, a new review of federal crash data shows that 303 people died after the air bags failed to deploy on two of the models that were recalled last month." In February 2014 G.M. announced that it was recalling 1.6 million cars worldwide due to the faulty switch which has been linked to 12 deaths, on the 2003-2005 Chevrolet Cobalts and 2003-2007 Saturn Ions.

[NYT 3/25/14 "Carmaker Misled Grieving Families On A Lethal Flaw" by Hilary Stout et al.] G.M. denied having proof but black-box data confirmed the defective ignition in 2009, the year G.M. engineers learned of a potentially fatal defect that existed in hundreds of thousands of cars yet G.M. told families of accident victims that it didn't have enough evidence of the defect. In one case, G.M. threatened to come after the family of an accident victim for legal fees if they didn't drop a lawsuit. In another instance, it dismissed a family with a terse form letter. When Neil Kosilla sent in the paperwork after his daughter, Amy, died in a Cobalt accident in 2010 (her air bags failed to deploy), the company said there was nothing to the claim. Christopher Hamberg, 18, died in a Cobalt. Since the 2009 meeting of G.M. engineers, 26 people have died in accidents linked to these defects. [NYT 5/18/1] "GMs ignition problem: who knew what when?" Danielle Ivory. "At issue is a faulty ignition switch that can turn off if it is bumped, shutting off the engine and disabling the air bags. G.M. has linked 13 deaths to the defect and has recalled 2.6 million cars." It was further revealed that there was evidence on October 29, 2004 that the switch was defective. In February 2005, a G.M. engineer stated that the switch was close to impossible to modify. In March of 2005 the inquiry at the company was closed: "The tooling cost and piece price are too high….none of the solutions represents an acceptable business practice."

Comment: G.M.s actuaries figured out that those whom G.M. sent to their deaths were not worth the money.

Chrysler Corporation has also been implicated in deaths as a result of negligence in design and testing of its vehicles. [The New York Times October 9, 1997]:"Jury finds

Chrysler liable for …" Associated Press. In 1997, a jury found Chrysler liable for $262.5 million in the death of a six-year-old boy when he was thrown from a minivan with a defective rear latch. "Nationwide, at least 37 passengers were killed in accidents in which they were ejected when the rear liftgates opened on Chrysler town and country vehicles." On November 19, 1997 the Wall Street Journal reports "Chrysler destroyed early films of minivan crash tests, design documents and computer records." Author not listed. "Engineers considered an additional method of strengthening the latches on new models for as little as $.25 apiece in 1990 but didn't do so because the move would have undercut Chrysler's position with safety regulators that there was no problem with the latches." In attempting to quash government attempts to recall the vehicles, a vice chairman at Chrysler told the Chairman and President in a memo: "if we want to use political pressure to try to squash the recall letter we need to go now." The tactic succeeded.

On January 5, 1993, the Wall Street Journal reported: (Public Affaires Quarterly contains the article P. Werhane) "A proto-type of Ford Motor Company's Bronco II lifted a front wheel off the road while rounding a test track in Dearborn Michigan in 1982. The lift off was witnessed by the Company's head of automotive safety, his immediate superior and Ford's top in-house lawyer." The same day, Ford ordered the handing over to its lawyers of copies of all Bronco II engineering and safety records. "The purpose of the document roundup was to prepare for safety-related lawsuits that Ford expected after the Bronco II entered the marketplace." "It reflected Ford's concern that the Bronco II…. tended not only to tip but roll over completely at relatively moderate speeds." Subsequently, "more than 260 people have died in accidents in which Bronco flipped over—several times greater than any similar vehicle." "Ford knew in 1981, it could stabilize the vehicle considerably by switching to a much wider chassis but, running behind in a race to market with General Motor's Blazer, it didn't do so." More than 50 documents that should have been included in the 1982 roundup where instead destroyed, including films of roll over tests and memos to top management about Ford's marketing concerns. "Ford's own analysis of federal accident statistics in June 1988, as introduced in the later lawsuits, projected 141 roll over deaths for every one million Bronco IIs on the road.

These unconscionable tactics directly contributed to the demise of the American auto industry. Unbridled capitalism isn't particularly interested in anything beyond short term shady profits. Human beings are expendable.

Sacrificing American soldiers in Iraq to squeeze out extra profits

[NYT 1/23/09]: "Soldier's Electrocution in Iraq Was Negligent Homicide, Army Concludes" by James Risen. A Green Beret electrocuted in a shower in his barracks in Iraq was the victim of negligent homicide in a case involving the largest American contractor in Iraq according to a written statement from one investigator. Sgt. Ryan D. Maseth's death led to investigations that uncovered widespread safety problems caused by shoddy electrical work. At least 18 American personnel members have been electrocuted in Iraq. KBR, based in Houston, was targeted in the Army's complaint but a decision has not yet been made on formal charges. His family pushed for answers.

Big Business in Foster Care

The New York Times [May 4, 1997] "Deletion of a word in welfare bill opens foster care to big business" by Nina Bernstein: highlighted the up and coming role of big business in foster care. As a result of Washington lobbying, a tiny change in the federal law "opened the way for for-profit orphanages to compete for the billions of dollars that the government spends each year to support poor children who are taken away from homes judged unfit." Historically, only nonprofit institutions were eligible for this money but in the welfare legislation law passed in 1996, the word "nonprofit" was deleted, "sweeping national companies traded on Wall Street deep into the sector traditionally left to religious and philanthropic groups." "The corporate giants benefiting from this change included the one billion-dollar Magellan Health Services and youth care chains like the 2500 bed Youth Services International, started five years ago by the founder of the quick oil change franchise, Jiffy Lube." "It's the fox guarding the chicken coop said Mark E. Courtney, a University of Wisconsin scholar at the Institute for Research Of Poverty." He pointed out business's incentive to maximize profit at the expense of the children in care.

A case in point was the Au Clair School: three employees "spoke of youngsters who suffered broken noses, black eyes and missing teeth in suspicious circumstances that went uninvestigated." An internal memo of the school states: "put the energy where the dollars are," and, "blueprint the company's efforts to form ties with influential public officials." It also ordered a reduction in staff caring for the disturbed children and called for employees who were "cost effective." (the same propaganda buzz-words used currently to exhort and justify rationing of health care). The Times goes on to state: "... the booming market is another example of how the welfare overhaul has opened up opportunities in the business of poverty." Lockheed Martin and Electronic Data Systems are bidding to privatize state welfare services. Magellan has a division to take advantage of what it called "the emerging market in public contracts for vulnerable high-cost populations", such as abused, neglected and retarded children. "Youth services international has $150 million in revenue and a stated strategy of reducing labor costs by making juveniles do more work." "A New York City inspection team, after a delay of six years, visited the Au Clair School to check on children in the $429 per day program and found them in trailers that reeked of urine and feces." "One deaf boy, weeping silently had lain there for hours in an immobilizing wrap mat restraint that had cut off his circulation, they said." "I cried all the way back on the Amtrak recalled one of the two child welfare officials." The school's manual instructed staff in the use of electrical shocking devices that were illegal in the state. According to the Times, lavish parties for government officials who held the purse strings including one individual who controlled $1 billion in funds and later went to work for Au Clair School.

The New York Times [July 15, 1998] headlines "Profits at Juvenile Prison's come with a Chilling Cost" by Fox Butterfield: (referring to Tallulah Correctional Center for youth in Louisiana run by Trans American Development Associates). With wages and services at a minimum, profit was maximized while taking in as many inmates as possible; in fiscal year 1996-97 Tallulah still listed no money for recreation or for planning to return inmates to society. Showers and urinals were opened to the rooms, allowing boys incarcerated for sexual assault to attack other inmates according to the Justice Department.

Regarding males who were subjected to rape, the prevalence of homosexual rape in the American prison system, in general, casts doubt on the notion that we live in anything faintly resembling a civilized society. Everyone knows that incarcerated young men are victims of systematic rape by sexual predators yet no one seems to care (after all they are just the poor). 40% of male inmates had participated in sexual encounters with another man according to Brent Staples of The New York Times. In 2000, the Human Rights Watch organization issued a grisly report titled "No Escape: Male Rape in U.S. Prisons," rape and "horrific violence."

Abuse of the Elderly

[WSJ 2/12/2008] "High-Interest Lenders tap Elderly, Disabled." Ellen Schultz et al.. Lenders are increasingly targeting recipients of Social Security and government benefits: "These people always get paid rain or shine....every 30 days," says a former manager of payday loan stores. Many of these lenders are forging arrangements with banks to send recipient's benefits directly to the lender. "As a result, these lenders, which pitch loans with effective annual interest as high as 400% or more, can gain almost total control over Social Security recipient's finances."

8

Unbridled Capitalism in the Armament Industry

The Military – Industrial Complex

"Oderint Dum Metuant" – [Caligula]: Let them hate so long as they fear

The ethics of the armament industry in our study of current economic realities is also worthy of scrutiny. Of course, The United States should have the strongest defense possible against foreign aggressors, but military budgets are growing exponentially for America, a nation continuously at war. Writing for Fortune, Jan 11, 2008, Lawrence Lindsey, White House economist for the Bush administration, states: "The bill for the Iraq war the past five years is now approaching a cumulative $500 billion." However, Linda J. Bilmes, a former chief financial officer at the Commerce Department (now at Harvard) and Joseph E. Stiglitz, a professor at Columbia, writing in the Washington Post, March 9,2008, estimate the total cost of that war will exceed $3 trillion. The latter estimate considers the cost to help future veterans and money to refurbish a depleted military ($1.5 trillion). Because the Bush administration cut taxes for the rich, the cost of the wars in Iraq and Afghanistan are on borrowed money. Figuring in cumulative interest on the borrowing, another $1 trillion will have been added. The authors contemplate what $3 trillion could have done for health care, education and improving the quality of life for people in this country.

No one is celebrating the supposed end of the second Iraq war. What has the blood of American soldiers accomplished except to create a vacuum for Iran and, even worse, revitalize Islamic extremists, destabilizing further our planet? As of this writing, both Iraq and Afghanistan are falling into chaos. Grand schemes of "nation-building" may conceal political agendas.

As for the general "defense" budget, expenditures are dazzling: in 2001, $305 billion, in 2002, $343.2 billion, in 2003, $396.1 billion, in 2004, $399.1 billion, in 2005, the military budget for the United States was $420.7 billion (not including the extra costs for the Iraq war). The 2005 budget, at the time, was almost half of the world's total military expenditure and eight times the Chinese military budget, the second-largest in the world (although the Chinese are able to exploit slave labor) [WSJ 1/3/2007] "Pentagon redefines emergency" Jonathon Karp. The regular 1997 defense budget was $436 billion but did not include the "war-fighting budget" of an additional $99.7 billion on top of $ 70 billion in war funds which had been approved. The 2008 pentagon defense budget approached $470 billion, not including "war-fighting" funds. There are also "emergency funds" to replace equipment and upgrade to newer models "for the overall efforts related to the global war on terror."

[NYT 9/28/2006] "Air Force jet wins battle in congress" Leslie Wayne. The cost of the 183 F-22 raptors is estimated at $350 million per plane (if development costs are included), total cost about $64 billion for an advanced fighter that has no equivalent foe in the world because no other country could afford such a weapon. The Air Force says that it should have 381 F-22's (scaled back from 750). The battle for the F-22 was won in congress in defiance of the Pentagon and President. Senator Saxby Chambliss, whose district includes an F-22 assembly plant, spearheaded the multi-year contract. The F-22 is, of course, in addition to the F-35 Joint Strike Fighter earmarked for all three services. The Republican administration (2006) planned to spend $2.2 trillion on the military over five years – and this as the Congressional Budget Office projected a federal deficit of $477 billion in 2005. Shipbuilding includes $11.1 billion to support procurement of nine ships including one "Virginia" class nuclear attack submarine ($2.6 billion). The Navy had had plans for the Seawolf submarine at an initial cost of $67 billion for 30 such submarines but these plans apparently were scaled back. Russell Baker who formerly wrote for the New York Times entitled his then column: "Boat Here Needs an Enemy". Is China the next excuse for the armament industry? In 2022, The House of Representatives passed a military budget of $768 billion. China, our archenemy's budget is $267 billion. Granted, their slave-labor costs are miniscule but the U.S. armament industry is a profit driven threat all its own.

Update: In July of 2014 I read that the F-35 has been grounded for safety concerns.

The New York Times [Nov. 30, 2008, "Military-Industrial-News Media Complex"] by David Barstow. describes an example of one former general's ties to corporate interests: General McCaffrey commands platforms in the news media (widely employed as a news consultant for NBC News) while also a government advisor on military matters, including White House meetings with former president Bush. He "has consistently advocated wartime policies and spending priorities that are in line with his corporate interests. But those interests are not described to NBC viewers." He has received up to $10,000 a month from contractors like Defense Solutions and at least $500,000 from Veritas Capital, "a defense industry power-house" to name a few "linkages."

Many are wondering about the high-tech enemy we face that could afford to match such a scale of military "modernization?" Many informed critics have written about the staggering waste and redundancy in the realm of military spending. A few years ago, the Brookings Institution concluded a four-year study showing that $5.48 trillion was spent on nuclear weapons since 1940 and, whereas the nuclear arsenal was probably the single greatest deterrent to another world war, were 20,000 nuclear weapons really necessary, far in excess of military requirements? The authors concluded that pork barrel politics was responsible. William Greider, author of "The American Military and the Consequences of Peace," pointed out that not only does the new weaponry cost a fortune to develop, build and maintain, but it renders current state-of-the-art weaponry obsolete. The American government then sells the "old weapons" for pennies on the dollar in the world bargain basements. Moreover, the production of military weapons which ultimately become obsolete contributes little to a country's future growth or vitality.

Eisenhower, a military man in the mold of George Washington, warned about the malignant potential of the military-industrial complex. Eisenhower's warnings are particularly relevant today given former president Bush's eight year policy of preemptive war (with the Democratic President Obama, until recently, a zealous runner-up). There is little doubt now that the basis for the Iraq war was spun out by the propaganda machine of a profiteering armament industry. As of this writing, well over 7,000 American young men have lost their lives in Iraq and Afghanistan. Many thousands more are maimed and disfigured. Tens of thousands of poor Iraqis (the Pentagon stated that it is not in the business of calculating civilian casualties) are dead. Remember the arrogance of how Americans were exhorted to hate the French.... "old Europe" ... "freedom fries" "....be patriotic, pour out your French wine"? President Trump rightfully warned about pouring more blood and money down a middle-east rat-hole. His generals, however, have his ear, and America will continue a hopeless war in Afghanistan ad infinitum and at great expense.

Consider the consequences: "Mourning her dead son, an Iraqi woman smeared herself with his blood yesterday...". "A Marine Struggles to Be Worthy Of a Comrade's LifeSaving Sacrifice." "Wounded GI's hurt again by privatized healthcare – This is all a charade to protect profiteering scoundrels.": The military journal Army Times reported that the disgraceful conditions (at Walter Reed Army Hospital) are linked to the decision several years ago to privatize operations at the hospital leading to a dramatic drop in personnel and resources to care for wounded soldiers. The private company wanted to maximize profits [Chicago Sun Times 3/27/07]. "Army Reports Suicide Rate Reached Highest on Record" [WSJ 5/30/08]. "For Wounded Veterans and Their Families...The search for care is a maddening exercise in self-help" [NYT 3/24/08] by L. Downes. "Tracking a Marine Lost at Home" [NYT 3/31/08]: by Damien Cave. "Becky Hall's son had experienced a flashback, fleeing a relative's home after sensing that Iraqi insurgents had surrounded him." He was

24 and endured repeated surgeries after he returned home. The bomb which injured his leg also killed his close friend. He was proud of his marine uniform but felt that he no longer fit in: "Everyone is moving on. Look at me. I'm not." He woke up screaming and slept with a pistol under his bed. A manhunt set out to find him. They discovered his decomposed burned body in a drain ditch.

[NYT 5/3/08 "Overkill and short shrift"] Bob Herbert writes of David McDowell, an Army Ranger, 30, father of two, who died in Afghanistan after being deployed to Iraq and Afghanistan seven times.

Profiteering from war under the Bush-Cheney Administration

Private contractors are doing the job that historically was the government's responsibility and making billions doing it. Thomas Frank [WSJ 6/25/08] notes the exorbitant cost-fraud perpetrated on the public by private companies given lucrative no-bid contracts by the Bush Administration. "Journalist Tim Weiner estimates that by 2006, about half of the people working for the CIA and the National Counterterrorism Center, were contractors, former CIA personnel accountable not to the American public but to their employers." Former federal employees quit their jobs to work for private contractors to do the same job as before for twice the pay.

[NYT 6/17/08]"KBR losing exclusive hold on Iraq contracts" by James Risen. Charles M. Smith, senior civilian overseeing the multi-billion dollar contract with KBR, the company that provided food, housing and other services to American troops, says that he was ousted from his job when he refused to approve paying more than $1 billion in questionable charges to KBR, until recently a division of Haliburton, where former Vice-President Cheney was chief executive. Army auditors determined that KBR lacked credible data for more than $1 billion in spending. So far KBR"s contract has cost $20 billion. The U.S. House of Representatives Committee on Government Reform, Minority Staff Special Investigating Division conducted hearings on KBR practices and issued a report on June 27, 2005, concerning $1.4 billion in unsupported costs from KBR, including charges of $45 for cases of soda, $100 to clean 15 lb. bags of laundry, charges for meals never served, billings for unnecessary equipment, "inflated," "excessive," "duplicate costs," torching $85,000 trucks rather than doing minor repairs, estimates of cost of operations at Baghdad Int. Airport of $12.8 million when the government's estimate was $1.9 million.

As we all now know, the Bush administration lied about "weapons of mass destruction" to justify starting a war. Claims of "liberating" the Middle East and "bringing freedom to the world" are reminiscent of the propaganda that Hitler and Stalin used prior to their imperialist military excursions. Knowing the ethics of the military-industrial complex and the historical proclivities of unbridled capitalism, it is likely that oil was the real reason for starting the Iraq war. Central Africa has no oil so it isn't a candidate for liberation. Some

American companies will profit from the destruction and reconstruction wrought by this military venture but America as a whole has paid a terrible price in blood.

George W. Bush was a puppet of the plutocrats whose unbridled greed led to an economic maelstrom. With the slogan "change you can believe in," President Obama was elected, but, unfortunately, proved to be a disappointment. The plutocracy won't willingly relax its stranglehold on the economic wealth of the nation any time soon and it will employ every means at its disposal to extend its control. The Republican Party establishment evolved over time into a tool of the super-rich and the interests of the .01%. Currently, the Democrat establishment has outdone the Republicans by far in this regard.

The military-industrial complex is alive and well. The Afghanistan war was justified by resurrecting the old domino theory previously used to rationalize escalating the Viet Nam war. Ben Friedman of the conservative Cato institute [CNBC, 3/26/09] stated that the Bush baseline military budget for 2010 was $523 billion (not including war costs). But the Obama budget was $533 billion for that same year and $750 billion when military research, veteran's costs etc. are added in. Mr. Friedman notes that we have troops in 90 countries and that the U.S. spends ten times what Russia spends on defense. Why are American troops in Europe, in South Korea, when those countries are rich and can defend themselves? Mr. Friedman points out that the military budget went up 50% since 1998, adjusted for inflation, and that did not include the war costs. He reasons that reducing it again by 50% is not an unrealistic goal. The armament industry is doing well. They also made some spare change in the recent Libyan conflict….and now comes Syria and then….. According to The Washington Post, 2/9/16, "This remarkable chart shows how US military spending dwarfs the rest of the world" Adam Taylor. The US military budget had increased to $598billion (not including add-ons).

The Pentagon sounded the alarm about the "Chinese Military Rise" by Thom Shanker [NYT, 3/26/09]. The Chinese dictators have, however, found a more practical and lucrative way to bring America to its knees courtesy of American corporate monopolies that have fueled a consumerist debt-spiral in this country and sacrificed the American worker to globalization. America's trade deficits with China (that now controls a few trillion dollars of American debt) stems from the fact that American workers can't compete with Chinese laborers earning 3% – 10% of an American worker's wages. Tariffs were, until President Trump's overdue measures, off the table because American companies profited by out-sourcing American jobs to China (their profits if left oversees can't be taxed). Its unbridled capitalism at its worst. The attitude is: So what if the American middle class is destroyed and American workers can't find a job? While The Pentagon pours trillions into potentially obsolete weapon systems, the Chinese have been scooping up resources around the globe. Is the United States paralleling the bankrupt policy that forced the collapse of the Soviet Union? In 2001, The U.S. gave China the right to join the World Trade organization and access to American markets while at the same time having the right to protect their own markets because they were a "developing nation." As Thomas L. Friedman points out [NYT 6/7/17], this allowed China to become an economic powerhouse at the expense of the United States. Chinese companies grew in strength and were protected from foreign competition while U.S. companies could gain access to Chinese markets only if they took on Chinese partners and shared highly sophisticated Silicon Valley technology with them. "Today, Allibaba can set up its own cloud server in America but Amazon or Microsoft can't do the same in China." The world leader in industrial robots, the German company Kuka Robotics was just bought by the Chinese company Midea; Beijing would never allow the U.S. to buy one of China's industrial gems like that." I would add that this serious threat to the U.S. is the handiwork of American global corporations who salivated at the prospect of profiting from Chinese markets and were willing to be blackmailed into turning over American technology to a foreign dictatorship to accomplish that.

American multi-national corporations are the sole reason that the Chinese dictatorship has become a powerhouse on the world stage (at the expense of the American middle class). Addressing and correcting the trade imbalance with China would be more beneficial than another aircraft carrier. Yes, there could be a trade war.

A country is strong when its people prosper. But the American people have been deserted by the politician-puppets of the super-rich. The robber barons don't care what happens to the individual. To them, the 57,000 young Americans – many barely out of boyhood – who died in Vietnam, in an immoral and demonic war, are forgotten statistics, but those who loved them will never forget what happened to them. Jeff Gurvitz [The New York Times 5/5/2000 "Home videos: war widows relive Vietnam by Peter Nichols] sent his wife Barbara a tape which arrived in the mail shortly after the news of his death in Vietnam: "I feel as if I were a bystander at my own life, calmly watching myself do things I never expected or desired to do." It was only 20 years later that his wife could bear to play and hear it for the first time. That's what the politicians and armament merchants have done and are still doing to real people of flesh and blood. America's soldiers, brave though they be, are not "dying for their country." They are being exploited by politicians for reasons that are financial, not ideological. The 40 million-dollar inaugural festivities for former President Bush, suggests "dancing on graves." America is closing in on 7,000 young American deaths in Iraq and Afghanistan. Look at the faces in The New York Times, March 25, 2008 ….many more have died since!

Think back….Adam J. Muller, 21, Pfc.,Army; Underhill, Vt.; 10th Mountain Division (Light Infantry). He died in Iraq. Remember him???

Am I re-inventing the wheel? Are these facts ho - hum "common knowledge"?

My reason for compiling data from the public record is to clarify the behavior of powerful corporate interests in the marketplace. The foregoing may be "common knowledge" yet this knowledge isn't influencing the voting records of captive congressmen. The public, whose senses are dulled by moronic "entertainment" and diversionary "news," is silent, while those who have let the scales fall from their eyes are without a forum. The transfer of wealth, trillions of dollars, into the hands of a plutocracy is accelerating and the public is told over and over again that no money is available for the people. Joseph Goebbles, Reich Propaganda Minister, taught that if you repeat a lie often enough, the public will come to believe it. Hitler instructed in "Mein Kampf" that big lies are especially successful. Hopefully, repeating the truth can serve as an antidote ...if the truth is allowed a forum. The increase of corporate power is alarming. Unbridled capitalism, when not constrained by law, is governed by one and only one guiding principal: self-enrichment. Human life, children, and the defenseless elicit no pity in the eyes of the plutocracy and the only thing that stands in the way of slave labor camps are counterbalancing forces: law, the threat of force, punishment, and, most important of all, an enlightened electorate. Unbridled capitalism has much in common with other totalitarian systems: fascism, Soviet style communism, "oriental despots." Ultimately they come to resemble one another, aiming as they all do, for total control of the individual and the fruits of production. As Lord Acton said: "Power tends to corrupt and absolute power corrupts absolutely." Take heed of his warning that the final endpoint of a political ethic based solely on power is the creation of a ruling gangster class. But let us continue to study present day economics and the matrix of values which have profoundly corrupted our culture and, along with it, present day psychiatry.

9

Unbridled Capitalism's Corruption of the Political Process: Selling out the Country

The legendary politician, Mark Hanna, observed almost a century ago: "There are only two important things in politics. The first is money and I can't remember the second." The Bipartisan Campaign Reform Act of 2002 was signed into law by George W. Bush on March 27. The law bans unlimited donations to national political parties, known as "soft money." Ironically, however, the tidal wave of money continues to surge through the corridors of Congress. The two major political parties are raising more money than ever before. What happens to a society's value system when a plutocracy whose only priority is money and power controls the legislative process? Statistics show that Congressmen of both political parties are increasingly beholden to and corrupted by the unlimited financial resources of a plutocracy of billionaires who dictate the law of the land and own the organs of propaganda. The goal of this plutocracy is total control, culminating ultimately in a dumbed – down dehumanized public, hoodwinked and impotent. The white middle class had always been a force to be reckoned with…but no more. Eliminating critical thinking and introspection is part of the oligarchy's agenda. Official psychiatry which has now become a tool of big business has its subservient part to play as well.

It is a rare politician indeed that money cannot reach

[www.motherjones.com/news/special reports/2004/04/100MJ]: in the presidential election of 1860, Abraham Lincoln, outspent his opponent, Steven A. Douglas by a two-to-one margin. Lincoln was substantially supported by the railroad industry and it was during his tenure as president that the federal government issued the railroad land grants allowing the companies to acquire the most acreage in US history. In 1932, Democrat Franklin Roosevelt favored the repeal of prohibition and restoring liquor control to the states. By years end, the 18th amendment was history. In the 1936 election, brewers and distillers gave Roosevelt's Democratic Party $73,000 and only $6,000 to the Republicans. In recent history, during the Clinton presidency, major Democratic Party donors were rewarded with overnight stays in the White House Lincoln Bedroom and Camp David. The party also accepted millions of dollars in illegal campaign contributions from overseas donors, many of whom met personally with the president. When President Bush signed into law The Bipartisan Campaign Reform Act of 2002 on March 27, there was no White House ceremony and no speech by the president. "A White House spokeswoman told curious reporters that the manner in which the President signed the campaign finance reform into law was consistent with his views on the legislation."

The new rules on the use of soft money by political parties aside, businesses have more tools than ever to influence elections, including the use of 527 Organizations, Political Action Committees (PAC's) and lobbyists. A 527 Organization is a special type of political committee that can raise unlimited amounts of money and influence elections. They are part of the Internal Revenue Code and can claim a tax exempt status. PAC's fall under the Federal Election Commission and until 2010 had been regulated by the FEC. A 527 Organization can accept funds from any source and can spend these funds on anything pertaining to the election except direct contributions to the candidates. More than 20,000 committees have filed as a 527. Republican 527's included (past and present) American Resolve, Club for Growth, Progress for America, Americans United to Preserve Marriage and Swift Boat Veterans for Truth. 527 committees supporting the Democrats are America Coming Together, Thunder Road Group, and Texans for Truth. Soft money can still indirectly benefit candidates if it is spent on travel, polling and other events.

And there is also hard money which can only be given by individuals and is used to directly influence elections. A PAC represents organizations such as corporations, labor unions and trade associations. Prior to 2010, a PAC could only spend $15,000 per political party, $5,000 per candidate per election and $5,000 per PAC, but one PAC can give money to another PAC. In 2010, however, The Supreme Court decreed that "corporations are people" with unlimited super PAC money to spend. As "people" the court deemed corporations protected under the first amendment and the government cannot limit the money they spend for political purposes. The Supreme Court again came to the rescue of the billionaires and their mouthpieces.

Lobbyists have a role to play as well. A lobbyist is one who communicates with someone in a public office to try and influence legislation or regulations. Companies, organizations and special interest groups hire lobbyists.[New York Times 7/29/1999 "Tab for Washington lobbying" David Stout.] companies, labor unions, and other organizations spent, for example, $1.42 billion on lobbying Washington in 1999.(Lobbyists are required to file semi-annual reports with the Senate and House identifying their clients and the amount of income they receive. Companies have to report their overall lobbying expenditures and the names of any lobbyists employed). In the year 2000, the communications/ electronics industry spent $204 million on lobbying. Other examples for that same year /

include: the energy industry, $159 million, finance, insurance and real estate $229 million, the health industry $209 million, defense $80 million etc..

Two years after the passage of the Federal Election Campaign Act (McCain/Feingold act in 2002) special interest cash continued to find its way into the campaign coffers of Republicans and Democrats in record amounts.[CorpWatch.org: Financing the Election, Bill Mesler, July 22, 2004]: "As of May, the two campaigns had raised over $364 million more than Bush and Gore had raised by this point in the 2000 campaign when soft and hard money were allowed." "The soft money of past elections has simply morphed into new avenues of political influence." A process called "bundling" accounts for the largest sums of corporate cash flow to candidates. Elite fundraisers circumvent spending limits on donations by collecting money from family, colleagues, and employees. These donations are than "bundled" under a single name, ensuring the recognition and influence equal to the money they raised. The total cost of the 2016 campaign, presidential and congressional was $6.5 billion [Washington Post 4/14/17 "Somebody just put a price tag on the 2016 election" by Christopher Ingraham.. The Federal Election Commission Chair, Bradley Smith, charged with enforcing McCain/Feingold expressed his disdain for the legislation. He called any limits on campaign contributions to be violations of the First Amendment rights to free speech and states: "The most sensible reform is a simple one: repeal The Federal Election Campaign Act." The Supreme Court did just that and gutted the legislation under the guise of 1st Amendment rights, the final decimation of attempts to control corporations from rigging the election process was achieved in the 2010 Supreme Court ruling.

Lifting up the rock

Thomas B. Edsall of the Washington Post, August 25, 2002, took a close look at "Progress for America" which was operating from the downtown offices of a company run by Tony Feather, the political director of the Bush Cheney 2000 campaign and a close ally of Karl Rove, President Bush's top political aide. PFA has raised millions of dollars which it uses to promote Bush's agenda of tax cuts, Energy legislation, judicial appointments and free trade. "Although it takes unlimited donations from corporations and individuals, it discloses neither its contributors nor its expenditures." Mr. Adelman who is the group's chairman, said he knows neither the organizations budget nor its sources of financial support: "I can't tell you off the top of my head." He also could not remember the phone number. The address provided, the high rent Lafayette Center complex in downtown Washington, gave no listing for Progress for America but did list the offices of Mr. Feather.

Payback

[The Center for Public Integrity, March 21, 2005] "Lobbyists Bankrolling Politics" by Alex Knott reports on registered lobbyists appointed to former President Bush's transition teams. Representative examples include Jason Campbell appointed to the Department of the Interior team, affiliated with Public Lands Council, lobbying expenditures of $27,113,226; Randall Johnson, Department of Labor team, affiliated with Chamber of Commerce of the USA, lobbying expenditures $22,840,000; Gary Gasper, Treasury Department team, affiliated with Ernst and Young, lobbying expenditures $20,400,000; Barney Skladany, Commerce Department team, affiliated with Akin Gump Strauss Hauer & Feld, lobbying expenditures in $19,004,000; Karl Feldbaum, Health and Human Services team, affiliated with Biotechnology Industry Organization, lobbying expenditures of $11,306,000.There are dozens more (consult The Center for Public Integrity for up to date facts and figures).

Detailing recent and ongoing historical patterns of corporate influence in government

The Bundlers

Money from bundlers poured in so quickly that the 2004 Republican campaign invented a new title, "Rangers," for bundlers that gave over $200,000. "Of the $296 million George W. Bush had raised from 1998 to 2004, at least one third of that total came from a mere 642 of the super donors, according to data accumulated by Texans for Public Justice, an Austinbased watchdog group." Among them are 370 corporate executives, 148 of whom have been associated with corporate scandals, including Enron's Ken Lay. These big bundlers are affiliated with 102 companies that received a total of $82 billion in contracts from the Federal Government over the previous fiscal year. "Campaigns are under no legal obligation to disclose who the bundlers are or how much they have bundled."

While influencing legislation is probably their primary goal, bundlers also move into political positions inside the administration. 24 pioneers or Rangers from the 2000 campaign had been appointed ambassadors to such key countries as Austria, Belgium, Saudi Arabia (which went to an oil executive from Harken Energy) and France. 47 were appointed to the transition team. Two, Homeland Securities Secretary Tom Ridge and Labor Secretary Elaine Chao, were appointed to Cabinet positions.

Tim Shorrock and Michael Scherer, reporting in Mother Jones, May 1, 2004, state in reference to the Energy industry: "…over the past two years, the administration has rewritten the clean air rules in almost exactly the manner industry representatives suggested, often using language from corporate memos verbatim." The president of the trade group Edison Electric Institute became a pioneer in 1999, urging donors to include his campaign issued tracking member on their checks so that "our industry is credited". In 2003 he earned an invitation to an August barbecue at President Bush's Crawford ranch. In 2001, representatives from the Edison Institute participated in at least 14 discussions with members of Cheney's Energy task force, pushing for looser air pollution controls. The task force also met with representatives of First Energy and Southern Company whose top officials are Pioneers and Rangers. The latter two companies are being investigated by the environmental agency for clean air violations.

The pharmaceutical and insurance industries:

Lobbyists, the K street connection, are big bundlers. "In 2003, the pharmaceutical industry, spearheaded by its powerful trade lobby, The Pharmaceutical Research and Manufacturers of America, launched the most expensive lobbying campaign in American history. [This lobby] spent nearly $109 million and hired more than 800 lobbyists to ensure the passage of the Bush administration's 535 billion-dollar Medicare/Prescription Drug Bill." This bill prohibits the American government from negotiating drug pricing with the pharmaceutical industry. In the past PhRMA has given about 80% of its donations to Republicans. Just two [months after the passage of the Medicare/ Prescription Drug Bill, PhRMA offered one of its top jobs to the powerful chair of the House Energy and Commerce Committee (which has jurisdiction over the drug industry), Rep. Billy Tauzin (R.-Louisiana), a key player in the passage of the bill. [Mr.Tauzin,"Top house Republican becomes chief US drug company lobbyist" 12/18/04 World Socialist Website by Patrick Martin,] was offered an annual salary of about $2 million. On December 15, 2004, Rep. Tauzin was named president and CEO of PhRMA. Capital Eye Of the Center for Responsive Politics reported that this congressman raised over $218,000 in his campaign account from pharmaceutical manufacturers over the past 15 years. The New York Times 9/1/16 "Rising drug prices put big pharma's lobbying to the test" Gina Chon. In the past decade drug companies spent $2.3 billion on lobbying.

Meanwhile, Thomas Scully, under Mr. Bush, the highest ranking administration official in charge of Medicare and a point man on the legislation, received an ethics waiver allowing him to secure a position with the prominent law firm Alston and Bird, which represents a variety of drug manufacturers and other healthcare industry concerns.

Public Citizen, April 5, 2000 [www.citizen.org/pressroom] reports that managedcare groups and the member companies of the Health Benefits Coalition (who opposed the patient's Bill of Rights legislation) had given nearly $21 million in federal campaign contributions since 1995, 75% to the Republican Party and its candidates. The Blue Cross and Blue Shield Association dispatched its national PAC coordinator, Brenda Becker, to help develop major Republican Party fundraising events. "She has played a leading role in at least eight key Republican leadership fundraising activities since 1997," including the annual GOP House-Senate fundraising dinner, the party's biggest fund raiser of the year.

The Congressional Budget Office estimates that the government could save $112 billion over the next decade if Congress gave Medicare the ability to negotiate drug prices.

The media conglomerates:

[NYT David Carr, "Stealthily, Comcast Fortifies Its Arsenal"; 2/17/14]:
Comcast, a gigantic provider of cable TV has reached a deal to acquire another giant, Time Warner, creating a super-sized monopoly that will have a stifling stranglehold on cable TV and high-speed internet services. Comcast already had a win in their acquisition of NBC Universal in 2009. One of the Federal Communication Commission's regulators who approved the NBCUniversal takeover was Meredith Attwell Baker, who now works for Comcast as a lobbyist. "Since that deal, there has been a change in leadership at the commission, and it is now run by Tom Wheeler, who was previously a chief lobbyist for the cable industry." Comcast wrote checks for $18 million for lobbying in 2013 alone. Brian Roberts, chief of Comcast, has golfed with President Obama and hosted him at his residence on Martha's Vineyard. David L. Cohen, who oversees the company's relationship with regulators in Washington, has been a big bundler of donations for the president and staged a $1.2million fund-raiser for him at his home. "In recognition of those close ties, Mr.Cohen was one of the guests at a state dinner at the White House for the French president, Francois Hollande, last week." [Monopolies, of course, exist for one purpose and one purpose only: price gouging].

The end of net neutrality

Mr.Wheeler, the current FCC chairman, also announced his intention to allow such conglomerates as Comcast or Verizon to negotiate prices separately with content company – like Netflix, Amazon, Disney or Google and charge different amounts for priority service, increasing the costs for the consumer.

The tobacco industry:

CorpWatch, July 28, 2004, Chris Berdik, details the tobacco industry's lobbying: "According to the Center for Responsive Politics, in the previous election cycle, the tobacco companies gave more than $6 million in soft money, mainly to the Republican Party. Between 1995 and the end of 2002, Phillip Morris alone put up more than $10.7 million (about $9 million to Republicans)." Common Cause compiled figures which show the tobacco industry contributing more than $4.2 million to 527 groups between August of 2000 and April 2004. In addition, every year, tobacco companies pay tens of millions to Washington lobbyists who push their agenda. "In 2003, tobacco interests spent $21.2 million on lobbyists." "And when tobacco companies can't find allies, they simply create them in the form of front groups." For example, Consumers for Responsible Solutions in 2002, attempted to discredit a workplace smoking ban in Florida with a weaker countermeasure. "The group was bankrolled by Phillip Morris and disbanded after its funding source was exposed." Camouflaging its real agenda, Phillip Morris changed its name to Altria and began running television ads about its charitable donations.

In California, Assembly Bill 2997 which would have outlawed smoking in cars with a passenger six years old or younger, failed by four votes. The state legislators who voted against the measure received more than four times the average amount of tobacco company contributions than those who voted in favor of the ban. The revolving door between tobacco company lobbyists and legislators is a matter of record. Daniel Boatwright, an Altria lobbyist formally registered to the Kraft Foods subsidiary (which paid him $260,000 in lobbying fees), was a California legislator for nearly a quarter century, chairing the Senate Appropriations Committee, the Assembly Ways and Means Committee etc. Karl Rove, President Bush's trusted political strategist, was once a political consultant for Phillip Morris. Mississippi's governor, Haley Barbour was a highly paid tobacco lobbyist for years. Scott Fisher, an Altria executive, is currently vice chairman on the private enterprise board of directors for the American Legislative Exchange Council, a group of lawmakers and big business executives who meet regularly to craft "model legislation" that can then be introduced in state legislatures.

The finance and credit industry:

On March 14, 2005 The Center for Responsive Politics analyzed the Senate vote on bankruptcy legislation which was supported by the finance and credit industry, which made it more difficult to escape from debt through bankruptcy protection: "An analysis of the contributions shows that senators who voted to pass the bill raised an average of nearly twice as much between 1999 and 2004 from the finance and credit industry as those who voted against the bill."

No industry, however, had produced as many top fundraisers for former President Bush as the finance sector. [New York Times 10/33/03 "Once at arms length from Bush, Wall Street is now his biggest donor" Glen Justice. The bundling worked like this: Merrill Lynch CEO Stan O'Neill, a Ranger, sent letters to 300 of his top executives, urging them to give to the Bush campaign. By March of 2004, Merrill Lynch employees and their families had already contributed more than $458,000, making the company Bush's number one source of campaign money. Certainly the elimination of taxes on dividends, capital gains and estates along with attempts to privatize Social Security were most welcome to Wall Street and the billionaires. They promoted the now infamous policy of deregulation that nearly brought down America's financial system.

The U.S. Chamber of Commerce (Big Business):

The Center for Responsive Politics, February 18, 2005, reports that business associations sent 84% of their individual and PAC contributions to Republicans in the 2004 election cycle. The US Chamber of Commerce spent more than $16 million in lobbying the federal government in 2003. The net result was passage of the Class Action Fairness Act, forcing cases with plaintiffs in multiple states into Federal courts, where large damage awards are considerably less common.

Corporate money flow's shifting sands

In past election cycles, the corrupting influence of Washington's big trade groups was split evenly between the two parties. Then, according to the Center for Responsive Politics, about two thirds of lobbyist money (prior to President Obama's first Presidential victory) flowed to Republicans, a testament to the power of the GOP's aptly named Kay St. Project, the brainchild of conservative strategist Grover Norquist, founder of Americans for Tax Reform and convicted former House Majority Leader Tom DeLay (R.-Texas)."

Of course, these facts should not be construed to conclude that it is only Republicans who are beholden to Big Money. The Democrats, with a few exceptions, have already shown themselves equally compromised. As of December 2011, Mr. Obama had gotten more Wall Street money for the 2012 Presidential campaign than all of the front running Republicans combined. Goldman Sachs was his #1 contributor. Michael Moore being interviewed by Piers Morgan on CNN wonders if "Wall Street has their man?"

By 2020 the billionaires, reconsidered the political landscape and launched the new Democrat party which now has become their subservient tool.

The Center for Public Integrity, researched by Wendell Potter, February 11, 2013 and updated May 19, 2014, reports the following lobbying expenditures by companies trying to influence federal legislation from 1998 through 2012: the pharmaceutical industry $2.6 billion; oil and gas companies $1.4 billion; defense and aerospace industry $662 million; the insurance industry $ 1.8 billion.

10

Globalization - Free Trade

Our investigation into the psychology of unbridled capitalism: we behold the startling phenomenon of American corporations sacrificing the American public to globalization and "free trade." The propaganda cheerleaders for globalization (and illegal immigration) include the editorial staffs of the so-called "liberal" media. "Free trade" is hailed as the nation's lifeblood, essential for survival, notwithstanding the fact that millions of American jobs are being eliminated as a consequence and the standard of living for Americans as well as the country's pre-eminence in the world is in decline. How is an American worker supposed to compete with a Chinese laborer whose average salary is 3% of his American counterpart? American multinationals exploit dirt cheap labor in foreign lands while they abandon their homeland workforce. Shouldn't these companies exist primarily for the benefit of Americans? Why aren't they being taxed on their astronomical foreign profits so that Americans can, if necessary, be retrained? Every day one reads that American corporations are "flush with cash" (Apple Computer's $100 billion in cash, for example) and hold vast non-taxable profits abroad. Yet mainstream Republican politicians, with the exception of Tea Party rebels, bemoan corporate taxation – most of whom, because of loopholes, pay no taxes at all.

[NYT 12/28/2007 Paul Krugman "Divided over trade"]: Wages in Mexico are only 11% of the U.S. level and only about 3 – 4 % in China (although Chinese wages have supposedly crept up a bit recently). Mr. Krugman states that whereas a small minority of highly educated people may benefit from growing trade with third-world economies, the vast majority of Americans, lose. It is no wonder that African – American unemployment is double that of whites, who also are losing. The assertion that Americans "don't want those illegal immigrant jobs" pretends to ignore the fact that if corporations paid decent wages, there is no question that Americans, black and white, would take those jobs in a flash.

Mark Krikorian [The Wall Street Journal, 3/25-26/2017] "The real immigration debate: who should be let in and why". writes that an authoritative study published in 2016 by the National Academies of Sciences, Engineering and Medicine (NAS) found that immigration creates a small net economic benefit by lowering the wages of Americans competing with immigrants by $500 billion but in turn benefiting businesses by $550 billion. The native-born disenfranchised working class have the most to lose from the politics of unbridled immigration. Low-skilled immigrants command low wages, pay little in the way of taxes, yet are the recipient of extensive government medical and welfare benefits. The NAS examined the balance between services used by immigrants and taxes paid and found that the fiscal drain to be as large as $299 billion a year. Mr. Krikorian also points out the need in any culture for stability, cohesion, a sense of solidarity and fundamental affection for our fellow citizens that we do not share with those of other countries. He highlights Harvard political scientist Robert Putman in his book "Bowling Alone" (2000) and in his subsequent research, that showed the decline in connections between individuals and a multifaceted decline of social trust. Dr. Putman studied Los Angeles which he calls "among the most ethnically diverse human habitations in history" as well as having the lowest level of social trust among all the communities studied.

An unbridled influx of immigrants who have little interest in integrating Western values leads to cultural instability and chaos [see also the epidemiological studies in Part V that show increased incidence of intolerable stress and serious mental illness when the cultural with which one identifies becomes fragmented and foreign].

"Outsourcing" and "offshoring" (the exporting of American jobs) ensures windfall corporate profits, but American workers lose their jobs when companies shut down factories in the U.S. and move to Mexico or third world Asia. Even highly educated Americans, those trained in sophisticated computer technology, lose employment security when their jobs move to India etc. [WSJ 3/28/2007]: "Offshorable Jobs" Arnold King. Alan Blinder, President Clinton's economic advisor, estimates that upwards of forty million American jobs may be vulnerable to extinction.

It is a sad fact that many of America's richest capitalists are only patriotic to their profits. America could become a minor satellite of China for all the plutocrats care, so long as they make money in the process. McDonalds Corporation, expanding in China, was part of China's biggest cheering section in the last Olympics, running a "Cheer for China" television ad. The phony Big Business refrain that they "welcome diversity" is a cover-up for globalization and cheap illegal labor. The real goal is to make obedient slaves of us all. Read on….

"How U.S. Lost Out On iPhone Work" [NYT, 1/22/12] by Charles Duhigg et al "The iPhone: Designed in the U.S…Made Overseas…Assembled in China." Apple Computer exclusively relies on Chinese companies whose workforce can be exploited using methods not yet legal in the U.S.. A case in point: Apple had redesigned the iPhone's screen at the last minute, forcing an assembly line overhaul. Immediately, the Chinese foreman roused 8,000 workers inside the company's dormitories. Each worker was given a biscuit and a cup of tea and within half an hour started a 12 hour shift. Presto! In 96 hours, the plant was producing 10,000 iPhones a day. "Companies once felt an obligation to support American workers, even when it wasn't the best financial choice", said Betsy Stevenson, the former chief economist at the Labor Department. "That's disappeared. Profits and efficiency have trumped generosity". (Apple declined to comment for this article, which was based on interviews of 3 dozen current and former employees and contractors – many of whom requested anonymity to protect their jobs). An Apple executive said: "We don't have an obligation to solve America's problems." Apple is no exception, most other American electronics companies have already gone abroad. Unions that would otherwise be able to safeguard working conditions don't exist in China and the central government has free reign to maximize competitive trade advantages in a way that would have earned the deep respect of 19th century robber barons. Giant supply chains have been created. On-site dormitories make workers available 24 hours a day. The Chinese government underwrites costs for numerous industries. Apple, for example, had a warehouse filled with glass samples free of charge. The iPhone is assembled at Foxconn City where 230,000 employees work six days a week, twelve hours a day. "[O]ver a quarter of Foxconn's workforce lives in company barracks and many workers earn less than $17 dollars a day." Foxconn has factories in Asia, Eastern Europe, Mexico and Brazil and assembles 40% of consumer electronics for Amazon, Dell, Hewlett-Packard, Samsung etc.. In Apple's case, the first truckloads of cut glass arrived in the dead of night. Managers woke up thousands of workers "who crawled into their uniforms….and quickly lined up to assemble by hand…" In 3 months, 200 million iPhones were constructed.

Consider also that if survival depends on Globalization, why has Germany done so well economically? It maintains a high standard of living for its people pretty much without sacrificing German jobs. The German government, so far, hasn't permitted corporate interests the unrestrained latitudes that exist in the U.S.. Unions still exist, have a say-so in Germany, and sit on CEO compensation boards. Switzerland is doing very well too but that hasn't prevented the Swiss from recently enacting laws to curb excessive corporate pay which now must be subject to shareholder approval. The Swiss have also prohibited huge windfalls for accepting positions at corporate headquarters and have made Golden Parachutes illegal.

The term "free trade" itself is a lie. The plutocrats are greedily buying up one another's companies for the express purpose of creating monopolies to control prices, all with the blessing of federal agencies which, by the way, they have also infiltrated and control.

Protectionism is made to sound like a dirty word (adding "ism" makes it so) but aren't all people created equal? Are only the ultra-rich to be protected?

"Is U.S. Government Outsourcing Its Brain?"

[WSJ 3/30/2007] by Bernard Wysocki Jr,. Post-9/11, the U.S. government has increasingly turned to private contractors, in particular the hundreds of companies in Tyson's Corner, Va., that operate some of the government's most sensitive and important undertakings.

"The risk of this approach in the words of Warren Suss.... expert on federal computer outsourcing, is that the government could wind up 'outsourcing its brain.'" The number of private federal contractors has soared to 7.5 million, four times bigger than the federal civilian work force. The problem is keeping tabs on these activities. Democratic Rep. Henry Waxman of California, chairman of the House Oversight and Government Reform Committee, has castigated the Department of Homeland Security for lax oversight. A case in point is the Coast Guard's $24 billion fleet modernization which was given to Lockheed Martin and Northrop Grumman Corp. The top decision makers were contractors, while the Coast Guard was demoted to the role of "advisor" on technical matters with no say so on subcontracts. As a result, cost overruns were enormous. Boeing has been given the contract for part of the $30 billion electronic fence project along the Mexican border, a project that doesn't work. These policies guarantee notorious ...cost overruns and design failures "much of which takes place under loose or ineffective government scrutiny." Contractors hire other contractors without competing bids. Booz Allen, another giant contractor, came under congressional scrutiny: "Among its more controversial projects was Total Information Awareness, a Defense Department plan for a grand database..." It was scraped after being criticized as an invasion of privacy. Orwell's "1984" is hardly fiction.

11

Unbridled Capitalism in the Market place of Medicine

My first introduction to "Managed-Care" (corporate controlled health care) was at a state hospital in Illinois in the seventies. I had just returned from 4 1/2 years of Wanderjahre in Europe, and sought to resume my work as a doctor. During those frugal years abroad, my savings from the military freed me of the need to work and I explored realms beyond medicine and psychiatry. On my return, I thought it would serve me well to gain experience treating very sick people in a state hospital setting. During that year and four months, a policy of "deinstitutionalization" was launched. One of my former professors, a psychiatrist, had taken a job there working under the industrial psychologist who was the administrator in charge of the hospital. Shortly thereafter, word came from the state medical director that patients were to be discharged into the "community" ("community psychiatry").

It soon became apparent, that regardless of the clinical condition of the patient, I was supposed to sign my name to the discharge order. Imagine my astonishment, as well, on witnessing the ethical abdication of my former professor who became part of a "death squad" that toured my ward and others regularly, demanding discharges of these hapless people, many of whom were minorities. I refused to comply with these inhumane policies, however, since I knew the potential harm that would befall patients for whose care I was responsible. My integrity as a physician was not for sale. As an employee, I was subject to an administrative psychologist, the "section chief," who exhorted me to be "innovative and creative," terminology that is always a dead giveaway for politically and financially motivated ends (examples of which include former President Obama's Health Reform law and the then Republican administration's dagger pointed at healthcare overall).That patients were floridly psychotic, delusional and hallucinating, potentially violent and suicidal, didn't enter into the calculations of administrative policy.

Administrators are not especially gifted in matters of the heart or The Golden Rule. They are, in general, bloodless bureaucrats who are guided by political expediency. Their jobs are, as in this case, dependent upon adhering to political decisions based solely on money, so-called "cost effectiveness." That seems to be a quality that administrators and politicians share in common, namely that the individual can always be sacrificed on the altar of control, money and power. Throwing patients out of state hospitals, of course, became the grist for statistics purporting to show that short-term hospitalization was just as good as long term care, if not superior. After all, they had been discharged, hadn't they? In reality, of course, the legions of the homeless mushroomed and along with that statistic, the exponential increase in violence and mayhem attributed to the mentally ill. The situation today has only worsened far beyond what I would ever have believed possible in a society that considers itself civilized.

And what about those "snake pits" of yesteryear?

Oliver Sacks, the renowned neurologist who recently died, wrote an article in the New York Review of books "The lost virtues of the asylum" [9/24/09] which I found remarkable for its courage and compassionate humanity, an article long overdue given the cruel and dishonest times we live in.

Dr. Sacks recalled the story of Anna Agnew (as Lucy King recounts in her book "From Under the Cloud at Seven Steeples"), judged insane by a court in 1878. She had made increasingly distraught attempts to kill herself and had tried to kill one of her children. In her words, after her admission to a state hospital in Indiana: "Before I had been an inmate of the asylum a week, I felt a greater degree of contentment than I had felt a year previous. Not that I was reconciled to life, but because my unhappy condition of mind was understood, and I was treated accordingly....And at the same time, I too, was treated as an insane woman, a kindness not hitherto shown me." Her psychiatrist acknowledged her "insanity" but added: "..we intend to benefit you all we can and our particular hope for you is the restraint of this place." "Anna spoke ...of how crucial it was, for the disordered and disturbed, to have the order and predictability of the asylum."

While conditions at asylums did indeed deteriorate in the 1950s, the original goal in the 19th century, before the era of psychotropic drugs, was to create a moral treatment for the whole person, "not just a malfunctioning part of the brain." Dr. Sacks described the early institutions as often palatial buildings with spacious grounds that were usually self-sustaining, where patients would work in the fields and dairies, "work being considered a central form of therapy for them ...Community and companionship, too, were central – indeed vital – for patients who would otherwise be isolated in their own mental worlds, driven be their obsessions or hallucinations." The asylum was to provide protection to patients "from the ridicule, isolation, aggression, or abuse so often visited upon them in the outside world." Although, generally, patients lived in these institutions long term, these places afforded at least some patients "to live through their psychoses and emerge from the depths as saner and stabler people."

As adequate funding disappeared, squalor and wretched conditions tarnished the original idealistic goals, but some good aspects of asylums could oftentimes be maintained: gardens, livestock, recreation rooms, swimming pools, music with patient orchestras, art and sculpture and, through work therapy, the opportunity to learn skills of daily life never previously acquired. In the 1960s, Dr. Sacks personally witnessed the prohibition of work opportunities under the guise of "patient's rights" – "based on legalistic notions of patient's rights and not on their real needs." "For many patients, who previously enjoyed work and activity, there was now little left but sitting zombielike, in front of the now-never-turned – off TV."

"The antipsychotic medications that ushered in this wave of deinstitutionalization often turned out to be much less miraculous than originally hoped." Dr. Sacks pointed out that it was not wholesale closings of state hospitals that was needed but fixing.

"There is, under the manias and grandiosities and fantasies and hallucinations, an immeasurably deep sadness about mental illness…"

He courageously signaled the failure of the exclusive chemical models of schizophrenia that "may leave the central human and social experience of being mentally ill untouched." Dr. Sacks understood that schizophrenia is not necessarily incurable I quote liberally from Dr. Sacks and would only hope that there could be more than a few psychiatrists with as much knowledge, insight, and humanity as this expert on the brain.

The current situation

One is witnessing the absolute destruction of outpatient psychotherapy. A typical ruse of the managed care arm of the insurance company, under the guise of "quality care," was to deny further treatment no matter what is said. Telephone negotiations with the designated insurance representative were always unsuccessful. Reports that documented potentially serious consequences including suicidal risk that justified ongoing intensive psychotherapy, were of no avail. For legal purposes, and to cover themselves, another "three sessions" might be allowed. Within the past year, Medicare has broken with its historical mandate to recognize the need for ongoing intensive psychotherapy for those afflicted with emotional problems. Under the ruse of dishonest pompous verbiage, it has denied this coverage for desperately sick people. Regardless of the dramatic need for help (including the risk of potential suicide), it now deems intensive supportive and insight oriented psychodynamic/psychoanalytically therapy "medically unnecessary." Official psychiatry, in its abdication to "its all an immutable inborn brain problem," has added and abetted a gangster approach to the human condition. And, of course, the reason is: follow the money.

Republican party spokesmen think it is the American way to subject future Medicare enrollees to vouchers

Medicare participants vouchers can be used to play cat and mouse with the trillion dollar private insurance industry. And if the stakes are life or death? So what! Turning to present day inpatient treatment policies (including those practiced by prestigious hospitals), current politics are such that even if a seriously sick psychiatric patient requires anything more than a few days in the hospital, one is hounded to sign the discharge papers (the whole "team" is in on it). Electroshock therapy is also making a strong comeback with the claim that it is safe, effective and "does not cause brain damage." The resultant memory problems it causes, even if "transitory," prove that brain damage at some level occurs. Oftentimes the memory loss can be devastating and permanent.

The New York Time's editorial board is irate about "Back in the Hospital Again" [4/16/09]. It asks: Why are hospital readmissions so common among Medicare patients?

There is an answer to their "Why?" It's because these patients are discharged too soon. Medicare reimburses hospitals with fixed lump sums regardless of an individual patient's needs. Hospitals lose money if the elderly are given the inpatient care they require. Hence, recurrent relapses are the rule. Nowadays, doctors generally don't treat their own patients in the hospital anymore. Hospital profit centers have installed salaried "hospitalists" to take over inpatient care causing unavoidable disruption of the doctor-patient relationship and continuity of care. The hospitalists rotate every few days and need to be briefed anew regarding the patient's history. Facts fall through the cracks.

Many doctors will no longer accept Medicare patients because government reimbursement is too low. "Fee for service" has been seized upon as the sin that drives up costs. That fee for service encourages overtreatment when "quality not quantity," to quote former President Obama, should be the watchword, is spinning its way through government mouthpieces and their media organs. Yet, If doctors over-treat in order to offset their financially flagging practices, why must patients wait weeks, if not months, for an appointment? To the extent that overtreatment exists, surely defensive medicine in our current culture of frivolous malpractice suits is an undeniable factor even though The New York Times says it isn't. Eliminating fee for service is a fine idea but why not include everybody: Plumbers, lawyers etc..

We are witnessing the demise of the doctor – patient relationship. A dehumanizing pestilence has taken root in our culture

The corporate takeover of medicine is not without its defenders. "Liberal" newspapers (which, of course, are also owned by Big Business) planted numerous articles in the late 1990s that wholeheartedly upheld the right of Big Business to make life and death medical decisions, medical decisions for which corporations could not be sued or held responsible given current federal law, leaving doctors holding the bag. The New York Times found managed-care's approach quite compelling: "In Managed-care, Consumer Laws Benefit Doctors", "Patients Seen As Losing" Peter Kilborn. [February 16, 1998]: "Politicians and lobbyists say that in the back rooms of law making, the debate is only tangentially about consumers. Mostly, they say, it is about protecting the incomes, jobs and turf of the biggest and richest vested interests" [note that the "richest vested interests" here are doctors not the insurance industry or multi-billion-dollar corporations]. It's "all under the guise of consumer Bill of Rights," the article goes on. "This is physician protection, not consumer protection." Furthermore, "by imposing businesslike disciplines on health services, managed-care has wrung excess from the system, stopped the rising cost of care." Contributors to the article were the Executive Vice President of the Illinois Association of HMOs and a chief lobbyist for the HMO Association who stated: "We're not about to die on the cross of specialist physicians rights..." (pretending to be cut from the same populist cloth as William Jennings Brian).

[The New York Times October 26, 1993]: David Rosenbaum calls the U. S. health care system an economic outlaw: "Doctors, in their greed for money, prescribed unnecessary tests to unsuspecting patients." [malpractice awards and defensive medicine had nothing to do with it?].

Medical newspapers have also supported managed-care. The politician officers of medical organizations have a different set of priorities than physicians involved in direct patient care. [Psychiatric News, May 21, 1999]: Barry Herman claims: "Holding HMOs liable for treatment decisions could hurt quality of care." "The current angst about managed-care is fueled by the popular press." He employs laughable pseudo psychoanalytic mumbo jumbo such as: "The HMOs have become our collective split-off Kleinian bad object."

Other articles by various apologists for Big Business intone: "The reason is not the bottom line (corporate profits), it is quality of care." (Note the similarity to the tobacco industry's propaganda as they tried to defuse the cancer factor in cigarette smoking). [The American Medical News September 12, 1994]: Dr. Eddy, a senior adviser at Kaiser Permanente HMO and a prominent "cost effectiveness" analyst states: "Physicians will have to learn to take the pulse of the population-not just individual patients-to succeed in the health system of the future." The reason, he concludes, is "burgeoning capitation" (the widespread managed-care practice of giving a doctor a fixed amount of money for each patient in a group for which he is medically responsible, regardless of the amount of treatment any one individual requires.) "Done right", Dr.Eddy goes on, "refocusing care on broad populations can improve access, outcomes and save money, providing more for less." (too bad if you are the individual they pull the plug on. You are being harmed for the greater good!).

Clinical experience, however, shows that Dr.Eddy's views are at variance with economic realities. Doctors who are forced to treat difficult patients without sufficient remuneration will, on average, deliver substandard medical care to these people, (for example the shamefully inadequate care available for the poor). It has become increasingly apparent that corporate controlled health care has one and only one top priority: profit. Low HMO insurance premiums for subscribers are compatible with business profits but only for a given population of the young and healthy. As the population ages and health problems emerge, the HMOs abandon their subscribers as they have abandoned the elderly in Medicare (unless, of course, the elderly are tricked into subscribing to HMO-Medicare plans). Profits can evaporate so managed-care companies increasingly employ tactics to squeeze doctors and patients alike, dictating that physicians see more and more patients in ever shorter office visit intervals. Hospital stays are aborted regardless of the clinical condition of the patient. Time is money.

Big Business propaganda continues. Writing in the Psychiatric News, January 16, 1998, Dr. Craig W. Maumus says: "Embracing Change Said To Be Key to Future Strengths." He quotes Dr. Kimberly Merenkov, editor of the Illinois Psychiatric Society's "Mind Matters" who states in pseudo compassionate tones: "Change in general is a difficult concept that can both exhilarate us and threaten our security." "It pushes us out of our world of comfort, passivity, familiarity or suffering." "It can come as quickly as the sudden death of a young princess.... or..." She mentions being "humble and open-minded." Then Dr.Maumus gets to the real point of "how we can adapt.to the changes in the healthcare delivery systems: Since 75% of all medication prescriptions are written by primary care physicians, psychiatrists should "collaborate to better inform primary care physicians, as we must become indispensable to our primary care physician colleagues, teaching them about the identification and treatment of mental disorders." Apparently, Dr. Maumus suggests that little training is necessary in treating psychiatric disorders. Pills alone will suffice. After all, that saves corporate America money.

Dr. Gerald Piaget, chief executive officer and director of the Consortium For Clinical Excellence (a corporate front) states: "One common misconception is that managed-care companies are basically in business to save money and reduce the number of sessions a psychiatrist can have to see a patient, but they are also interested in quality" (the same rhetoric that Mr. Obama used and which is, of course, a lie. Iimiting the treatment itself and "quality" treatment are not compatible). Standard Medicare, until now, does not limit the number of psychotherapy sessions per week nor the duration of treatment and the Canadian health care system pays for both psychoanalysis and intensive psychotherapy. Of course, the soon to be empowered federal "commission" provided for by the new Health Reform Law will change all that. Rationed care will be justified by Evidence Based Treatment Guidelines that pretend to uphold quality but which will be solely motivated by cost. "Studies" will be quoted. Under the current administration's Medicare policy, medical progress notes will be investigated to see if ongoing psychotherapy is warranted and cost effective. Is money being squandered on the poor, elderly, disabled, and mentally ill? After all, hasn't science shown emotional problems in those categories to be inborn and genetic?

Michael M. Weinstein writing in the New York Times dismisses allegations against managed-care companies as "anecdotal evidence," an unwholesome tendency that could jeopardize cost-saving. Mr. Weinstein [the New York Times May 31, 1998] suggests that the public is being hoodwinked under the guise of "consumer friendly names" like "Patient's Bill of Rights", "almost certain to do the opposite of what consumers say they want." Dr. Susan Love, a breast surgeon, [the New York Times June 7, 1998], abhors HMO bashing and is tired of "sob stories," the concoction of "lobbyists and public relations firms." She offers "preventive medicine" plus "acupuncture and biofeedback" ("preventive medicine" and "wellness" usually translates as sanctimonious guidelines for doing it on your own in combination with hokey, cheap, pseudo treatment). She feels that we shouldn't quick fix legislate or pine after "the good old days" but "improve quality." Dr. Love was getting her MBA at UCLA. She obviously had her sights set on working for a managed-care company....maybe she started her own or is now an appointee of President Obama.

A New York Times editorial [September 11, 1996] states that managed-care's practice of charging a fixed fee no matter how much or little is done for the patient could have bad consequences, but "so far studies show that typical managed-care programs have not compromised on quality of care and in fact have brought forth quality-improving innovations" (the "studies" are heavily tainted with corporate money and are biased toward the Big Business agenda). The editorial warns against state legislatures that have "overreacted by shackling managed-care plans, driven by potent lobbying by physicians and insurers (?) who profit from traditional systems." It is a shame that such a "liberal" newspaper could so blatantly serve as a mouthpiece for unbridled capitalism. It is particularly ludicrous to claim that the none-HMO insurers are allied with the doctors.

Writing in the Wall Street journal, April 14, 1993, Richard Vatz, another mouthpiece for unbridled capitalism, says: "blanket mental health coverage is crazy." He warns that former President Clinton's plan for parity for mental health treatment would inflate costs by tens of billions. For Mr.Vatz, the contention that "mental illness is like any other illness "is just a favorite cliché." He concludes that most of the public seen as mentally ill are "just have problems in living" and the so-called "medical treatment" is just counseling, costly counseling. Talk therapy just leads to "spurious claims."

Poor Corporate-America, depicted as innocent, practical and sensible, is the helpless whipping boy, while doctors are greedy powerhouse behemoths. That explains, I imagine, why business executives are making medical decisions and why most physicians these days are forced to work for hospital conglomerates or lose their practice and patients.

Comment:

Most politicians and Big Business plutocrats share the same top priority: power and control. In their universe, what happens to flesh and blood human beings can be written off as collateral damage, nothing to lose sleep over. They are the sociopathic manipulators in our society. The term "psychotherapy" is widely used, but psychotherapy as practiced by whom and to what end? Serious emotional problems for the most part begin in childhood and cannot be "fixed" in three to five "sessions," not even in 20 sessions, even though the first diagnostic session may very well clarify the problem and its origins. At a minimum, adequate treatment entails one therapy session weekly for at least a year. Intensive analytically oriented psychotherapy and psychoanalysis entail multiple sessions weekly over a number of years. Treatment should provide the support and understanding necessary to resolve the central presenting problem. Medication may or may not be utilized. In my clinical experience, intensive psychotherapy diminishes the need for large doses of medication as the alliance between doctor and patient is, in itself, healing. People who call themselves "psychotherapists" but have not undergone rigorous training are basically ignorant at best. Psychiatrists or psychologists who have not had a personal psychoanalysis cannot understand patients because they do not understand themselves.

The erroneous assumption is made that if psychotherapy were made available to everyone, the costs would be prohibitive. In reality, however, only a relatively small percentage of the population is motivated to seek serious treatment. Most people are afraid to confront their problems and in this society, they certainly are not encouraged to do so. Their resistance is reinforced by a culture that discourages critical thinking and denies the value of memories, while at the same time upholding power and money as the solution to all problems in living. Of course, if people were given a real opportunity, many more might seek serious treatment. Would this be bad? Hardly. Were the government and the establishment to demonstrate true concern for the welfare of the people and for their innate potential, the ensuing explosion of productivity would more than justify the cost of the investment. If people thought the system REALLY cared about them, an outpouring of the creative energy that fear and depression had suppressed would revitalize all of society, an explosion of human energy that would do for society what splitting the atom did for physics, but be infinitely more important. For the first time in history, enlightenment and true civilization would emerge from a barbaric night.

12

The Cost of Mental Illness and Treatment, the Efficacy of Psychotherapy

Psychodynamic psychotherapy, which is based on psychoanalytic concepts, focuses on understanding and resolving emotional problems that are a consequence of past and present life experiences. Psychoanalysis aims to resolve unconscious psychological conflicts that have their origin in repressed childhood trauma.

The 2003 Jefferson Center annual report states that the World Health Organization found that mental illness is the number one cause of disability in the United States and is the most prevalent health problem in America today. The New Freedom Commission on Mental Health, established by President Bush in April of 2002 concludes: "Mental illnesses are shockingly common. They affect almost every American family" The Center for Health Policy, University of Missouri School of Medicine, June 2003, cites the National Institute of Mental Health: The annual cost of untreated mental illness averages $300 billion a year in the United States.

A case study in Connecticut documented that a 30% reduction in mental health services at a large corporation, triggered a 37% increase in medical care use and sick leave by employees (Yale Bulletin and Calendar, September 20-27, 1999). Susan G. Lazar, M.D., in the 1997 supplement of Psychoanalytic Inquiry published by the Analytic Press states that despite concerns that the "worried well" would abuse unneeded outpatient psychotherapy and psychoanalysis benefits, the reality is that, when coverage for weekly outpatient psychotherapy is 100%, only 4.3% of the population would use it. Psychotherapy is hard work and most people, unless they were enlightened to do so, avoid looking into the nature of their own emotional problems, even if it were free.

An interesting comparison between the Australian and New Zealand mental healthcare delivery systems shows a 44% lower-cost per capita in Australia where there is much more readily available outpatient psychotherapy and insurance coverage than in New Zealand, which has a hospital-based system and little outpatient treatment (Andrews, 1989).

In this country, a study of the CHAMPUS system (the insurance program for military dependents and retirees) demonstrated that instituting utilization review of inpatient care plus a great expansion of outpatient psychotherapy between 1989 and 1992 led to tremendous savings in hospital costs of four dollars for every dollar spent on outpatient treatment (Zients,1993). In Ontario, where psychoanalysis has been fully covered, the length of treatment is no different from that of patients in New York City where virtually no insurance covers psychoanalysis at a comparable level (Doidge et al.,1994).

Studies show the superiority of psychotherapy in the treatment of psychiatric disorders:

Journal of the American Academy of Child and Adolescent Psychiatry "The efficacy of psychoanalysis in disruptive children" Jan. 1994. Target and Fonagy.

1. for many children, especially those suffering from severe psychiatric illness, intensive psychotherapy is more effective than short term approaches (Target and Fonagy,1994);
2. for children with anxiety and reading problems, more intensive psychotherapy has been demonstrated to be associated with greater improvement (Heinicke and RamseyKlee,1986; Target and Fonagy,1994); 3) J. of child and adolescent psychopharmacology "Psychopharmacology of child and adolescent major depression" psychotherapy is especially important for depressed adolescent patients since suicide is a leading cause of death in male teenagers and antidepressants do not have their usual efficacy in depressed adolescents (N. Ryan, 1992), [In 2004, studies have shown that treating depressed adolescents with antidepressants alone actually increases the risk of suicide]; 4) preferably 2 1/2 years of intensive psychotherapy is necessary for borderline patients to improve work functioning and decrease recurrent hospitalizations (Heard, 1994); 5)The New York Times, February 26, 2005, "As autistic children grow so does social gap" by J. Gross. reports that many autistic children, prior to the age of six, when provided with a 40hour-a-week home program of one-on-one individual behavior therapy on an ongoing basis, can make a normal school adjustment.

Consumer Reports in 1995 published an article which concluded that patients benefited very substantially from psychotherapy, that long-term treatment did considerably better than short-term treatment and that psychotherapy alone did not differ in effectiveness from medication plus psychotherapy. PubMed "The effectiveness psychotherapy".

Evaluating the statistical significance of the Consumer Report Study

Martin E.P. Seligman, Ph.D, University of Pennsylvania, who was a consultant on the Consumer Reports Study analyzes in detail its significance [Effectiveness of Psychotherapy, E.P. Seligman ME Am Psychol 1995 Dec; 50 (12):965-74]. In particular, he addresses the standard claim that there is no proof that long term psychodynamic treatment is effective because controlled double-blind studies are lacking.

Dr. Seligman, a research-psychologist who has published extensively ("learned helplessness") and an expert in the application of statistics, evaluates two different methods that measure psychotherapy outcomes: efficacy vs. effectiveness.

In efficacy studies, patients are randomly assigned to some kind of therapy or to a control group with no therapy. Placebos ("nonspecific") are included to control for such influences as expectation of gain and sympathetic attention. Treatment is manualized and highly explicit. Videotaping insures adherence to the manual. Patients are seen for a fixed number of sessions, usually 12.Target outcomes are specifically linked to the DSM diagnostic categories. Raters are blind to which group the patient comes from. The patient meets the criteria for a single diagnostic disorder and is followed after termination of treatment for a fixed period with an assessment battery.

Dr.Seligman states that he had been a firm believer that efficacy studies were the "gold standard" to evaluate psychotherapy outcomes. He still finds them very useful, "but my belief has changed about what counts as a 'gold standard.' And it was a study by Consumer Reports (1995, November) that singlehandedly shook my belief. I came to see that deciding whether one treatment, under highly controlled conditions, works better than another treatment or a control group is a different question from deciding what works in the field." He concludes that efficacy studies are not necessarily the best measure of what treatment works in the field. He has come to believe that "effectiveness studies" of how patients fare under the actual conditions of treatment in the field can yield credible "empirical validation."

It is usually argued that for long-term dynamic therapy [which includes psychoanalysis] and other therapies to be considered in an efficacy study would require control groups receiving no treatment for several years, an equally credible comparison treatment of the same duration that has the same non-specifics – rapport, attention, and expectation of gain – but is actually inert; a step-by-step manual covering hundreds of sessions, and the random assignment of patients for years.

There is, however, a much better argument against the inertness assumption: "The efficacy study is the wrong method for empirically validating psychotherapy as it is actually done, because it omits too many crucial elements of what is done in the field. Some of the properties that characterize psychotherapy in the field but are absent from efficacy studies include the following:

1. Psychotherapy (like other health treatments) in the field is not of fixed duration.
2. Psychotherapy can very techniques depending on the need of the patient.
3. Patients in psychotherapy usually have multiple problems and the therapy is geared to solving interacting difficulties. Patients in efficacy studies are rigidly selected to have but one diagnosis.
4. Psychotherapy in the field aims to improve the general functioning of patients rather than focusing on specific symptom reduction.

Dr.Seligman concluded that effectiveness studies can be empirically validated but it requires a different method: a survey of large numbers of people who have undergone such treatments. He proceeded to describe the Consumer Report Survey about psychotherapy and drugs in 1994.7,000 subscribers responded to 100 mental health questions. Of these, 3,000 just talked to friends, clergy etc. and 4,100 sought a combination of mental health professionals, family doctors or support groups. Of these 4,100, 2,900 saw a mental health professional. The respondents were mostly middle class and highly educated. The survey questions were detailed (see article).

Results:

1. "Treatment by health professionals usually worked. Most respondents got a lot better."
2. "Long-term therapy [longer than six months] produced more improvement than short-term therapy. This result was very robust, and held up over all statistical models."
3. Mental health professionals did better than marriage counselors. Family doctors did well in the short run but worse in the long run.
4. Respondents who were limited in their choices by their insurance coverage did worse.
5. CR is unbiased. They do not accept advertisements. "They are not pursuing government grants or drug-company favors. They do not accept advertisements. They have a track record of loyalty only to consumers. So the study comes with higher credibility than studies that issue from drug houses, from either APA, from consensus conferences of the National Institute of Mental Health, or even the halls of academe."

Comment: Dr. Seligman provides an in-depth analysis of the CR study. Readers can see the article for further details. I find it a welcome antidote to the politics that discredits the findings of long term treatment. Recently I heard a presentation of an investigator whose study promoted a family-oriented treatment for "pediatric bipolar disorder." In no more than 12 sessions, either individual or group oriented, positive results were claimed that persisted on a six month follow-up. The presentation boasted algorithms, graphs, and boxes brimming with wordy investigative details all of which was supposed to lend an air of scientific rigor. I suspect that government grant money, however, was the real motivating factor for meaningless pursuits of this kind. It takes years to raise a child to maturity. How could 12 sessions solve longstanding emotional disorders practically overnight? How could one even take such an approach seriously?

[Children of Depressed Mothers 1 Year After the Initiation of Maternal Treatment: Findings From the STAR*D-Child Study; Pilowsky, Wickramaratine, Talati et al. Am J of Psychiatry; Sept 2008; Vol 165: No.9, p. 1136-1137]: "Maternal depression is a consistent and well-replicated risk factor for child psychopathology." "Continued efforts to treat maternal depression until remission is achieved are associated with decreased psychiatric symptoms and improved functioning in the offspring." The children themselves did not receive treatment.

As a resident in psychiatry at the University of Chicago, I spent two afternoons a week for six months at Bruno Bettelheim's Orthogenic School. Whatever one may think of his personality, his philosophy of treatment, which was predicated on the need for complete care (psychological, intellectual and physical) of very disturbed autistic children, from early childhood through high school, did get results. Children who had suffered seemingly irreparable damage, oftentimes seemed, as I observed, indistinguishable in their outward behavior from their "normal" peers.

There are many more studies available from a variety of sources. Susan Sherkow, M.D., a psychoanalyst at Albert Einstein College of Medicine recently reported very encouraging results in the treatment of six children suffering from autism or "on the spectrum" of autism [Psychiatric News, March 6, 2009, The American Psychiatric Association's newspaper]. The children ranged in age from 2 to 9 and were in analysis anywhere from two to four years. Her clinical approach was to reach the child by interpreting to the child how their behavior was a manifestation of their feelings (anger, upset etc.). The mother was present during these analytic sessions. Dr. Sherkow states: "...By the end of the first year of analysis they had developed empathy ...They can socialize with other children and communicate their needs. They can say 'I'm angry,' 'I'm sad,' 'I'm hungry,' ...They look like a child without a diagnosis....they all arrived at that...Some have even gone on to mainstream schools." One of her patients who had started analysis at age nine had already had speech therapy which did nothing to help his grave speech difficulties. But now, after analysis, "he is understandable...You can actually have conversations with him." The press that autism is always incurable ".....is just not true," she states.

Unfortunately, however, the opponents of psychotherapy and psychoanalysis will not be persuaded no matter how many studies verify their validity. If a study affirms the value of psychoanalysis, that is dismissed as "anecdotal", while drug industry financed "studies" are "objective." Unbridled capitalism, disdainful of the doctor-patient relationship and human relationships in general, realizes that analytically oriented treatment just gets in their way: Individuals who value human relationships want to write their own script in life rather than act out the one handed to them by the system, and they will be much less vulnerable to the plutocracy's siren song of bread and circuses. Freethinking individuals don't fit into the billionaire's game plan that aims for Pavlovian programmed puppetry. The pretext for dismissing the accumulated in-depth clinical findings of trained experts, who have worked in the real world with patients, is the assertion that these findings are not backed up by randomized controlled trials, the so-called gold standard for scientific research. In defense of expertise, Jamie Homes [NYT Sympathy For the Dentist; 11/27/16] quoted a spoof scientific article that maintained that we don't know if parachutes really work because we have no randomized controlled trials of them.

Frankly, even some of the pronouncements from the psychoanalytic quarter are puzzling. By the time the official politicians in the psychoanalytic establishment (what's left of it) finish obsessively categorizing who can or cannot be analyzed, few patients are left that fit the criteria for analyzability. Because of ignorance, lack of clinical experience, and abdication to reigning politics, many "psychoanalysts" pontificate that schizophrenics cannot be analyzed and that homosexuality is inherited. Casse studies reveal otherwise.

As for worrying about exactly how many therapy sessions will be allowed patients, treatment deadlines are destructive. Where is the unequivocal advocate for the individual? As long as patients are benefiting from the treatment, it should continue. Suicidal potential is not the only yardstick for measuring the need for treatment (and managed care doesn't worry about losing someone to suicide anyway). Wanting a happier life is a valid goal.

If there is any doubt about the inherent superiority of long term psychodynamic/psychoanalytic therapy over short term treatment, a recent study should clarify the facts: [Effectiveness of Long-term Psychodynamic Psychotherapy (LTPP) – A Meta-analysis; Falk Leichsenring, DSc; Sven Rabung, PhD; JAMA (The Journal of The American Medical Association), 2008; 300 (13):1551-1565]. Studies of LTPP, lasting at least a year, or 50 sessions, published between 1960 and May 31, 2008, were identified. Randomized controlled trials were considered. Twenty-three studies involving a total of 1053 patients were included along with 11 randomized controlled trials and 12 observational studies. Complex mental disorders including complex depressive, anxiety and multiple mental disorders with a chronic course were included.

Results: After treatment with LTPP, patients with complex mental disorders were better off than 96% of the patients in the comparison short term treatment group (P= .002). (see article for details). LTPP yielded large and stable effect sizes and was significantly superior to shorter-term methods. Dr. Leichsenring noted that patients in LTPP internalized their therapist's methods and were able to go on working on their problems even after the therapy is terminated.

Dr. Jonathan Shedler, a psychologist at the University of Colorado, Denver School of Medicine, has extensively investigated the published research regarding the effectiveness of psychotherapy in scientific studies. American Psychologist, Feb.2010, "The efficacy of psychodynamic psychotherapy".

He notes that meta-analysis is a widely accepted method for comparing the findings of independent studies by converting findings into a common scale, the effect size. Smith, Glass, & Miller,1980, found an effect size [see glossary] of 0.85; Lipsey and Wilson (1993) tabulated a median effect size of 0.75; Robinson et al.,1990 Psychological Bull. "Psychotherapy for the treatment of depression" found an effect size of 0.73. These are relatively large effects.

By contrast, it was reported in the New England Journal of Medicine that the Food and Drug Administration, between 1987 and 2004 found the overall effect size for antidepressant medication was 0.31(Turner et al. 2008), a relatively small effect (see article for additional details). A rigorous metaanalysis of psychodynamic therapy, published by the Cochraine Library "Short term psychodynamic psychotherapy" (Abbass et al., 2006) found an effect size of 0.97. The effect size increased to 1.51 when patients were assessed > 9 months post treatment.

The "Evidence-Based" Drumbeat

Dr. Shedler has analyzed the methodology of "evidence-based therapy" claims promoted by insurance companies and government that strive to ration psychiatric treatment: "Where is the Evidence for "Evidence-Based Therapy?" The Journal of Psychological Therapies in Primary Care, Vol.4, May 2015: pp.47-59:

Evidence based therapy has become a code-word for manualized, brief, cognitive behavioral therapy (CBT)." Treatment follows a manual that leaves little room for understanding patients as individuals.

The contention is that psychodynamic/psychoanalytic therapy belongs to the dark ages of unscientific therapy and claims "evidence-based" therapy to be scientific. The media chimes in as well: The Washington Post (Baker et al.,2009) likened traditional therapy to pre-scientific practices like blood-letting.

Yet, research shows that evidenced-based treatments are weak treatments with trivial benefits that don't last and that people don't get well.

In the NIMH study. the primary outcome measure was the 54-point Hamilton Depression Rating Scale.

The difference between the CBT and the control groups was 1.2 points. The 1.2 point difference is trivial and clinically meaningless.

75 % of the patients did not get well.

Dreissen et al. 2013, studied 341 patients randomly assigned to either 16 manualized CBT or 16 manualized [brief] psychodynamic therapy. Only 22.7% of patients achieved a remission. These researchers concluded that such patients require more than time-limited therapy to achieve remission.

Dr. Shedler, in this article, also takes a look at research practices behind "evidence based" therapies. The following issues are addressed: 1) most patients are never counted in the research studies, 2) the control groups are shams, 3) manualized "evidenced based" therapy has not shown superiority to any other legitimate psychotherapy, 4) data are being suppressed.

1. In the typical randomized controlled trial for "evidenced based" therapies, about two-thirds of the patients are excluded from the studies because they are considered unstable in some way, or may be suicidal. Of those who get well, we are down to 11% and for those who get well and stay well, we are down to 5%.
2. The control group is usually a sham. A case in point was a NIMH-funded study of post-traumatic stress disorder (PTSD) that claimed that CBT was superior to psychodynamic therapy (Gilboa-Schechtman et al., 2010, p.1040). The therapists providing "psychodynamic" treatment were graduate students who received exactly two days of training in psychodynamic therapy from another graduate student.
3. Wampold et al.,Oct. 2011 "Psychotherapy works, here's why" Amer. Psycho. Assoc. did a comprehensive review of 2,500 abstracts in a search to compare "evidencebased" therapy with a legitimate alternative therapy in the treatment of anxiety and depression. There were only 14 studies that included controls receiving anything approaching real psychotherapy. (Wampold et al., 2011, p. 1311).
4. Negative results (publication bias) never get published, the so-called "file-drawer" problem. Research shows that the benefits of CBT are exaggerated by 75% (see Dr.Shedler's examination of the "funnel plot" in statistics that can ferret-out what is hidden in the "file-drawer").

As ... for cost estimates of intensive "psychotherapy, Hay-Huggins, on actuarial firm hired by the American Psychoanalytic Association recently found it would cost about $2-$5 a month in the average person's premium to cover psychoanalysis (200 sessions a year). Clinical News [November 1992] reports that in 1992, Duke University provided $15,000 a year in outpatient coverage for those affiliated with Duke and paid 80% of the monthly premium of $360 as well. "This startling information certainly suggests that insurance carriers can afford to cover dynamic psychotherapy and psychoanalysis." This excellent coverage obtained for the faculty of Duke was instituted when the president of the university was a psychiatrist, someone who was obviously aware of the debilitating effects of disability and lost productivity due to mental illness, and the benefits of treatment.

13

Managed Care Compromised the Quality of Care: The Case for Criminal Racketeering

It is claimed that Big Business controlled healthcare has not jeopardized the quality of medical treatment in the United States. The facts, however, dispute this claim. As 1999 came to a close, five health maintenance organizations (HMOs) faced lawsuits from 32 million patients. They are accused of offering bonuses to physicians who restricted patient's access to expensive procedures, treatments and tests. Pacificare Health System, Foundation Health System, CIGNA Healthcare, Prudential Healthcare and Humana are accused of violating anti-racketeering laws. In the investigation of these issues, in addition to corporate managed care, it is important to include all medical care systems whose primary goal is financial cost saving through rationing of medical treatment, including Medicare and Medicaid, since the billionaires who buy Congressman influence all of these healthcare delivery systems. Of course, healthcare expenditures such as elective cosmetic surgery, total body scans and radical surgery on people in their nineties etc. cannot be justified. Doctors guilty of fraudulently exploiting the system should be prosecuted. They are cut from the same cloth as their Big Business counterparts. On the other hand, the alleviation of suffering both emotional and physical, in a country as rich as the United States, is the responsibility of society.

Fact-finding has turned up a pattern in managed care practices. Let's investigate the historical details by highlighting examples as reported in the popular press.

Psychiatric News of the American Psychiatric Association, August 18, 1995, reports that the Rhode Island State Department of Health fined United Behavioral Systems, owned by United Healthcare Corp. $100,000 and mandated removal of the Company's medical director, a psychiatrist, because of complaints mostly involving delays or denials of hospitalization for seriously mentally ill patients. There were also allegations that this medical director had received incentive bonuses contingent on the firm's financial performance. A company spokeswoman admitted no wrongdoing but implied that they only needed to enforce better documentation.

Bob Herbert, The New York Times, "In America Hidden agenda" July 15, 1996 reported that a hematologist specializing in the treatment of sickle cell anemia had evaluated a teen-age girl and realized the need for frequent blood transfusions to prevent the risk of a stroke. The mother then joined an HMO and her daughter's treatment was transferred to an HMO doctor who had little experience treating sickle cell patients. He stopped the transfusions in spite of compelling scientific evidence to the contrary. A second specialist supported the first hematologist. The HMO would not relent. "The kid went on to have a stroke and died." As Mr. Herbert points out: "Who doubted for even the merest moment that financial incentives to deny medical treatment would result in widespread denial of medical treatment?"

Forbes magazine, June 10, 1991 states: "Pacific Bell recently found that employees enrolled in HMOs filed more mental health-related workers comp and disability claims. Why? HMOs may not provide specialized mental health treatment promptly enough, so some patients get sicker."

The Psychiatric Times, October 1991, reported that the New York State Commission on Quality of Care For the Mentally Disabled issued a report condemning psychiatric discharge procedures in state facilities after a series of suicides and homicides occurred.

The New York Times, May 26, 1999, "Desperate for treatment and battled every step" reporter Randy Kennedy exposed the cruel policy of Aetna U.S. Healthcare that, like many HMOs, found a neat excuse to deny coverage for drug rehabilitation, pretending they are justified in discriminating against psychiatric treatment for the addicted (those dirty little problems).Robert Peyton, 42, "a tall athletic Manhattan lawyer with dark brown eyes and a fast bright smile," graduated magna cum laude from Boston University but he had an emotional problem, a drug problem. In January 1998 he overdosed on a mix of alcohol, cocaine etc. and lay unconscious for two weeks. When he awoke "he knew he was lucky to be alive and he wanted to start fighting his addiction. But first, it turned out he had to fight something else: his managed-care company, Aetna US Healthcare which would not approve his request for inpatient drug rehabilitation." "Eight months later, after Herculean efforts with hundreds of phone calls in documentation, he won coverage, but Mr. Peyton was not there to get the letter. He had died three weeks earlier, of another accidental overdose."

The State of Illinois recently gutted its mental health coverage for those patients on Public Aid – Medicaid – and turned these poor people over to Aetna and other HMOs.

The American Medical News, November 9, 1998, reports the case of a man 68, Fort Worth Texas. Merit Behavioral Care Corp., later acquired by Magellan Health Services, supervised the patient's medical treatment. He became suicidal after he was diagnosed with prostate cancer and lost his job of 11 years. He was admitted to a hospital. After one week, a lawsuit alleges, an osteopathic psychiatrist, working for Merit told the patient's psychiatrist that he had used up his hospital days, even though the HMOs limit had not been reached. Upon discharge, the patient went home and drank a half gallon of antifreeze and died. The article also reveals that nationwide, spending for mental health care benefits in the preceding 10 years had fallen 54% to $69.61 per person, compared with a 7.4% drop for general healthcare benefits, according to a 1997 study by the Hay group for the National Association Of Psychiatric and Health Systems.

The New York Times, December 10, 1997, Peter T. Kilborn states: "Mentally Ill Called the Victims of Cost-cutting." Dr. Robert Dorwart, a professor of psychiatry at Harvard, and Mark Schlesinger, on economist at Yale, report that hospitals discharge mental patients prematurely and sometimes reject the mentally ill patients simply by denying admission.

The New York Times, December 22, 1995, reports: "A federal court ordered study co demns the State run psychiatric hospitals in Illinois" AP. "The judicial study revealed that patients in the 10 psychiatric hospitals run by the State of Illinois are subjected to conditions so filthy and harsh that they sometimes lie in their own excrement and are victims of physical assault." "Patients also receive inadequate psychiatric treatment, it said, because the staff frequently depends on medicine when other treatment is needed." "Ann Patla, Director of the Mental Health Department, described the study as 'impressionistic and filled with anecdotes.'" "It is a pretty useless report," she said. Webster's dictionary defines "anecdote" as "a short narrative of an incident of an interesting or amusing nature." It is a common practice to dismiss evidence of the abusive exploitation of people as "anecdotal". Using this ploy, they imply that anecdotes are fanciful whimsy having little to do with the facts. It seems however, that observations are only as good as the training and honesty of the observer, whether it involves broad statistical studies or in depth individual cases. 10,000 or 100,000 "anecdotes" tabulated by trained professionals are not so easily dismissed, if one is honest. Furthermore, statistical studies in the healthcare field funded byBig Business, have reeked of corruption and bias.

The Wall Street Journal, October 15, 1996, adapted from George Anders book: "Health Against Wealth: HMOs And the Breakdown of Medical Trust", highlights the following: "What governed Health Insurance Plan of Greater New York when it came to its subscribers who suffered from heart disease and needed open heart surgery?" "The answer is: money." HIP would begin steering thousands of members to North Shore University hospital in Manhasset New York in return for sizable discounts. North Shore was assured an extra 4 million in extra annual revenue. "The only losers were HIP members with heart disease." For 10 years the patients had gone to New York hospital, one of the best heart surgery centers in the United States, with a mortality rate of just 1.7% on their heart bypass cases. North Shore's adjusted death rate was nearly 2.7% in 1993. HIP Took the View: "It's our job to get the best terms for our members and that includes financial terms." Mr. Anders also describes a situation with Good Samaritan Hospital in Los Angeles: "They completely revamped their surgical floor to create a heart surgery assembly-line that could handle more than 1000 cases per year." The hospital offered big discounts to managedcare plans in return for volume. Medicare patients, however, who received bypass surgery, suffered.

Death rates went up from 6.7% of patients within 30 days of discharge in 1989 to 8.2% in 1990, a full percentage point above HCFA's expected range. For 1991 to 1993, "the 30-day mortality rates for Medicare patients climbed to 10.4%, one of the highest in the region."

To offset money incentives to managed-care insurance companies, hospitals embarked as well on general cost trimming: "scaling back postsurgical tests, reducing nursing levels, hurrying patients out of costly intensive care and into more lightly staffed general recovery units." Dr. David Perkowski, a Laguna Hills California heart surgeon, notes that hospitals are cutting budgets to the point that one nurse is managing 10 patients: "That's nothing but crowd control." (It used to be one nurse for every three patients). Also, bypass patients go home in just four days after surgery, down from a 10 days stay.

Those who are wary of cost-cutting in pursuit of managed-care contracts, are losing business.

Turning to pediatric heart surgery, Dr. Kathy Jenkins, a Boston cardiologist studied 7000 heart surgeries performed in 1992. After adjusting for riskiness, she found that patients with regular commercial insurance were less likely to die than those with HMO coverage. "In many states, results for HMO patients were no better than those children covered by the governments Medicaid programs for the poor….and, in Illinois, they tended to be worse." Dr. Stuart Kaufman, a cardiologist in New Jersey, sees hundreds of children with congenital heart defects. He states: [Managed-care companies] "just go on the basis of what is cheapest." The cardiologist then detailed the horror stories.

[7/4/97 NYT "A chance to survive"] Bob Herbert, former columnist for the New York Times, wrote about an advertising salesman's, 29 years old, with metastatic malignant melanoma. Dr. Jonathan Finlay at Sloan-Kettering Cancer Center had some success with an aggressive chemotherapy program and modified bone marrow procedure. The patient's HMO refused to pay for the treatment. Dr. Finlay states: "Insurance companies are in the business of making money. They will use any excuse to deny payment of what they perceive as more expensive therapy."

Dean Baquet and Jane Fritsch writing in the New York Times, March 5, 1995, exposed the situation of newborn babies in New York public hospitals where brain damage and deaths have resulted because of mistakes made by midwives, nurses and inexperienced doctors. For example, Velma Martinez, a 25-year-old Brooklyn factory worker, "languished in the delivery room of Woodhull Medical and Mental Health Center in Brooklyn for 14 hours in July 1993 as nurses first struggled to deliver her baby then desperately searched for a doctor." The father "watched in horror as a monitor showed the baby's heart beat fade, then stop. In the end no doctor came. The New York Times ascertained that for babies weighing more than 5.5 lbs., the death rate in public hospitals in the first month after delivery was 80% higher than in private hospitals.

In addition, Big Business, with audacious cunning, attempts to clothe managed-care cost-cutting in the respectability of pseudoscientific statistics and outcome studies. [The New York Times April 12, 1994]: "Companies assess psychotherapy by the numbers" by M. Freudenheim. Managed-care companies use a "new" system to pretend to give "broad coverage for mental health but only if patients use therapists who have agreed with the company to use the new outcome studies approach." This approach is based on computer models fed certain data. The resulting guidelines emphasize the briefest therapy possible. One company, Integra Inc., a behavioral health company in Pennsylvania reported that Sterling Winthrop, a pharmaceutical maker in New York, "increased the level of mental health coverage when it adopted the new system and still realized cost savings over the previous year." Sterling is a unit of Eastman Kodak with 4200 employees. 659 workers asked for help in one year and, by using the Integra system, the number of therapy visits averaged 3.5 per patient down from 5.5 visits two years ago. Spending on mental health and substance abuse which had increased 15% in 1990 and 17% in 1992, dropped 47% in 1993 after the company introduced managed-care on an outcome model. The benefits director of Sterling said: "We feel that with the new system we have not only started to improve the quality of care, we've also saved a ton of money." (It is, of course, dishonest to label 3.5 sessions "treatment").

These same inhumane policies are also prevalent at the State Government level. Melody Petersen writing in the New York Times December 26, 1996,"Prisons cut costs by managed care" reports that Governor Christine Todd Whitman dismissed the prisons' doctors and nurses and hired a private managed-care company to care for New Jersey's 26,000 inmates, "saving" taxpayers at least $14 million in the first year. New York City was to follow suit. These new entrants into the field of medical care "set stricter rules on when doctors can call specialists or use expensive tests or send inmates to the hospital." "Few people are listening to complaints from prisoners." Some correction officials have, however, ended their managed-care contracts after inmates have died and investigations showed that the private companies at times have dangerously limited medical care to save money. In Florida, Sheriff Everett Rice terminated a contract with EMCA correctional care after Melanie Bird, a 24-year-old prostitute, died. Nurses feared she was having a heart attack, but the medical director did not agree to send her to an emergency room until 13 hours later. "The Sheriff later discovered that the company sometimes paid the medical director a $250 bonus for keeping inmates out of the emergency room." Company nurses came forward to say that they had been pressured to avoid sending inmates to the emergency room because of the expense.

Consider the case of "John", reported in the Psychiatric Times, June 1993, by Sarah D. Atkinson, M.D.: "Caught in the System". John was a paranoid schizophrenic, a six-foot 6 in. noisy young man: "People out there, they come to find me at night, he said. "The bowel trap only works in the dark of the night in the full of the moon." John bore the scars of repeated knifings received while roaming the streets looking for a safe place to sleep. He had a doctoral degree and once had private insurance. Because of his illness, he lost his private insurance and was admitted to a State hospital where he stayed five months, "apparently making steady progress." Then the unit closed due to funding cuts. Although he needed continued hospitalization, "his days had run out on his hospital allowance." He had 26 admissions. Various programs were instituted but did not recognize the fact that he needed ongoing care and an ongoing psychotherapeutic relationship. Dr. Atkinson last saw John as a senior psychiatry resident when she signed his death certificate. He had frozen to death. She states: "a vast amount of time was devoted to moving John's case through the mental health system, while little time was ever spent actually treating his illness."

Clinical Psychiatry News, July 1991, reported typical managed-care abuse of psychiatric patients. The focus was on MCC managed-care firm which manages health care nationally for more than 4 million people. Dr. James C.Bozzuto, a psychiatrist in private practice in Hartford Connecticut, charged that MCC sells its services at substantial cost savings by reducing costs of psychiatric care to any level desired for the bottom line. "Enrollees in the plan who want to receive psychiatric care must first come in for an assessment by a team of managers. This step alone saves 25 to 35% of psychiatric care costs." Patients are understandably fearful of such abusive tactics. "If psychiatric care is approved, the patient is directed to care deemed appropriate by the firm: the company scours the community for the most financially troubled undereducated practitioners and makes deals with them to offer limited services to patients referred by the firm. Patients are referred to physicians rarely and then, only for medication." Examples included a 35year-old woman with depression. In the waiting room she could overhear patient's names and diagnoses in telephone conversations. The diagnostic reviewer smiled at her responses and repeatedly mentioned cost containment. The patient later described the incident as the most degrading experience of her life. A 68-year-old man with pedophilia was told his diagnoses excluded treatment "because it involved a willful choice on his part." A managed-care assessor told a 45-year-old woman who had been discharged from a hospital for depression that she was dependent and psychotherapy would make her more so. She was referred to group therapy as part of cost containment. "The mother of a 10-year-old boy with severe behavioral and emotional problems, including impulsivity and preoccupation with violence, was told he had a social problem. The reviewer suggested a peer socialization group and questioned the need for a psychiatrist." A 25-yearold woman with a long history of bulimia was told that 8 sessions of psychotherapy would be enough to cure her condition. If not, the assessor told her, there was something wrong with her or her therapist.

The American Medical News, November 11, 1996, reports on a family who claimed wrongful death against Aetna Health Plans of California the claim was allowed of the ninth US Circuit Court of Appeals: Cynthia Ardary suffered a heart attack in May 1993. She was taken to a small hospital without cardiac care facilities. "Despite her doctors repeated requests the suit said, Aetna's administrator refused to authorize an airlift to a university medical center. The patient died. Aetna pleaded that government administrators should decide the case rather than a jury and only for the amount of benefits withheld, a privilege shared by all conventional employer sponsored plans. Imagine going to the expense of a lawyer but only being able to sue for benefits actually withheld – too bad if the patient dies allegedly due to big business medical decisions. Follow the money.

The Journal of the American Medical Association, [October 2, 1996,vol.276 no.13 John E.Ware, Ph.D, Bayliss et al]: "During the study period, elderly and poor chronically ill patients had worse physical health outcomes in HMOs than in fee for service systems;" (a four-year study of 2235 patients, 18 – 97 years of age, who suffered from hypertension, diabetes mellitus, acute myocardial infarction, congestive heart failure and depression).

Managed-care employs words like "quality care" and "limited resources" and then bends its clinical decisions towards its real objective: money and the ongoing enrichment of its executives. In the Harvard Mental Health Letter, Harvard Medical School, vol. 2, no.7, January 1995, James E. Sabin, M.D., Associate Director of Teaching Programs at the Harvard Community Health Plan and Assistant Clinical Professor of Psychiatry at the Harvard Medical School, explains the philosophy of managed-care through a few patient examples. Dr. Sabin asked the question: When is a course of psychotherapy indicated according to managed-care principles?

Case #1: A patient, in his early forties, states that he feels lost and diffusely unhappy. He says that his marriage seems stale and his professional work meaningless and that he is confused about his goals. Dr. Sabin concludes: "Certainly he is suffering and the proposed therapy might help, but it is not clear that he has an illness or disorder." Dr. Sabin notes that "expansive attitudes toward psychotherapy is no longer acceptable under managedcare." Dr. Sabin's brand of "honesty" is to tell the patient: "You are clearly unhappy and feel lost but you do not appear to have a psychiatric illness. Psychotherapy can often help in situations like yours and health insurance sometimes paid for it in the past. But your present insurance only covers illness, and you do not appear to be ill. Let's consider some alternatives": Examples would be psychotherapy at the patient's own expense, vocational counseling, a men's mutual support group or a program like Marriage Encounter." Dr. Sabin notes that patients should be helped "with the least possible expenditure of the therapist time."

Comment: Of course, again the sophist apologist (and a Harvard professor) for managed-care rationing has already made his clinical decision in advance and it is based on Big Business profits, not medical need. This patient is indeed suffering. He is depressed and needs an honest psychiatrist.

Case #2: Another patient "functioned well until he lost his engineering job three weeks ago. At that time, he briefly contemplated suicide and he remains excessively self-critical and discouraged about the future." "The therapist recommends 10 sessions of individual psychotherapy concentrating on the rigidity of his self-imposed standards and depressive thinking." "The goal might be to help him recover his confidence so that he can find another job and to understand what button that job loss pushed so that he can be less vulnerable to other disappointments."

Comment: More sophistry. There is no attempt to understand this patient but merely dishonest hypocrisy pretending to masquerade as wisdom and "treatment." As I pointed out earlier, even suicidal ideation doesn't dissuade managed-care from its money agenda.

Case #3: a homosexual craftsman feels "dead inside." He has a life long history of serious depression. Dr. Sabin approves of a so-called therapy program where the patient and therapist meet 10 times over the next two years. (And if the patient disappears between appointments, whose the wiser?).

Clinical Psychiatry News, August 1992, reports of an HMO sued after a patient kills her children. Annamaria Rescott of Maryland who killed her two boys and attempted suicide in October 1988 was hospitalized in February 1988 after seeking help from a clinical psychologist. In 30 days she was discharged because of a limit set by her HMO, Columbia Freestate Health System. A plan to re-hospitalize her because of her deteriorating mental condition in April 1988 was reversed because the HMO, the claim charges, did not want to pay for more inpatient care.

A publication of the Chicago Medical Society, January 21, 1994, Health Reform Report, discusses a reprint from the Wall Street Journal, 1994, concerning the methods of HMO Kaiser Permanente Foundation Health Plan. Although this HMO is brimming with references to "quality care" and other buzzwords, already, at 1.3/1000 doctor-patient ratio, it is one third of the national average for health care systems. Other cost-saving tactics include a rotating cast of doctors, nurse practitioners instead of physicians, and endless waits for appointments. "There isn't as much of an incentive for you to stay well as there is for them to stay profitable" says Richard Mattingly, a San Diego branch manager For Robert F.Driver & Co., a giant in the field of employee benefits consulting.

Here is what happened to Angela Farnham, 38 years old: she noted some trouble in her breast in 1985. Her Kaiser physicians dismissed the problem as a benign condition. Her symptoms persisted and she requested a mammogram. Her doctors said there was no basis for the test, "even chastising her for her hypochondria." Only five years later, after she found dimpling in her breast, was she able to obtain authorization for an MRI. The results showed that a cancer had metastasized throughout her body. In 1992, she won a $500,000 settlement from Kaiser. Kaiser's CEO, David Lawrence asserts: "There are a lot of common myths about routine screening."

Data compiled by the national ambulatory medical care survey confirmed that HMOs and other managed-care plans are less likely to authorize high-tech testing. For MRIs and CT scans, the difference is a factor of two to one. Walter Lawrence of the American Cancer Society says that the problem is the culture doctors operate in, "a culture in which every decision is assessed in terms of statistics and probabilities and dollars, including the year-end bonus to doctors for doing less treatment."

The Psychiatric Times [September 1993,vol. 10,no.9] reports on a Rand Corp. study authorized by William H. Rogers Ph.D., a psychiatrist Kenneth B. Wells, M.D.et al., showing that seriously depressed patients treated by psychiatrists in pre-paid plans have worse outcomes than those served by fee-for-service psychiatrist. "Among psychiatrist's patients, those initially receiving pre-paid care acquired new limitations in role/physical functioning over time, while those receiving fee-for-service did not." Researchers also concluded that the outcome difference was not due to the severity of the illness saying that the managedcare plan patients were, if anything, less sick than the fee for service patients. 600 patients were surveyed over a two-year period from 1986 to 1988. (Is this also "anecdotal?")

Lucette Lagnado, The Wall Street Journal Oct. 30, 1997 and May 30, 1997 "Columbia chief says reforms could take time", reports on Columbia/HCA Healthcare Corp. that, at that time, assembled a vast chain of 343 hospitals and increased earnings while competitors faltered. How did they do it? 33-year-old Mark Gardner says he knows how. He was a manager at three Columbia hospitals over three years: "I committed felonies everyday." Mr. Gardner describes Columbia HCA's voracious appetite for profit, including allowing doctors to buy shares in hospitals where they worked, shares that would rise in value as earnings did, extra thousands to doctors who could boost traffic. Each of its hospitals had a scorecard that tracked costs ranging from supplies to the number of surgeries performed. Medicare charges were inflated. Columbia was Humana on steroids-20 times more aggressive," he says. As a vice president of a subsidiary of Columbia, Mr. Gardner was given a target to increase earnings by 50%. Medical directors who admitted children with public aid or who were uninsured were threatened with expulsion he says. Although admissions rose 34%, staffing decreased 7% in 1995. Mr. Gardner fired 15 nurse managers and cut back on regular nurses in favor of L.P.N.'s who earned half as much. Cheaper supplies were mandated. Unionization attempts were outmaneuvered by outsourcing. An obstetrician gynecologist was given a contract with a set "production budget" calling for 52 surgeries, 10 deliveries and 150 office visits each month. If the surgeon did 78 surgeries each month, she would get a bonus of 30%.

George Anders and Laurie McGinley [The Wall Street Journal (pre – Rupert Murdock), June 15, 1998] "Actuarial firm takes unpopular role of trimming patients' hospital stays" detail one of managed-care's leading allies in the battle to increase profits and lend an air of legitimacy to the politics of drastically rationed medical care. The actuarial firm based in Seattle of Millman and Robertson Inc. publishes seven volumes of adult care guidelines covering everything from sore throats to heart surgery. One of the firm's favorite lieutenants is a pediatrician based in Houston. They are ready to publish his work as volume eight, a 400 page book of guidelines designed to cut down lengths of stay in the hospital for children. Using the typical managed-care marketing script, the actuarial firm states that "better medical quality is at least as important to them as saving money." The thick gray books provide detailed road maps for people who must ration care, allowing insurance companies to "simply refuse to pay for treatment that takes longer than the timelines spelled out in the books." Some of the firm's earlier controversial ideas included allowing elderly patients with bilateral cataracts surgery on one eye only (but it later withdrew this proposal). Volume eight, as the article points out, "ventures into uncharted territory." Thus, children with bone infections are accorded as little as two nights in the hospital and then sent home to complete their course of intravenous antibiotics. The pediatrician supported his guidelines by referring to a study of 50 children in Finland. (As it turned out, however, the children in the Finnish study averaged a much longer 11 days in the hospital). As for life-threatening endocarditis – a heart valve infection – the model would hospitalize the children for three days and then send them home with intravenous antibiotics. "Dr. Thomas Cleary, an infectious disease expert at the University of Texas, terms that unrealistic and an invitation to trouble." What about asthma attacks so severe that children need bedside oxygen? "Try to send these youngsters home after two days as well." [Think of all the money corporate America will save, money that will enrich their CEO's by tens of millions a year.] [Bridge JA et al. "Suicide trends among youths aged 10 to 19 years in the United States, 1996 – 2005" JAMA, 2008;1025-1026]: After a decade long decline in the suicide rate among youths aged 10-19 years in the United States, there was an 18% increase in suicide rates in 2004 with an upward trend continuing in 2005. Lack of caring treatment is the obvious reason for these sad statistics.

Other popular cost savers for insurance companies are worthless but cheap stress management and meditation classes. One may be familiar with these approaches after reading about the Columbine high school killers who were ordered by a court into some kind of "anger management" class which proved, as we all know, rather less than effective. Nancy Ann Jeffrey, a reporter for the Wall Street Journal, July 9, 1997, writes that Procter and Gamble and Harvard Pilgrim Health Care offer a six-week course entitled "Personal Health Improvement Program" which is designed to cheaply substitute for psychotherapeutic treatment of costly psychosomatic ills, including headaches, physical aches and pains related to stress. This is offered to three dozen health plans.

One such class had a woman suffering from stress headaches, standing in the center of a circle of patients who call her names and criticize her while a "clinical nurse specialist" points out how the patient's shoulders tense up in response to stress. Employing terms like "holistic" or "spiritual meditation" is often a cover-up for ludicrous and shallow programs devoid of any therapeutic merit. Eliminating costly cancer treatment by calling it "experimental" yet covering yoga and massage therapy administered by an army of charlatans at dirt cheap rates is an answer many insurance companies have hit upon.

"The big trend is for health plans to cover holistic type alternative medicine such as chiropractic care and massage therapy" said Karen Ackley, vice president of Bolton & Co., an insurance agency in Pasadena California." That's the new wave. More and more plans will cover 15 or maybe 20 visits a year for these kinds of treatment." Oxford Health Plans, an HMO based in Norwalk Connecticut, now gives full coverage of chiropractic, acupuncture and nontraditional naturopathy based on vitamins, herbal medicines plus yoga. Midwives are also covered. Alan Kittner, president of consensus health, a San Francisco-based consulting firm that helps HMOs set up networks of alternative care providers, recalls that his former employer "created the perception" it was expanding benefits for employees in its health plan when in reality it was scaling back. He noted that a company took back its previous coverage of one visit per week of mental health benefits for an "employee-assistance program," an in-house program under the direct control of the Company. Naturally, there is an inherent conflict of interest in such an approach. What if, for example, the Company's dehumanizing treatment of the employee is a large part of the problem? Such programs always exist to circumvent expensive medical treatment and they always hire people with little training whose job depends upon satisfying the company first, not to mention the exposure of an employee's personal records to "Big Brother."

Elizabeth Rosenthal, the New York Times March 16, 1997, points out that the words "prevention saves money," "has become a refrain of managed-care (and of former President Obama) repeated in ads and by HMO executives so often, that it has taken on the aura of truth. "Investing in preventive care is a cornerstone of our business because of the tremendous returns it provides," says U.S. Health-Care annual report. In reality, Ms. Rosenthal points out, the hitch in all this: while preventive care is good for your health, it often does not save money, since early detection of many diseases like high cholesterol and HIV infection, often necessitates a lifetime of costly treatment. The self-interest of HMOs does not lead to top-notch prevention. Wall Street's demands for the short-term bottom line, doesn't care about savings later on. The preventive care touted is usually the low-cost type like rebates on the purchase of bike helmets. "Moreover, preventive programs advertised in glossy brochures sometimes have little substance." "The stop smoking program at one large HMO consists of a prescription for a nicotine patch-the cost of which is not covered by the plan and 12 follow-up letters." An accompanying photo shows an HMO sponsored stress control session with people sprawled out on the floor with their arms flung out. They are "relaxing." It's cheap and it's incredibly cost-effective.

Nancy Ann Jeffrey, The New York Times, January 5, 1998 reports that after spiraling upward in the 1980s, mental health costs have come way down from greater than 15% of many total healthcare costs to around 5% according to Coopers & Lybrand. One increasingly popular cost saver for HMOs is the "Case Rates" method whereby the therapist, perhaps already a low-cost social worker, is given a flat fee say 200 or 300 dollars, for example, to hold up to 10 sessions with a depressed patient. "If the patient's problems are resolved after just one or two appointments, the therapist gets a windfall. But if the therapy costs the maximum number of sessions, the therapist suffers a loss." A California psychologist who asked not to be named, said he recently saw an 18-year-old young woman who had just been released from an intensive care unit after a suicide attempt. Merit Behavioral authorized eight sessions for a flat $200 fee. But he utilized only four sessions because "it cost me $50 an hour to keep the office open." Mr. Stone, an officer at Merit Behavioral, says "quality control programs ensure that providers are not under-treating patients," also, Mr. Stone says practitioners are resistant until they see that these methods help them "predict their own income.

[NYT 3/16/09] "Massachusetts faces costs of big healthcare plan" Kevin Sack. Alex The state of Massachusetts mandated universal medical coverage for its citizens, but apparently doesn't want to make Big Business or the super-rich help pay for it.Blue Cross, working with the state's payment "reform" commission, suggests that doctors are the real culprits and welcomes eliminating fee for service treatment in favor of a flat fee per patient for their total care. Of course, these are the basic tenets of HMO managed care plans. Also "...the state and federal government may need to place actual limits on health care spending which could lead to rationing of care." What kind of "care" is this? Obviously it will result in a grossly inferior rationed care system. Would the several proposed trillions pouring into the bank and brokerage companies' bailout have served better ends had it benefited the health and education needs of Americans?

[NYT 2/10/10] "Long-Term Care Hospitals Proliferate Without Much Scrutiny." Alex Berenson, a consequence of Medicare rules, whereby traditional hospitals lose money when Medicare patients require longer stays, traditional hospitals have a financial incentive to discharge patients to so-called long-term hospitals, which then receive new Medicare payments for admitting the patient. Healthcare entrepreneurs rushed in to take advantage of these profit opportunities where profit margins are greater, a difference of 12% compared to regular hospitals. Margins are greater in part because there is not always a doctor on duty and other staff positions are reduced.

One such operation is Select Medical which has 23,000 employees and cared for 42,000 patients in 2009. Its two top executives, a father and son, made about $200 million from salary, benefits and share sales since founding the company in 1996. Select has no physicians on its board or management. It hired a physician, Dr. Jarvis, for a new position in 2007 but he devotes only about ten hours a week and has no management responsibility.

Dr. Jarvis states that long-term care patients "need gentler care that will enable them to recover on their own." Its corporate medical officer is a nurse. Numerous derelictions of treatment of patients were detailed in the article: "In a scathing report after Ms. BellJackson's death, Medicare inspectors found that the hospital did not have enough nurses on the night she died and that the volume on her monitor was turned down." "Medicare inspection reports…describe preventable patient injuries and deaths, and portray Select's hospitals as understaffed and with a high turnover." In 2006, patients developing serious infections in long-term hospitals was over three times the rate of traditional hospitals.

Dr. Jeremy M. Kahn of the University of Pennsylvania who investigated these hospitals states: "They can pick the most profitable types of patient." He furthered: "[that Medicare has never] taken steps to curb the perverse financial incentives" that drove the long-term hospital explosion ($4.5 billion in 2006).

One may have noticed that the referenced articles on managed-care abuses are somewhat dated. Little seems to have been reported on the subject in recent years that is, until very recently. It is far more likely that the corporate media have acquiesced to their bosses and that we are now all supposed to assume that this is the way it is and just accept it. A schizophrenic patient of mine gave me an analogy that might be apropos in his recipe of "how to cook a frog": Put the frog in the bottom of a deep kettle of cold water. Very slowly turn up the heat until the point is reached where it is too late for the frog to escape.

Democrats and Republicans are resurrecting managed care for our times.

14

"No Money for Medicare" – "Health Care Costs Out of Control!" "You Cannot Tax the Plutocrats. Rape the Middle Class and Poor Instead."

The Return of Managed Care

Republicans say they are desperate to safeguard the "wonderful" private health insurance system. President Obama and the Democrats passed a health care reform law and say they want to promote health insurance for everyone but how can they find the money for it? The hypocrisy of both parties demands adequate scrutiny. The truth is that they are both united in their resolve to safeguard the ill-gotten gains of "the gangster class," as Lord Acton so aptly described the plutocracy.

There are, of course, some glaring distortions in the current fee for service system that should be corrected. Reimbursement to physicians could reflect time spent with patients rather than the current practice of egregious payments because some procedure was performed (after taking into consideration length and cost of specialty training as well as overhead expenses, including malpractice premiums). Nevertheless, most professional people and businesses who perform a service for the public charge a fee for services rendered. Is "fee for service" responsible for physician "over-treatment?" Most internists are swamped with patients. It is doubtful that they are desperate to drum up more business. Their work is also verifiable in contrast to the incredible scams of lawyers who get away with billing a half hour for a two minute telephone call and who concoct itemizations that have zero transparency if not in great measure made up, a practice that has the blessings of the courts. The charge is also made that physicians reap windfalls by ordering unneeded tests. But a doctor who orders an M.R.I. or blood work doesn't profit from such tests since he or she doesn't own the testing facility. Of course, performing unnecessary cataract surgery on everybody in the nursing home is another story, and that is a criminal offense.

Politicians and corporate media mouthpieces apparently have little use for the medical profession and claim the high ground in the health care debate. Their mandate that doctors should agree to treat a patient's chronic illness with a flat lump sum of money ă la H.M.O.s, no matter how much work that patient will eventually require, guarantees rationing of medical care and second tier quality of care. It is unlikely that physicians will exhaust themselves unless they are paid for it, nor should they be expected to do so. After arduous years of training, burdensome debts, ridiculously high malpractice premiums, and swarms of frivolous lawsuits on the part of sociopaths out to make money, physicians are entitled to be appropriately compensated. Other professionals also seek compensation. I read today that teachers in Washington D.C. will be scheduled for maximum $145,000 salaries and, in Illinois, government employees were, up to now, eligible to retire at 55 with top pensions of over $100,000 yearly (police and firemen may retire at 55 with close to 80% of their salary). The minions of the super-rich typically admonish others to belt-tighten and self-sacrifice "because it's for the good of the country." Their masters, the upper one tenth of one percent, comfortably lounge in their hundreds of millions and billions knowing that both major parties wouldn't dream of taxing them as social fairness and common decency would demand.

The basic costs of medical care are rising because of an aging population, a proliferation of expensive high tech treatment tools, care of illegal immigrants who have no money yet have unlimited access to the E.R. of top hospitals, defensive medicine because of the malpractice quagmire, and the corporate control of the practice of medicine. The pharmaceutical industry charges astronomical prices for the very same drugs that are but a fraction of the cost in Canada or Europe and their wasteful marketing outlays exaggerate all medical costs. Recently drug companies, as they have successfully eliminated the competition, increased charges on drugs, including generics, that previously cost pennies but now command hundreds if not thousands of dollars. A former hedge fund manager who runs a start-up, Turing Pharmaceuticals, in August 2015, acquired the 62 year-old patent for Daraprim, the standard of care for a life-threatening parasitic infection and, overnight, raised the price from $13.50 a tablet to $750. Prior to multiple buyouts, Daraprim cost only $1 a tablet several years ago, "Turing's price increase could bring sales to tens or even hundreds of millions of dollars a year if use remains constant." It's the business strategy of buying up old drugs and promoting them as "specialty drugs." Rodelis Therapeutics raised the cost of Cycloserine (used to treat multidrug-resistant tuberculosis) from $500 for thirty pills to $10,800. Doxycycline, an antibiotic, went from $20 a bottle in October 2013 to $1,849 by April 2014 [NYT 9/21/15]."Drug goes from $13.50 a tablet to $750 overnight" by A. Pollack. Two drugs sold by Valeant Pharmaceuticals Int. to treat cancer related skin conditions increased in price by about 1,700 percent over the last six years. Over all, retail prices of 19 brand-name dermatology drugs from various manufacturers quintupled from 2009. Some generic drugs almost quadrupled in price according to a study published by the journal JAMA Dermatology. Two drugs owned by Valeant increased by 18 times: a tube of Targretin in the treatment of cutaneous T-cell lymphoma rose to $30,320 from $1,687 in 2009 and Carac cream rose to $2,865, also 18 times the 2009 price [NYT 11/26 15] "Two Valeant drugs lead steep price increases" A. Pollack.

[NYT "Why Drugs Cost So Much," Peter B. Bach, M.D.; 1/15/15] Dr. Bach, a medical director at Memorial Sloan Kettering Cancer Center, commented on the practice of how drug companies buy up the rights to old inexpensive generic drugs, lock out competition, and raise prices. Albendazole, a drug for parasitic infections was approved in 1996. In 2010, its cost was $5.92 per day. By 2013, the price had risen to $119.58. Novartis, in 2001, charged $4,540 for a month's worth of treatment, in 2014 dollars, for the leukemia drug Gleevec, By 2014, the price had risen to $8,488. In France, Gleevec today costs $3,300 per month (see article for further details).

[NYT "In Pursuit of Liquid Gold" 12/28/17] David Segal. With drug abuse rising, companies have found new ways to turn a fortune. The Affordable Care Act offered insurance to millions more young people and the cost of urinalysis soared with clinics and labs commonly charging more than $4000 per test and testing clients two or three times a week. "...[T]he patients are basically just there to urinate, and management calls them 'thoroughbreds'" One young man's family received a bill for $260,000 a few months after he started testing. Pitches made to potential labs to enter the lucrative field promise $800,000 profit on 15 samples a day. The F.B.I. is investigating a billion-dollar fraud in Florida alone.

Doctors either have a gun to their head to maximize profits for the insurance industry and the corporate entities that own their practices or there are no trained physicians available at all as patients are supposed to get "even better care – studies show" by nurse practitioners who have only a fraction of the training that a medical education demands.

Big Business already has most physicians under its thumb and dictates via managed care contracts how much time can be spent with a patient and what treatment can be undertaken. Hospitals, because they receive a set amount of money from Medicare for any given diagnosis regardless of how long the patient stays in the hospital (including university hospitals), hound doctors to prematurely discharge Medicare patients. Hence, the revolving door problem with Medicare patients is really no mystery.

If doctors are to be denied a fee for services rendered, shouldn't all citizens be so subject (lawyers, plumbers, actors etc.)? Is it really fair for judges and politicians to retire after a few years work with pensions equivalent to 80% or more of their salaries? Couldn't that money be reallocated to healthcare? I read that a fire-chief's pension in California is nonother than $500,000 a year.

The New York Times blames physicians for spiraling costs, not surprising since the Times has never really swung away at the plutocracy. They are, after all, owned by Big Business interests themselves and doctors are an easy and vulnerable target. The Times also falls into line when it comes to supporting the government's agenda. They supported both the Iraq war and Afghanistan wars [NYT 5/4/10 editorial]: "President Obama made a convincing case last December for sending an additional 30,000 American troops to Afghanistan." (and the military-industrial complex has profited handsomely as a result. Not so, the thousands of American soldiers who have died or been maimed).

Bolstering the propaganda impact against practicing doctors, The Times publishes Letters to the Editor from M.D. academicians solemnly intoning the need to do away with fee for service care, academicians who work at a very strenuous pace, say two days a week, at exorbitant salaries, rake in big business grant money, sit on corporate boards, and don't bother seeing patients anyway. The other letter writers are the irate medical students who know all about everything and are all for healthcare "reform." They don't realize that they will find themselves being exploited by both corporate hospitals and the government and will never have known the difference. An economist academic writing in the Times [6/14/09] claims that "It's not the profits of the drug companies or the overhead of the insurance companies that make American health care so expensive but the financial incentives for doctors…" He admits, however, "that a Kaiser Family Foundation poll found that 67% of Americans believe that they do not receive enough treatment and that only 16% believe that they have received unnecessary care."

"Doctor's Salaries Are Not the Big Cost"

[NYT 5/18/14] Elizabeth Rosenthal, a reporter for The New York Times states that "Executives in the business of medicine make far more." She continues: "[T]here is a startling secret behind America's health care hierarchy: Physicians, the most highly trained members in the industry's work force, are on average right in the middle of the compensation pack…..the biggest bucks are currently earned not through the delivery of care but from overseeing the business of medicine." An analysis for The NYT by Compdata Surveys revealed that the salaries for insurance chief executives on average was $584,000, $386,000 for a hospital C.E.O. and $237,000 for a hospital administrator, compared with $306,000 for a surgeon and $185,000 for a general doctor. But these numbers understate the payment gap since top executives frequently earn the bulk of their income in nonsalary compensation. For example, Mark T. Bertolini, the C.E.O. of Aetna, earned a salary of about $977,000 in 2012, but a total compensation of $ 36 million, including stock options etc. Robert J. Del Mauro, a former president of Barnabas Health, earned a salary of just $28,000 in 2012, the year he retired, but total compensation of $21.7 million. The proliferation of hospital administrators here stands in contrast to other countries where top-ranked hospitals maintain the bare minimum of administrative staffs. Cathy Schoen, of the Commonwealth Fund, a foundation that focuses on health care, states: "At large hospitals there are V.P., V.P.s of this, that, and the other….[E]ach one of them is paid more than before, and more than in any other country." She said that in addition to Mr. Del Mauro, Barnabas Health listed over 20 vice presidents who earned over $350,000. Their new C.E.O. earned about $3 million. Barnabas Health's hospitals oftentimes bill more than twice the national average. In 2006, the hospital paid one of the highest Medicare fines ever to settle fraud charges. It is estimated that administrative costs account for 20-30 percent of healthcare costs leading to cost inflation.

An oft cited statistic of the "health-care costs-too much" circle and repeated by former President Obama in his speeches, is that the U.S. ranks 37th out of 191 nations in quality health care, just below Costa Rica, according to the World Health Organization's 2000 report. Greece is rated 10th. "Quality" is not determined, however, by treatment outcome but is skewed by criteria unrelated to treatment outcome. For example, a "Financial Fairness" factor is in the mix: It elevates countries in the ranking that spend the same percentage of household income on healthcare and downgrades countries that spend either a higher or lower percentage. A country where all healthcare is paid for by the government but delivers terrible healthcare will enjoy top ranking. The number of uninsured in America likewise skews ranking although that number includes 11 million illegal aliens. "Health Distribution" and "Responsiveness Distribution", also unrelated to medical treatment outcome, influence ranking. These factors measure inequality across the population. Thus, if care is equal for everybody, even if of poorer quality, that country will rank more highly. The W.H.O. criteria for assessing "quality" rewards uniformity. As for the lower life expectancy in the U.S. compared to other industrialized nations, I have yet to see it truthfully acknowledged that the reason for this statistical anomaly is the fact that the poor in this country receive poor medical care. African Americans, for example, are subjected to inferior medical care, inferior schooling, are more prone to lead self-destructive life style patterns or be victims of homicide and, as a result, die younger. The politicians have never really lost sleep over these realities (after all the super-rich are doing well aren't they?). It is no mere anecdote that foreigners head to the United States for the best medical care rather than risk dying in Canada or elsewhere waiting for surgery or a C-T scan. Americans have a higher survival rate than any other country in the world for 13 out of 16 of the most common cancers and by far the most Nobel Prize winners in medicine.

The Republicans talk about the threat of rationed medical care under "socialized medicine." I must remind them that insurance companies and large corporations have been brutally rationing medical treatment for decades via managed care and H.M.O.s. Unconscionably, they also deny coverage for "pre-existing conditions," even a minor hint of such (to his credit, Mr. Obama attempted to abolish this cruel policy). Insurance companies clearly are more in the business of collecting premiums, than fulfilling their obligations to the insured. To my knowledge, no insurance company has gone out of business because of what they paid out in medical benefits. Consider also that their CEOs rake in millions of dollars, if not tens of millions. These injustices, my esteemed reader, compelled me to embark on this investigation, witnessing as I did, the complete destruction of a humane psychiatry and the upending of the doctor-patient relationship.

Unfortunately, Democrats are comparable hypocrites. President Obama in addressing the American Medical Association (to repeated puzzling standing ovations), sternly educates the doctors about healthcare and throws in a few statistics which were supposed to give his lecture an air of authenticity (after all, he knows more about medical treatment than the doctors do). Firstly, he is all for "preventive care" and "wellness programs," as if physicians were to blame rather than corporate America for pushing consumption of junk food and pressuring doctors to see scores of patients at 10 minute intervals to fulfill managed care and H.M.O. quotas. "Wellness programs" sound good. They also don't cost anything.

[World Socialist Website Joanne Laurier 3/2/10 "The Dartmouth atlas of healthcare costs: Shoddy science in support of healthcare cuts"] The reason for increasing costs is not simply because of an aging population...", stated President Obama, "but the nature of the delivery." He quoted a Dartmouth study "Healthhcare costs and outcomes" that "You are less likely...no, more likely ... to die of a heart attack in a high spending area than in a low spending area" (note the Freudian slip). He decried "a model of care that rewards quantity of care rather than quality of care...".He found it deplorable that the pursuit of medicine has gone from a profession to "a business." Here I would point out that yes, it is a business, but that doesn't mean that the average doctor didn't go into medicine to help people. Then, after the niceties, he got to his real point: "Now, that starts with reforming the way we compensate our providers. We need to bundle payments so that you aren't paid for every single treatment you offer patients for a chronic condition like diabetes but instead paid well for how you treat the overall disease." "We need to give doctors bonuses for good health outcomes...but we are not promoting just more treatment but better care...working in underserved areas instead of more lucrative paths." He claimed to know that "too many doctors and patients are making decisions without the benefit of the latest research" which showed that cheaper treatments in many cases are just as good as expensive treatments. His reform included "evidence based guidelines," a Medicare Payment Advisory Commission, "started by Republicans," "to contain the cost of healthcare."

Translation:

Behind the despicable hypocrisy of "quality not quantity" lies the exact phraseology previously employed by H.M.O. and managed care propagandists, the fronts for the insurance industry and Big Business profit centers. Re-read examples of the actual practices of the health care conglomerates that are already detailed as a reminder of the real purpose of these policies: money. Aside from mouthings, quality medical treatment isn't even part of the equation.

No one is against scientific "evidence", but "evidenced based guidelines" are the ploy of administrative bureaucrats/doctors hired by insurance companies and the government for the soul purpose of forcing medical treatment rationing to increase profits and reduce cost. I defy anyone to find any "evidence based guidelines" that advocate more rather than less treatment. All is clothed in high sounding Orwellian double talk to cover up the fact that these policies will surely lead to rationed medical care and a two tiered treatment, one for the people and a second for the super-rich as is the case in Britain.

As for the Dartmouth study, who funded it?... the government? Furthermore, it is reported in The New York Times [12/23 09]: "Weighing medical costs of end of life care" by Reed Abelson. "...the Dartmouth end-of-life analysis...considers only the costs of treating patients who have died. Remarkably, it pays no attention to the ones who survive." "Because Dartmouth's analysis focuses solely on patients who have died, a case like Mr.Putrus's [a survivor] would not show up in its data....if you consider only the patients who die, there is really no way to know whether it makes more sense to spend more on one case than another." A focus of the article is The Ronald Reagan U.C.L.A. Medical Center, one of the Nation's most highly regarded academic centers. Its chief executive, Dr. David T. Feinberg states: "If you come to this hospital we're not going to let you die." That statement incensed Peter Orszag, the Obama budget director, because Medicare pays about $50,000 during the last six months of care at the U.C.L.A Center whereas at The Mayo Clinic, who are slow to bring in specialists, the figure is only $25,000. Mr. Orszag says more is not better.

"Health Reform" aims to reward hospitals like Mayo and perhaps penalize those like U.C.L.A. But Dr. Thomas Rosenthal, UCLA's chief medical officer, states: "There's a real risk of doing harm here – real harm." The question at stake is, what is excellence and what, excess? Recently, "U.C.L.A and five other big California medical centers published their own research results with a striking conclusion: for heart failure patients, the hospitals that spend the most seem to save the most lives."

The final year of life accounts for a quarter of Medicare's total spending. Are irate bureaucrats and economists stupefied that people get sick nearing the end of their lives? Do vote-grasping politicians, swindling insurance company CEOs and economists hold the higher ground when it comes to patient treatment than doctors? Was the accusation of "Death Panels" for the "counseling" of the elderly which Mr. Obama wanted to push through (doctors would be given bonuses for subjecting their patients to this) so off the mark, even if the language is a bit dramatic?

Ironically for Mr.Obama and his budget director, Mr. Orszag, In 2010, their poster child, The Mayo Clinic, will no longer accept new Medicare patients at their Glendale Arizona facility. The Mayo Clinic will conduct a two year pilot program that will determine whether Mayo will accept any more Medicare patients at any of its facilities. Last year, Mayo lost $840 million on Medicare patients.

Bonuses to physicians for "good treatment outcomes" is based on a lie and is an old HMO trick. It is a Trojan Horse to guarantee cheap and inferior treatment. The quicker the "treatment" is truncated, the more unbridled capitalism and the government will like you. You are bad, if treatment "goes on and on" (who cares what happens to the patient?). Believe me, my esteemed reader, I know from experience that conscientious caring for those suffering from long term illness elicits hateful attacks from those who control the marketplace. That, in spite of the fact that many with long term illness can go on to lead productive or, at the very least, meaningful lives and, yes, not infrequently can be cured when adequate treatment is available, not to mention the boost to morale and productivity of a nation if people really thought that the government cared about them.

The rhetoric about spiraling health care costs is unconscionably silent about an obvious truth: nothing is more important than the physical and emotional health of a people. The means at our disposal to control disease vastly eclipses what was possible 50 years ago. The increasing percentage of a nation's wealth devoted to healthcare and healthier lives, closely parallels the increasing wealth of that nation and can pay exponential dividends in increased future productivity. Poor nations spend little on healthcare but are hardly better off for it. In Asia, life is cheap. Wealthy China, that cynosure of capitalism, provides no social net at all for its people. Pay in advance at one of their hospitals or it's the street.

But we do not have to look to distant China for examples of callous neglect of a country's citizens as a consequence of "cost saving" based on a managed care template. American soldiers returning from recent wars have been subjected to falsified wait lists also linked to reviews of performance: [NYT "Doctor Shortage Is Cited In Delays At V.A. Hospitals.... 'Exploding Workload'"; 3/30/14 by Richard Oppel et al.]. The article cites "13-hour [doctor] workdays fueled by large patient loads that kept growing as colleagues quit and were not replaced....resulting in nurse practitioners handling far too many complex cases and numerous complaints from veterans about delayed care." Wait time data was falsified by hospital officials in order to excel in annual performance reviews used to determine raises bonuses and promotions.

Whistleblowers reported to the chairman of the House Veterans Affairs Committee that they would be threatened if they failed to alter data to make patient-access numbers look good for their supervisors.

In Jackson, Miss. Hospital administrators created "ghost clinics" that didn't exist to make appear that veterans were receiving timely care. In the Albuquerque V.A. doctors receives notice that 20 percent of their "performance pay" would be doled out to doctors who found a way to limit veteran's outpatient visits to an average of two a year.

It has been pointed out that part of the financial waste in the V.A. system is a result of hiring too many politically-connected administrators instead of doctors How to pay for healthcare ? Tax the super-rich at the time-tested tax rates of prior administrations:

an equitable seventy-five to ninety percent. The money is available: "Big Pay Packages Return to Wall Street" [WSJ July 2, 2009]."Big pay packages return to Wall Street by Aaron Lucchetti. "Pay Stretching to 10 Figures"; NYT, 4/15/13, Hedge Fund Titans…And Lavish Paydays: David Tepper.

$2.2 billion, Ray Dalio $1.7 billion, Steven A. Cohen $1.4 billion, James Simons $1.1 billion, Kenneth C. Griffin $900 million etc. etc..

As Andre Gregory says in the movie "My Dinner With Andre": "Maybe they (the public) are all brainwashed in an immense totalitarian conspiracy to control people's minds for money."

Congress passes "Health Reform"

"…for many Americans this is a major step toward the most fundamental form of equality: equal access to quality health care," writes someone "To the Editor" of The New York Times. The letter brings to mind two clichés: "ignorance is bliss" and "the devil is in the details." Universal health care of equal quality for everyone could usher in the beginnings of true civilization, but this law is more threat than salvation.

The New York Times champions rationed care for the middle class

Shockingly, The New York Times, a "liberal" paper, consistently supports managed medical care, corporate run medicine and the profit interests of HMOs. The priority of these agendas is money, not "quality care." For The Times, the propaganda leading up to President Obama's new law, is in much the same vein as its historical approach to these issues. An updated review:

[NYT 7/25/09] "Wealthiest hospitals got billions in bailout…" by Jesse Drucker. A few choice examples of the "superior care" offered at certain centers, where doctors are salaried, like the Cleveland Clinic, are highlighted. It is suggested that the care is perhaps "superior" by the very fact that doctors are on salary. Sen. Charles Schumer, a Democrat and friend to Wall Street, is sure that is "the right model."

Comment: Left out is the fact that The Cleveland Clinic receives hefty subsidies and grants from the Federal Government. What happens, however, when private doctors are eliminated and all physicians are conscripted into hospital conglomerate monopolies? Care will suffer when hospitals are given bonuses for showing patients the door and encouraging them to agree to an earlier death. Private practitioners won't be around to interfere.

[NYT 7/26/09 "Forget who pays the bills" David Leonhardt] The paper questions the value of patients trusting their doctor because "doctors order costly treatments with serious side effects and little evidence of their being effective…" What exactly are the unnecessary costly tests that are ineffective and dangerous and where is the proof of these claims? Patients are also exhorted to blame their doctor for rising medical costs: "…many people are inclined to blame forces that health economists say are far less important, like greedy insurance companies or onerous malpractice laws." [Apparently, economists, known for their honesty and medical omniscience, are well equipped to prescribe the right treatment plan for the public].

[NYT 7/26/09] An editorial: "It is true that the long-term goal of health reform is to get rid of the fee-for-service system in which patients often get very expensive care but not necessarily the best care." The high-sounding terms "research" and "pilot programs" are employed to assure the skeptical public that "reliance on treatments known to work best" will be the order of the day. [From my experience, [NYT 8/1/09] Fearful that their super rich friends (advertisers etc.) will be alarmed by calls for the super-rich to pay for universal health care, we read: "Obama's Pledge to Tax Only the Rich Can't Pay for Everything, Analysts Say." By Jackie Calmes.

[NYT 8/9/09] "The Massachusetts Model" Forehandedwa: A commission wants doctors and hospitals to receive fixed sums to deliver whatever care a patient needs over a year "with safeguards to ensure that they do not skimp on quality." [Politicians and fat cats never skimp on quality for themselves anyway. No rationed care here. ABSOLUTELY NOT! say the politicians.][NYT 8/10/09] "Effort To Rein In Pay On Wall St. Hits New Hurdle": "The resurgence of bonus guarantees underscores how difficult it is to control Wall Street pay,.." [It s just impossible apparently. Let's just forget about reigning in pay in any meaningful way. Besides, we can save money by hastening the death of the elderly in their last year of life].[NYT 8/25/09] "In Healthcare Debate, Bioethicist Becomes a Lightening-Rod for Criticism": Dr.Ezekiel Emanuel, White House adviser on health care, advises: "...those who are irreversibly prevented from being or becoming participating citizens should not be guaranteed the same level of treatment as others."

He cites an example: "...not guaranteeing health services to patients with dementia."

Comment: These proposals sound like they were drafted in the era of The Third Reich. Doesn't the individual have value? Do we exist only for the colony? Is this a liberal newspaper, a liberal President? "Dementia" is on a spectrum of grays. It isn't an either/or condition but bureaucrats will make it so. I (follow the money).

[NYT 11/20/09] "A Medical Culture Clash" by Paul Costello: refers to "The backers of science –driven medicine, with its dual focus on risks and benefits, have cheered the elevation of data in the setting of standards."

Comment: Objective "data" and "science" have little to do with these studies. They are profoundly biased and motivated solely by economics. The investigators are paid by the government etc. to lend an air of respectability to the coming rationing of medical care. Follow the money.

NYT 12/1/09] Dr. S. Jauhar writes: "To Curb Repeat Hospital Stays, Pay Doctors." He cites a study in The New England Journal of Medicine that found that one in three

Medicare patients discharged from the hospital were readmitted within three months. He blames doctors for lax aftercare. He grants, however, that hospitals receive a set payment from the government per Medicare diagnosis regardless of how long the patient stays in the hospital and "the pressure to reduce length of stay has probably increased readmission rates due to premature discharges." This also is the doctor's fault somehow. He quotes some anonymous colleague who admits that he keeps patients in the hospital just to make money (we are to believe that this anonymous doctor would make such an admission to an obvious big-wig at the same hospital). The writer suggests doctors be paid incentives not to keep patients in the hospital: "It is easy to say that doctors should adhere to higher moral standards, but it is naïve to think that money cannot or should not be used to influence their decisions."

Comment: What happened to "quality care," or am I just an idealist? I can share with my esteemed reader my own extensive experience treating psychiatric patients in the hospital. In the days when I was a resident at a university hospital, I could care for a schizophrenic patient six months at a time and achieve a good outcome. In the last decade or two, however, shortly after I admitted a patient, particularly patients on Medicare, the "team" would initiate unremitting pressure on me to discharge my patient, regardless of the patient's emotional state (the brain-oriented gerontology administrative psychiatrists were among the worst). Since I determined length of stay by the needs of the patient, I became, shall we say, rather a pariah. The doctor's signature is required to discharge a patient.

If the real motives of Mr. Obama's health care overhaul aimed at the elderly were not clear enough, note that the federal government will penalize hospitals that have high admission rates [The New York Times 2/30/2013] "How Medicare penalizes hospitals for being too careful" by Jordan Rau (read take money away from them). This new policy will add to the certainty of a higher death rate for senior citizens although it will masquerade as concern for "after care."

[NYT 12/4/09, 2/12/10, 3/22/10 "Health care showdown"] Paul Krugman, a respected economist, has blindly supported "health reform": "…the proposed health care reform links the expansion of health coverage to serious cost-control measures for Medicare. Think of it as a grand bargain: coverage for (almost) everyone, tied to an effort to ensure that health care dollars are well spent." He is sure that the "death panel" is just a Republican smear. He is not very knowledgeable about the practice of medicine, however. One would have expected him to be a little more insightful about the corrupting role of money in political decision-making, being an economist. Is taking money away from Medicare and, yes, from medically necessary treatment, the only way to pay for health reform?

[NYT 12/9/09 "Forget who pays the medical bills its who sets the cost"] David Leonhardt, another economist, notes that fee-for service is an "insidious" payment system [doctors are a vulnerable group to target as opposed to the super-rich and the billionaires who, as advertisers, are the main revenue source for The New York Times. The economist is fed-up with a "watered-down" Medicare commission because it would be hampered in its dictatorial decision-making power over what treatment the elderly are entitled to! He is irate about "scare tactics": "How do you respond to a lobbyist effectively accusing you of killing patients?" [puzzling as to who these lobbyists are for the elderly? Will this economist lose much sleep over who might die as a consequence of rationed care. Money, again, like Marx said, becomes the answer and justification for everything.

[NYT 12/23/09 "Last call on reforming health reform…] Mr. Leonhardt again makes the pitch for an "independent Medicare commission" that will decide what treatment the elderly are entitled to and what compensation doctors will get. It will literally be above the law: Congress may not "interfere."

[NYT 3/25/10] "The Fight Is Over, the Myths Remain" by Brendan Nyhan; states a political scientist at the University of Michigan. Always the scientist, he deigns to mention the 'death panel' claim but proves it is false because "…this claim was widely discredited in the press…." "This doesn't stop the "conservative pundits," he continues, from labeling future rationing "de facto death panels." [Ho-hum, that assertion doesn't impress the professor either]. As yet further proof that it's all a myth, he states without reservation, that it is. Even if the public remains skeptical, he goes on, it should be understood that that is just how the public is. [Would that the rather mentally-challenged middle class simply understood that Noblesse Oblige].

Comment: We all know how objectively honest the press always is. That's why The New York Times concluded that the weapons of mass destruction was a slam-dunk for starting the righteous war in Iraq.

[NYT 4/7/10] "In Medicine, the Positive Power of Learning to Say No": "How can we learn to say no?," asks the writer, David Leonhardt. He praises a government-run group that will compare different treatments, the "Medicare innovation center" and a Medicare oversight board that can set payment rates. Wanting more treatment is "ingrained in our culture"…"but it also has big downsides, including the side effects and risks that come with unnecessary treatment." He notes: Medicare "will bankrupt"; 15,000 are "projected" to die from overuse of C-T scans; "Men who would never die of prostate cancer have been left incontinent or impotent"; "Cardiac stenting and bypasses, with all their side effects, have become popular partly because people believe they reduce heart attacks. For many patients, the evidence suggests, that's not true"; "unnecessary care causes a lot of pain and even death." The writer puts on his humanist hat when he acknowledges "economic arguments are soulless" when compared to "a cancer patient looking for hope," so rather than sounding dictatorial about it, the government should bring rationed medical care to fruition by "changing the economics of medicine, to reward better care rather than simply more care." "When patients are given information about potential benefits and risks, they seem to choose less invasive care, on average, than doctors do, according to early studies." Then, he continues, the public can be helped to decline prostate cancer detection, cardiac stents, skip prenatal tests to see if their baby has Down syndrome, or opt out of intensive care for hospice care. Steering patients in the right cost-saving direction may be the answer, he says.

Comment: Is the writer a renowned medical expert? No. It is again the economist, Mr. Leonhardt, who arrogantly writes as if he knew all about the life and death issues of medical care, only confirming what Marx said in regard to unbridled capitalism: money is the ultimate authority. The economist's stated medical opinions are self-serving distortions that can be traced back to an underlying agenda: cost saving for the government at the expense of the middle class. If there is a question regarding cardiac bypass surgery vs. drug management, one ought to get a second medical opinion (rather than listening to an economist) or go straight to The Ronald Reagan U.C.L.A. Medical Center or the Cleveland Clinic. Generally, the 10 year survival rate after cardiac bypass surgery is 85%. As for prostate cancer, I recall a urologist writing into The Times who noted that since 3% of all men die from prostate cancer: "that seems like an awful lot of men to me." 30,000 men will die yearly of prostate cancer, the second leading cause of cancer deaths for men after lung cancer. The "15,000 projected deaths" statistic from C-T scan radiation is an invention, not fact. As for hospice, the overall aura smacked very much of blatant cost saving for Medicare rather than care. As for being "innovative, it is the favorite euphemism administrators use to justify abandoning the patient. Sincere concern for the patient's best interest is best served by getting a second opinion from a real medical expert, rather than the dictates of number-crunching Big Brother doctor-hacks who run government commissions. By the way, patient abandonment is always excused by some "study" whose data are selected to fit pre-ordained conclusions.

[NYT 3/22/10] Editorial. More of the same: "innovative cost reduction strategies".... "paying doctors and medical institutions based on the quality, not quantity, of services they deliver."...these approaches will spread ultimately from Medicare into the private sector... Doctors must face "the challenge of changing their ways." (hypocrisy)

Translation: Foster the interest of the plutocrats at the expense of the middle class all the while clothing the hypocrisy in sanctimonious double-talk. No mention of a viable alternative: Taxing the super-rich at a 90% rate, no loopholes.

The Government's Task Force On Mammograms: A Hint of Money-Saving Rationed Medical Care to Come

The United States Preventive Services Task Force, in November 2009, recommended that women not receive mammogram cancer screening until age 50 and that women ages 50 to 74 should have mammograms every two years rather than every year. In an editorial [NYT

11/20/09], The Times cautions against connecting these recommendations to "the partisan debate over health care reform." The editorial acknowledges that the "experts" of the task force are in conflict with the recommendations of the American Cancer Society etc. but "every-other-year screenings could provide 80% of the benefits of annual screening..." and, it continues, screening turns up lots "of slow growing cancers that would never progress to the point of killing a women...." The treatments (surgery, radiation, chemotherapy) "carry risks." "The scientific argument is that it is not worth taking such risks for the large number of women whose cancers grow too slowly to kill them." For women in their 40s, the "experts" estimated that 1,900 women have to be screened for a decade to save one life; in their 50s, 1,300 would need to be screened; in their 60s, only 377. "The panel also cites the anxiety and distress that many women experience when a mammogram finds something suspicious." The editorial somehow bemoans any chance that health reform will limit mammograms.

Comment: The editorial and related articles in the Times talk of the terrible "harm" caused women as a result of yearly mammograms, the anxiety stirred up because something "suspicious" but not really life threatening was found, unnecessary biopsies etc. "Only" one women out of 1900 will die as a result of postponing mammography to age 50 or, stated another way, "only" 1000 women will die out of 1.9 million, or "only" 10,000 will die out of 19 million. Unclear how many will only die as a result of every other year screenings beginning at age 50 instead of yearly screenings. A cartoon depicts a portly academic "expert" standing over a woman's tombstone and commenting how gratified she would have been to know the "anxiety" she was spared by avoiding unnecessary yearly breast screening. The Times pontificating on cancers that "will never amount to anything" is rather nauseating hypocrisy. Medicine does not have the diagnostic tools to predict which tumors will remain slow growing and which will become aggressive. Money is the only real consideration of the Health and Human Resources appointed task force. Adding the "United States"...task force to its title is supposed to make its findings very patriotically high-type indeed. I am currently treating a 49 year old young woman who is soon to undergo a bilateral radical mastectomy for recently discovered breast cancer. Breast cancer in young women is all too often a death sentence.

Dr. Jerome Groopman of Harvard Medical School, writing in the New York Review, February 11, 2010 "Healthcare, who knows best?" questions whether we really want government making medical treatment choices for us. The oncologists who head the breast cancer programs at Minnesota's Mayo Clinic and Utah's Intermountain Health described by President Obama as pinnacles of quality care disagreed with the task force. Dr. Robert Truog of Boston Children's Hospital acknowledged that mammography saves lives, but asked if it is cost effective.

Dr.Groopman states that cost-effectiveness is going to be a hard sell to the American people not only because of the great value placed on each life in the Judeo-Christian tradition, but because the federal government has devoted many hundreds of billions of dollars to the bail-out of Wall Street. To perform mammograms for all American women in their forties costs some $3 billion a year, a pittance compared to the money put into the bank rescue. Dr. Groopman thinks the American people are suspicious of the "quants," the math whizzes whose computer models were, in theory, supposed to accurately assess the value of complex monetary instruments but who in fact nearly brought down the world financial system. Are the medical statisticians any more trustworthy?

Comparing cost effectiveness of European medical models with American medicine is also twisting the facts. Mr. Obama says that other countries spend half of what we do by only paying for "what works." Dr. Groopman notes that this contention is not supported by evidence….Lower spending in countries like France and Germany is accounted for not by comparative effectiveness studies but by lower costs of treatment and reduced medical budgets. In Europe, prescription drugs cost 50-60 percent of what they do in the U.S.… insurance premiums are also tightly constrained [not to mention malpractice cost and defensive medicine costs]. In Great Britain, with rationing of expensive treatments, cancer outcomes are among the worst in Europe.

Mr.Obama convened a meeting at the White House on healthcare. Diane Sawyer of ABC News asked him some pointed questions.

Sawyer: "But a lot of people say… 'I'm very concerned that there's going to be a reduction in treatment someplace in all this.' And the question is if there is a board that is recommending, that's one thing. If there is a board that is dictating through cost or through some other instruction, that's another thing. Will it have the weight of law?…"

Obama: "…I don't think there's anybody who would argue for us continuing to pay for things that don't make us feel better. That doesn't make any sense..[Yet] that's the reason why, in America, we typically pay 50 % more for our health care than other advanced countries that actually have better health outcomes."

Translation: The slippery politician, as usual, conceals the facts with phony statistics. Read money, money, money, rape the poor and the middle class if you have too, but don't dare tax the plutocrats.

Also coming down the pipeline are "Accountable Care Organizations," government's push to force Medicare patients (and others) as well as physicians into HMO style conglomerates with the same money saving agenda.

Access to psychiatric treatment in the new law: the devil is in the details

The new law is supposed to offer access to treatment for mental illness for a much larger segment of the population. Yet, health care costs overall are supposed to shrink. How can this be? The law attempts to address supply issues by allowing care to be delivered by a variety of people defined as "mental health professionals." Dr. Stuart Gitlow, associate professor of clinical psychiatry at Mount Sinai School of Medicine, New York, said that these people would include someone with a graduate degree in psychiatry, psychology, school psychologists, psychiatric nursing, social work, marriage and family counseling, school counselors: In essence, said Dr. Gitlow, nurses or social workers could be listed as first tier providers offered to patients participating in a health insurance exchange plan. The psychiatrist would be relegated to a tertiary care clinician involved only in cases of treatment failure. "This essentially means that psychiatry as a specialty is finished." [Clinical Psychiatry News, April 2010].

Comment: Many may think "so what?" Unfortunately, however, a realistic understanding of mental illness and the mind requires exhaustive training and discipline. Medical School is not superfluous when it comes to teaching clinical responsibility and the special quality inherent in the doctor-patient relationship. Understanding the complexity of emotional problems necessitates undergoing a lengthy psychoanalysis for the psychotherapist, that is, four or five times a week for years. One may begin to grasp the complexity of treatment in reading psychotherapy case histories in a second book. Understanding nuclear physics requires training as a physicist. The mind is no less complex if not infinitely more so.

The real issue is again money. "Access to care" will mean cheap and worthless alternatives to the kind of psychotherapy that psychiatric patients really require. The insurance industry and their foot-soldiers in congress have only one priority: maximize profits. A case in point is the recent decision of the State of Illinois to herd all Medicaid (Public Aid) patients into managed care insurance plans, conglomerates like Aetna Health Care, Meridian etc.. My continued work with these poor people is already being stonewalled. Apparently, these poor psychiatric patients don't deserve to be treated like human beings as there isn't a plutocrat among them. "Obama Care" wasn't a bad idea except for the fact that the socalled care people will have access to was shifted over to managed care conglomerates from traditional government plans. People will die as rationing gains momentum. They will also be relegated the status of sub-humans which Huxley so presciently foresaw.

The New York Times implicitly supports Wall Street's billion dollar bonuses ("No money for health care")

[NYT Editorial 1/15/10] "Goldman Sachs where compensation for 2009 is expected to near the record $20.2 billion it paid out in 2000 has said its top 30 executives will receive their entire bonuses in stock that cannot be sold for five years. It has reassured regulators that cash will make up only a small share of bonuses for executives further down the ranks. Others are said...." "That's better than how the game had been played," says the editorial. "But we would find it more persuasive if the boards of banks disclosed clear guidelines on how performance-related bonuses are determined."

Comment: It is gratifying that the paper finds Wall Street headed generally in the right direction, or is it? Perhaps it is actually disappointing that a "liberal" paper ("liberal" in veneer only) would congratulate itself for offering up a few disingenuous pseudo-populist band aids while implicitly supporting bonuses of $20.2 billion to 30 Goldman executives. After all, the "gangster class," to quote Lord Acton, robbed and is still robbing the American people. Many Americans have been reduced to poverty and American soldiers are dying in wrongful foreign wars. Where are the headlines and the trillions for them?

Goldman Sachs suffers from "unbridled capitalist disorder"

A small step in the right direction was taken by President Obama and the SEC when the powerful Goldman Sachs investment banking and securities firm was charged with civil fraud in its mortgage deal schemes. Goldman sold bundles of risky collateral debt obligations to other entities who normally would rely on the firm's honesty to vouch for the quality of the securities it was selling, in this case, CDOs. The CDOs (credit default swaps that insured against default of the underlying mortgages) were allegedly secretly selected for failure and sold, knowing that the mortgages that underlay the mix were on the verge of default. Goldman allegedly secretly bet against the very derivatives it was selling without revealing that it was scheming. As Roger Lowenstein, author of "The End of Wall Street," points out [NYT 4/20/10]: "...credit default swaps greatly multiplied the subprime bet. In some cases, a single mortgaged bond was referenced in dozens of synthetic securities... [and] raised society's risk for no productive gain."

This investment banking firm, whose raison d'être one would expect primarily to consist of making loans to commercial businesses, in reality occupies itself 70% of the time with trading. The trading involves trillions of dollars of opaque "derivatives" that provide no meaningful value to society but reap billions in profits for the firm's traders and top executives. Goldman Sachs operates in reality like a giant hedge fund but with the added advantage that, as a "bank," it can borrow unlimited amounts of money from the government at zero % interest rate, gamble on those vast sums, all the while knowing that its trading bets will be insured by the federal government for any losses. That's the kind of injustice to which the American public is captive and which contributed to the near collapse of the American and world economies. The SEC decision to charge Goldman went along party lines. The Establishment Republicans voted against it.

I suspect, however, that this action on the part of the SEC will not stop the ongoing swindle of the public by the banks and the plutocracy that controls them. The real solution to this corruption is to remove the incentive for astronomical profits by taxing the superrich (for example, those whose incomes are in excess of $10-20 million a year) at a 90% + rate. Unlimited profit potential fuels unlimited incentives for wildly ruthless behavior. A case in point are the Mexican drug cartels.

The problem for Wall Street is "how to wrap eye-popping paychecks in a mantel of moderation.

Comment: The New York Times and the Wall Street Journal, one "liberal," the other "conservative," dutifully report the news, but, beyond that, do they really serve the same masters? True, the editorial board of the Wall Street Journal is nothing more than a mouthpiece for the super-rich and doesn't pretend otherwise. The Times, on the other hand, tries to secure its cachet as a liberal paper by front page spreads on minority problems and impassioned defense of illegal aliens (who are the best source of ultra-cheap labor for corporate America). Both papers report corporate crime but where are the headlines and aggressive editorials? It is fact that The New York Times has been a consistent covert supporter of the plutocracy. They have also cowardly supported both the Iraq and Afghanistan wars (and the profits of the military-industrial complex). In their editorial of 12/2/09 they state: "Overall, we found the president's military arguments persuasive." In April, 2010, The Department of Defense identified 4,381 American service members who have died in the Iraq war and 1,026 who have died as part of the Afghan war. There are many more dead, maimed and disfigured as of this writing.

The New York Times, giddy on Mr. Obama's victory in the struggle for healthcare rationing, ups the ante for the middle class

[NYT 3/23/10] "Next Big Issue? Social Security Pops Up Again": Jackie Calmes. "Now that landmark legislation overhauling the health insurance is about to become law, addressing Social Security's solvency could well be the next big thing for President Obama and congressional Democrats." With reductions in Medicare spending in place and expansions of Medicaid complete, that leaves Social Security. ".... it now stands as the likeliest source of the sort of large savings needed to bring projected annual deficits to sustainable levels,".

Translation: the next step is to squeeze the benefits of the middle class. The billionaires can get by very well without Social Security, thank you.

[NYT 3/23/10] "End Deductions for Mortgages". Agnes Crane. "...That's why it's a good idea to put elimination of the tax deductibility mortgage interest on the political agenda."

Translation: This planted article in The Times takes into account the fact that the plutocrats have no need of mortgage deductions. They can outlay $50 million apiece for a selection of nice villas scattered around the planet.

And, of course, the Republicans, the party of the rich, in 2018, outflanked the Democrats, as they rammed through "tax reform" which is destined to phase out mortgage deductions and property tax deductions for the middle class.

A curious coincidence in timing

On 4/21/10, President Obama was interviewed on CNBC, a mouthpiece for the plutocrats. After dutifully noting the "burden on the middle class," he went on: "that being said," social security entitlements will have to be looked at as well as a VAT (value added tax). [The VAT is a sales tax that hits all equally, whether they make $5000 a year or $5000 million]. Mr. Obama has already clarified that he is opposed to taxing the super–rich at equitable levels: "...and you certainly don't want to use the tax code to punish people." The Obama's reported an income of around $5.5 million in 2009. With all the book deals, speeches etc., there will be more to come ($20 million since 2005)

"The Bailouts Are Working"

[NYT 4/13/10] "Surprise! The Bailouts Are Working," writes New York Times columnist Andrew Ross Sorkin: "And what if after all that vitriol over the government risking hundreds of billions of dollars to rescue Wall Street from disaster, it turned out that taxpayers might actually lose nothing, or even make a profit?" The loss will be only $89 billion, not $250 billion according to reports, he states. Furthermore, he knows people on the board of AIG who tell him that even the $48 billion rescue of AIG may be recouped from assets that were "once considered toxic" and perhaps may not always be.

But others see things differently, like Gretchen Morgenson, the independent minded contributor to The New York Times [4/18/10]. The $89 billion figure leaked by the Treasury's Timothy F. Geithner is far below the $ 1 trillion or more loss estimates of some. For a complete picture, however, Ms. Morgenson points to the enormous transfer of wealth from investors to banks as a result of the near-zero interest-rate policy afforded the banks. Banks pay next to nothing on investor's deposits while they garner a windfall via the exorbitant interest rates on what they loan out. Current credit card interest rates average 14%. She quotes Christopher Whalen, editor of the Institutional Risk Analyst: "All interest-sensitive investors have been transferring what they should be receiving to Uncle Sam and the banking industry,...". The Treasury's current estimates also do not reflect a loss sharing arrangement set up by the F.D.I.C. whereby healthy banks take on the assets of failing banks. Mr. Whalen expects those losses to hit $400 billion. Washington also encouraged the banks to pay back their TARP loans rather than write down their toxic assets to realistic levels. As a result, future costs from crippled economic activity may run into the trillions, he states [the motive for paying back TARP loans was to justify revitalizing the billion dollar bonuses].

William D. Cohan, "You're Welcome, Wall Street" [NYT, 4/20/10] writes:

"-the Fed is crushing the rest of us, especially senior citizens on fixed incomes..."

Mr.Cohan's "premier platinum savings" account is earning a 0.15 % interest rate. "At $140 billion in compensation and benefits, the 2009 paychecks on Wall Street were the best ever." The top 25 hedge fund managers alone earned a total of $25 billion in 2009. As of April 2013, they are equally criminally bloated.

"Even if the rich were taxed at a 100% rate, the recouped monies would be insufficient," say the plutocrat's media

President Obama's (now defunct) tax increase called for raising the marginal tax rate to 39.6% from 36% on those earning $200,000 or more. But are those earning $200,000 really the super-rich? The Wall Street Journal BLOGS, 4/15/2010, quotes David Leonhardt in the New York Times Magazine that the top tax rate in 1960 was 91% for those earning $400,000 a year, equivalent to $3 million in today's dollars: "The top bracket last year started at $357,700. Any income above that – whether it was the 400,000th dollar earned by a surgeon or the 40 millionth earned by a Wall Street titan-was taxed the same, at 35 percent. This change is especially striking, because there is so much more income at the top of the distribution now than there was in the past."

John F. Miglio, writing for OpEdNews, 12/6/2008 notes that in the 1950s even working-class Americans could afford a house, two kids, a car, and a two week vacation on one income. That was a time of strict corporate oversight, strong labor unions, and a fair tax system. Today, the truly wealthy are supposedly taxed at a 35% rate. Loopholes insure, however, that they pay much less than that. Many of the ultra-rich live off their capital gains whereby they are taxed at a rate of only 15%.

The top 1% of income earners own over 40% of the country's assets. Forbes Magazine reports that from 2006 to 2007, the number of billionaires in the U.S. rose from 793 to 946 with a combined net worth of $3.5 trillion, a one-year increase of 35% in their net worth "during a time of increasing poverty and stagnant wages for ordinary Americans." The bottom line is that the wealthiest individuals are being taxed at a rate 55% less than they were in the 1950s.

Robert Perrucci, author of "The New Class Society," points out that large corporations in the 1950s paid 27% of the total tax load. Today they pay 10%. It is ordinary Americans who must make up the difference.

[Les Leopold, author of "The Looting of America"; "Why Are We Afraid to Tax the Super-Rich?" 4/15/10]: In a time of financial devastation for the average American, Warren Buffett wrote, "We've put a lot of money to work during the chaos of the last two years. When it's raining gold, reach for a bucket, not a thimble." Forbes Magazine adds, "many plutocrats did just that. Indeed, last year's wealth wasteland has become a billionaire bonanza. Most of the richest people on the planet have seen their fortunes soar in the past year."

Mr. Leopold notes that the IRS says that the top 400 richest tax filers actually paid a rate of just 16% in 2007. They took in on average $343 million each while 29 million Americans are without work or forced into part-time jobs. He adds that if we reduced their wealth to $100 million each yearly income, we would have enough money to set up a trust fund whose interest could provide tuition – free higher education for students at every public university in perpetuity.

As of this writing, the unemployment rate is below 4% but the underclasses have yet to see their share of the wealth effect. N. Gregory Mankiv, a Harvard economist, [NYT 6/17/18], puts the unemployment numbers in perspective: "Male employment remains anemic compared with what was seen in decades past." While more women have joined the work force since 1950, men exhibit the opposite long term trend. In 1950, 14% of men were out of the work force, but today that figure stands at 31%. Even when one considers only prime men, ages 25 to 54, in 1950 only 4% of prime-age men were not working or looking for work but today that figure is 11% (those who are no longer looking for work are not considered in the unemployment rate). Women have been forced into the work force because of price inflation. On 8/23/18, The New York Times, it was reported that as of 2016, the last year with solid data, the wealth of the median American household was 34% below where it was just before the Great Recession.

How the plutocrats hoodwink the unsuspecting public through their pseudo-liberal news organs

Mr. Obama was not a champion of the middle class. "Change you can believe in," he called it, but his actions belied his promises. A case in point were the recommendations of the President's Deficit Reduction Commission. There was uproar from both liberals and conservatives. The Times, ever thoughtful and sober, applauded the need for fiscal belt tightening and cut backs on bloated entitlement programs. The Commission recommends draconian cuts in Social Security and Medicare and paring back almost all domestic programs, the possible elimination of mortgage deductions (now a fact), raising the retirement age to 70, slashing corporate taxes (now a fact) and cutting the tax rates for individuals (a temporary pittance for the middle class) including the upper 0.1% who make hundreds of millions a year. This was a "bipartisan" commission. Not a word in The Times about bloated entitlements to the real welfare parasites, the plutocrats. Mr. Obama's proposed $500 billion (in 2012, $500 to $700 billion) cut-backs in Medicare expenditures over the next decade in his health reform law wasn't sufficient, apparently, nor the fact that U.S. corporations already pay less in actual taxes than any other western country, nor the crazy incomes of the super-rich. The billionaires, of course, have no need of mortgage deductions.

Let the laborers retire at 70 (if they live that long). The changes would erase nearly $4 trillion from projected deficits by 2020.

Will it take the guillotine to cut a fair deal for the poor and the American middle class?

The billionaires are getting anxious

Warren Buffett is alarmed about the widening wealth disparity between the plutocrats and the people. Confirming Mr. Leopold's statistics, he quotes the IRS that for the 400 highest individual tax returns, the average income for one year was $358 million. Multiplying by

400, gives $1.4 trillion combined yearly income. Their tax rate was under 17%, "the lowest it's ever been," says Mr. Buffett.

Plutocrat mouthpieces rail against increasing the tax rates on the super-rich (and please, let's not lump those earning $ 200,000 yearly with the truly wealthy). They claim that "these are the very ones who create jobs so you can't tax them, it's un-American!"

Where are the jobs they are creating? Are they in China? In Mexico? At the expense of Americans? One wonders how long the public will stay narcotized by the plutocrat's lies and propaganda. The country should consider the public benefit of expropriating this $1.4 trillion to shore up Medicare and Social Security: Presto!, "crisis" miraculously solved! Subsequent tax rates on the super-rich could be appropriately levied for the greater good. The plutocrats would still have trillions left over in their cheek pouches. The productivity of a nation is dependent upon the people having money in their pockets. It is the people who create demand and ultimately jobs.

The plutocrats have already signaled the desperate need to eliminate mortgage deductions, a deduction that has been in place since 1913. The plutocrat media assures us that the newly enacted tax reform law will have little economic impact. After all, the billionaires don't need mortgages.

Courtesy of the plutocrat media

The increasingly shrill propaganda to cut "entitlements" for the middle class and poor is approaching organized brainwashing of histrionic proportions. Any mention of taxing the ultra-rich has curiously disappeared from the media. The Republican establishment proposed slashing corporate taxes and eliminating deductions and they have succeeded in doing so. They would also favor instituting a flat tax across the board, whether one makes $50,000 a year or $ 50,000,000,000. In the past, the politics of "let them eat cake" fomented revolutions.

"Income Slides to 1996 Levels"

The Wall Street Journal [9/14/11]by Conor Dougherty. reports that the income of the typical American family is roughly where it was in 1996 when adjusted for inflation (the inflation rate is kept artificially low by the government). "For a huge swath of American families, the gains of the boom of the 2000s have been wiped out." "Earnings of the typical man who works fulltime year round fell, and are lower – adjusted for inflation – than in 1978." "The fraction of Americans living in poverty cliqued up to 15.1% of the population, and 22% of the children are now living below the poverty line…"

As for the "problem" with Medicare, there are ways to insure sufficient funding: 1) tax the salaries of the CEOs of HMOs, insurance companies and corporate executives at appropriate levels 2) rein in the salaries of the officers of hospitals 3) cap marketing and advertising expenditures of pharmaceutical and insurance companies to a reasonable percentage of revenues, say 5% instead of the absurd outlays of 30% and higher 4) repeal the recently enacted Medicare drug coverage bill and replace it with catastrophic drug coverage and price controls since, in its present form, it is more designed to destroy Medicare then bestow a benefit 5) repeal the provision that prohibits the federal government from negotiating with drug companies on pricing 6) reverse recent regulations that allow drug companies to advertise and market prescription drugs directly to consumers ("ask your doctor"). Drug companies waste additional billions of dollars in their attempts to manipulate the unsuspecting. 6) tax drug company profits, tax the super-rich, tax corporations oversees profits 7) end the Middle East wars and end absurd American troop commitments all over the globe like Europe) 8) consider making the pharmaceutical companies public utilities.

Honest efforts to resolve the crazy income disparity in America is, of course, the bane of entrenched politicians. In fact the pseudo-liberal media, when it isn't promoting the cause of illegal immigrants, cautions against imprudently putting the plutocrats in its crosshairs. Bill Scher [NYT, "How Liberals Win," 7/1/12] educates us in a strategy for future progress. The "great" liberals of the past didn't fight with corporations, they bargained with them (like Teddy Roosevelt?):"The necessity of forging coalitions with corporations is understandably difficult for progressives to accept," he intones, but that's how Mr. Obama is successfully getting his agenda through (the health care law … that the elderly will pay for by rationed medical care etc.).

The theory goes something like this: If you don't hang yourself first, they'll do it for you. Has great social progress really been made by forming "coalitions" with the ultra-rich?

David Stockman, a Republican, and President Ronald Reagan's budget director before he quit, brings up some troubling economic facts [NYT 3/31/13]: Since March 2000, real median family income growth has dropped 8 %, and the number of fulltime middle class jobs, 6 %. The real net worth of the bottom 90 % has dropped by one-fourth. The number of food stamp and disability aid recipients has more than doubled to 59 million, about one in five Americans. [Meanwhile, the incomes of the top 0.1 % has soared].

The media chortles that the stock market is flying high again via The Federal Reserve's money creation strategies and Americans are spending again. What Americans?

15

Unbridled Capitalism and the Corruption of Medical Research, Academia and Psychiatric Practice, A History

The current politics of psychiatry is heavily influenced by corporate America's economic priorities. That corporate agenda is not compatible with the alleviation of emotional suffering that is the psychiatrist's true calling, as a doctor. The goal of psychiatric treatment is the individual's self-realization and his ability to form mutually fulfilling human relationships, in short, the elements of a happy life. But present day society, controlled as it is by an oligarchy, substitutes bread and circuses and the siren song of power for fundamental human needs. Official psychiatry, now captive of Big Business, reflects the current state of dehumanization in its Frankenstein-mantra of "the brain" and its denial of the mind. Many of the researchers are in one way or another on the payroll of the drug companies. Research money from corporations or the government is not available unless it supports the gene and brain chemistry agenda. Biased "research" falsely promotes the view that the individual is "born that way." Mindless "born that way" individuals are more easily controlled and manipulated by Big Brother. The extent to which Big Business finances, controls and corrupts medical research is a matter of record. Let's take a look at the facts.

The Journal of the American Medical Association, January 22/29, 2003, Vol. 289, No.4: "Scope and Impact of Financial Conflicts of Interest in Biomedical Research: A Systematic Review," Bekelman AB. et al. reports that financial entanglements between big business, medical investigators and universities are widespread, leading corrupting conflicts of interests. A Medline search was conducted, 1980 – 2002. Eleven studies concluded that industry sponsored research tends to yield pro industry conclusions. A 1998 study compared authors' financial relationship with industry with their published position about the safety of calcium channel blockers. Authors who were dependent financially on pharmaceutical companies were significantly more likely to reach favorable conclusions than authors without such ties (51% versus 0%; P<.001). Similar skews were found in studies of the health effects of secondhand smoking. In another study of nonsteroidal anti-inflammatory drugs, the industry drug was found superior but only because the selected comparative agents were poorly absorbed.

One study found that lead authors in one of every three articles published hold financial interest in the drug being reviewed and two thirds of academic institutions hold equity in "startup" businesses that sponsor research performed by their faculty. Evidence shows that industry ties are associated with negative data withholding. Reports show alteration, obstruction or stopping publication of negative studies, The Wall Street Journal reports that a study by Eric Campbell of The Institute for Health Policy at Massachusetts General Hospital in Boston for Academic Medicine found that almost one half of medical faculty serving on boards that review patient safety in clinical trials were paid consultants to the health industry. Marcia Angell, M.D., senior lecturer In the Department of Social Medicine at Harvard Medical School and former editor in chief of the New England Journal of Medicine states that researchers that have financial ties to companies sponsoring their research become biased and universities, beholden to money, are permitting companies to have direct control, designing trials, controlling the data and writing the papers,

Dr. Angell's article In The New York Review of Books, July 15, 2004, "The Truth About the Drug Companies," presents an insightful overview of a chilling problem. She writes that the election of Ronald Reagan in 1980 was paramount to the rapid rise of big pharma. The Reagan administration shifted values and extolled great wealth as a virtue. She notes that before Reagan, people were inclined to view obscene wealth and "doing good" as rather mutually exclusive (for obvious reasons). Scientists and intellectuals had not yet been corrupted. Starting with Reagan, however, the wealthy came to be revered, (and I paraphrase), geniuses who deserved their hard-earned riches. The cult of power was in and the gap between the rich and poor widened at a breathtaking pace. [Review my data on incomes for the ultra-rich beginning in the 1990's]

Important business-friendly laws were passed. Thus the Bayh – Dole Act enabled universities and small businesses to patent discoveries emanating from research sponsored by the National Institutes of Health (the major distributor of tax dollars for medical research) and then to grant exclusive licenses to drug companies. Until then, taxpayer financed discoveries were in the public domain, available to any company that wanted to use them. But now, universities, where most NIH sponsored work is carried out, can patent and license their discoveries, and charge royalties. The NIH itself colluded with drug companies, transferring NIH discoveries to industry.

Dr. Angell describes how the law fostered small biotech companies, many founded by university researchers. Usually both academic researchers and their institutions hold equity in the biotechnology companies they develop .... all parties get rich on the public funding of research. Few of the big drug companies rely on their own research for new drugs. At least one third of drugs marketed by the major drug companies are now licensed from universities or the above described small biotech companies. Medical schools started to see themselves as partners of industry. Money became the priority. Dr. Angell explains how the power of the drug companies grew to the extent that if it didn't like something about the FDA, the federal agency that is supposed to regulate the industry, it could change things in its favor through its friends in Congress. Drug industry expenditures for research were consistently far less than profits.

It is beginning to dawn on Americans that they pay much more for prescription drugs than do Europeans or Canadians. One reason is expenditures on marketing. The biggest single item in the budget of drug companies is not R&D but something called "marketing and administration," something like 36% of sales revenues (two and a half times the expenditures for R&D). Dr. Angell points out the dearth in truly innovative drug discoveries. Instead, the industry spends billions of dollars promoting "me too" drugs as if they were miracles. In reality, the "new" drugs don't have to be better than an older drug already on the market that treats the same condition. According to FDA policy, the "new" drug need only be better than placebo.

[The New York Times, September 6, 2004, Janet Maslin]: For example, ScheringPlough's Clarinex is a me-too variant of the company's popular allergy drug Claritin whose patent expired in 2002. Clarinex is an improvement only because it was approved for the treatment of both indoor and outdoor allergies. "It was approved for the additional use only because the company decided to test for that use."

Dr. Angell points out that because of market monopolies, multiple tax breaks, and the rights to NIH research, "the pharmaceutical industry should be regarded much as a public utility."[The New York Review of Books, July 15, 2004, "The Truth About the Drug Companies"]

[The New York Times, December 6, 2004, Gardiner Harris: "At FDA, Strong Drug Ties and Less Monitoring"]: "... advocates for patients say that the agency's efforts to monitor the ill effects of drugs that are on the market are a shadow of what they should be because politicians forced a collusion between the agency and industry years ago for money. Under the 1992 agreement, the industry pledged to give the FDA millions In 2003, $200 million, but only if the agency spent a specified level of money on new drug approval.

Half of the budget for the agency's Center for Drug Evaluation and Research comes from industry.

[The New York Times, December 6, 2004, Stuart Elliott, "With or Without Vioxx, Drug Ads Proliferate"]: Seven years after the Food and Drug Administration ended decades of restrictions by allowing drug makers to advertise prescription products directly to consumers, spending on such ads has reached $3.8 billion. That is more than such companies as Coca-Cola, Pepsi-Cola and Cadbury spend combined each year to sell their soft drinks. Yet the drug companies justify their outrageously inflated drug pricing because they "spend so much on research and development."

[huffingtonpost.com 8/9/12]: The British Medical Journal reports that the pharmaceutical industry spends nineteen times more on self-promotion than on basic research.

[The New York Times, November 29, 2004, Barry Meier, "Contracts Keep Drug Research Out of Reach"]: In December of 2003, medical school researchers went to a professional meeting in Puerto Rico to review test data regarding the prescribing of antidepressants to young patients. Many of these researchers had published positive findings that persuaded doctors to prescribe antidepressants to children and adolescents. Federal drug regulators were reviewing unpublished data to see if the drugs increased suicide risk. However, the medical school researchers, could only get pieces of that information. Some drug companies refused to turn over data to the group, even though these researchers had helped come up with the data. Medical schools, in agreeing to run the tests, had signed agreements with the drug makers that kept the data secret.

[The Guardian, 10/1/2003. S. Boseley, "Lead author rethinks positive JAMA Zoloft article"]. Karen Wagner of the University of Texas medical branch at Galveston participated in more than a dozen industry financed pediatric trials of antidepressants and other types of drugs from 1998 to 2001. Dr. Wagner was associated with 12 industry sponsored trials in which antidepressants were tested against placebos for depression or other problems. All five of the reports claiming positive results were published. Seven other studies were inconclusive or negative. Two of them were never submitted to the Food and Drug Administration to support an application for the drug's approval. Results of her study of Zoloft for childhood depression, financed by Pfizer, was published in the journal of the American Medical Association. The study concluded that the drug effectively treated depression and received widespread publicity. However, academic researchers said that the difference in improvement that the study found between young depressed patients taking Zoloft and those receiving a placebo, 10 percentage points, was not substantial. Pfizer paid the Center $80,000 in connection with the Zoloft test. However, Dr. Wagner also received sizable payments from the company for work she did related to the study. A lawyer for the school disclosed that she received $20,500 during the course of the Zoloft trial.

[The Wall Street Journal, December 4, 2002, "Drug companies foot the bill" Scott Henseley] reports on extensive pitches to doctors at a luxury hotel touting a particular new and expensive drug under the guise of continuing medical education credits. Eli Lilly & Co. with its proposed antidepressant Duloxetine was highlighted: Doctors are goaded into prescribing expensive brand-name drugs but not about subjects from which manufacturers can't profit, such as psychotherapy. The educational firms that run many CME courses depend on the goodwill of the drug companies for their money says Arnold Relman, a former editor of the New England Journal of Medicine: ...education providers are not going to be paid if they don't speak well of the company's product. A whistleblower lawsuit now pending with the federal government as co-plaintiff has accused the Warner-Lambert company(now owned by Pfizer) of handpicking speakers and signing off on their presentations about unapproved psychiatric uses of Neurontin, an antiepilepsy drug, inappropriately costing Medicaid insurance for the poor hundreds of millions of dollars. Psychiatry is particularly targeted for industry sponsored courses. Direct industry commercial support of CME courses for doctors was 62% of the $1.18 billion total spent. Litigation spearheaded by the Washington Legal Foundation, a front for the drug makers and other manufacturers successfully curtailed FDA efforts to restrict drug company communication with doctors. [The New York Times, June 27, 2004, Gardiner Harris, "As Doctor Writes Prescription, Drug Company Writes a Check"]: "The check for $10,000 arrived in the mail unsolicited. The doctor who received it from the drug-maker Schering-Plough said it was made out to him personally in exchange for an attached "consulting" agreement that required nothing other than his commitment to prescribe the company's medicines." Other physicians received similar offers (some 20 were interviewed). "Those checks and others, some of them said to be for six-figure sums, are under investigation by federal prosecutors in Boston as part of a broad government crackdown on the drug industry's marketing tactics." "Pfizer agreed to pay $430 million and pleaded guilty to criminal charges involving the marketing of the pain drug Neurontin by the company's Warner-Lambert unit. AstraZeneca paid $355 million last year and TAP pharmaceuticals paid $875 million in 2001; each pleaded guilty to criminal charges of fraud for inducing physicians to bill the government for some drugs that the company gave the doctors free." Furthermore, regarding Schering-Plough's drug for hepatitis C, Dr. Chris Pappas, director of clinical research for St. Luke's Texas Liver Institute in Houston, said that Schering-Plough "flooded the market with pseudo trials."

The New York Review Books, Richard Horton, March 11, 2004 reviews a book by Sheldon Krimsky, "Science in the Private Interest: Has the Lure of Profits Corrupted Biomedical Research?" Dr.Krimsky is a physicist and policy analyst at the Tufts University School of Medicine. The book reviewer (who is also editor of The Lancet) reveals that when the well-known physician David Healy raised concerns about the risks of suicide among those taking one type of antidepressant, his new appointment as clinical director of the University of Toronto's Center for Addiction and Mental Health was immediately revoked. The point is made that even scientific journals are owned by publishers and scientific societies that derive and demand huge earnings from advertising by drug companies and from the sale of commercially valuable content.

Another scandalous example is the case of Dr. Nancy Olivieri who worked at the University of Toronto and at the city's Hospital for Sick Children on a drug to treat the rare blood disorder, thalassemia. Her work was sponsored by the Canadian Medical Research Council and a pharmaceutical company called Apotex. When the drug appeared to have serious adverse effects, she indicated her desire to publish the findings and inform the patients in her care. The company threatened her with legal action. The hospital began an inquiry that, according to Dr. Krimsky, failed to give her a fair hearing or due process. She was fired. All the while, the University was itself engaged in discussions with Apotex for a $12.7 million donation by the company to the University of Toronto.

The New York Times, November 22, 2002 reports: "Madison Ave. Plays Growing Role In the Business of Drug Research." By Melody Petersen Although federal investigators had rejected the conclusion that a new drug Bextra offered superior relief to acute pain following dental surgery, dentists found a study in the Journal of the American Dental Association that made that very claim. Pharmacia and Pfizer were stressed to sell it as an advance over Celebrex, their earlier entry. Following the new study, Bextra's sales soared 60% in the following 3 months. But the research was not conducted by academics, reports Melody Petersen, but by Scirex, a research firm owned partly by Omnicron, one of the world's biggest advertising companies. TV ads have turned Viagra and Vioxx into billion-dollar bonanzas and the science of drug development is next. "The three largest advertising companies-Omnicron, Interpublic and WPP have spent tens of millions of dollars to buy or invest in companies like Scirix that perform clinical trials of experimental drugs." Separating their advertising and marketing from the science is not possible said Dr. Arnold S. Relman, professor of emeritus at Harvard Medical School.

Some ad agencies own companies that ghostwrite articles for medical journals. Doctors are coaxed to prescribe drugs for unapproved uses. [NYT Melody Peterson 11/22/02 continued from above] Novartis, the Swiss drugmaker, was desperate when its competitors came out with a longer acting version of Ritalin for Attention Deficit Disorder (12 hours versus its own 8 hour pill). Intramed, a medical education company owned by the global ad giant WPP suggested they would take an article commissioned from two university professors that objectively surveyed a wide range of drugs and rewrite it. "We would like to help you draft this manuscript," Marcia Zabusky, a vice president of Intramed,, told the doctors at a conference call, according to a transcript of the conversation obtained by the New York Times, "and then submit to you …for your editing and for approval." "Shane Schaffer, a Novartis marketing executive, told the doctors that the company wanted 'a quick, down and dirty' article." "The lack of research findings should not be an obstacle," he said. "Of course, inferences can be made." The doctors of the Medical University of South Carolina agreed, adding that they were quite clear on what the next manuscript should look like. A ghost writer for Intramed produced the new manuscript in a few days.

Dr. Linda Logdbergher who subsequently quit Intramed, said that the typical procedure would entail sending the manuscript to the drug company for prior approval before sending it to the doctors, who were paid to be listed as the authors. She said the marketing companies will drop a doctor if they don't think he will be particularly malleable, marketing masquerading as science. The article states that in the early 1990s, 75%of drug industry's clinical research dollars went to universities. By 2000, 34% did and the rest went to private research firms like Scirix. Omnicron paid $20 million for a percentage ownership of Scirix in 1999.

Forest Laboratories, a drug company, invited 20 psychiatrists to dinner at Daniel, one of Manhattan's most expensive restaurants, to promote Lexapro, a new antidepressant. Included with the dinner was $500 for each doctor attending. J.P. Morgan called Forest's Lexapro introduction "an instant success". Forest is trying to persuade doctors to switch to Lexapro (an altered version of its Celexa) because its Celexa patent expires in 2004. Forest can claim only one study that Lexapro offers patients an advantage over Celexa – a study Forest paid to have published. Dr. Gorman, the author of the article, receives payments as a consultant from a dozen other drug makers as well. The FDA's new chief counsel, who fought restrictions on drug promotion as a private lawyer, is reviewing regulations that limit the marketing of drugs.

[NYT 12/13/2008 Duff Wilson "Wyeth's use of ghostwriters questioned"] Wyeth, the pharmaceutical company paid ghostwriters to write medical journal articles endorsing its hormone replacement therapy Prempo., A federal study found the drug raised the risk of breast cancer. Doctors were recruited to put their names on papers for publication.

[Melody Petersen, writing for the New York Times, "Undisclosed financial ties prompt reproval of doctor" 8/3/2003] reports on the case of The Chairman of the Department of Psychiatry at the Emory School of Medicine in Atlanta, Dr. Charles Nemeroff. Doctors Robert T. Ruben and Bernard J. Carroll faulted the policy of the journal "Nature Neuroscience" and that Chairman's article for not disclosing financial ties to three therapies he mentioned favorably. Nature Neuroscience is part of the Nature Publishing Group, including the highly respected journal, "Nature." A patch that delivers lithium that was promoted in the article is one for which Dr. Nemeroff holds the patent. He also found "impressive studies" of Mifepristone for psychotic depression. Dr. Nemeroff was given an option to buy 72,000 shares of Corcept Therapeutics for less than $25 total, the same company trying to develop Mifepristone. He also kept secret the fact that he is on the board of Cypress BioScience whose sole product is Milnacipran in the treatment of fibromyalgia which he found more effective than some other antidepressants. Cypress paid him $36,000 in consulting fees the prior year and he would receive $100,000 if he helped Cypress succeed with the drug.

[WSJ, 2/26/09 "What did Emory tell NIH about Dr. Nemeroff's big pharma pay?" Sarah Rubenstein]. Dr. Nemeroff and Emory University are also being investigated by federal officials and Sen. Charles Grassley to determine if the school misled the National Institutes of Health regarding payments made to the researcher from drug companies. A NIH funded a grant to study five GlaxoSmithKline antidepressant drugs. During the 2003-2008 period,

Dr. Nemeroff failed to report $800,000 he received from Glaxo from 2000 to 2006. Emory received $251 million in NIH grants in 2008 alone.

Sara Rimer, reporting in The New York Times, April 16, 2003, reviews a book by Dr. Derek Bok, former president of Harvard University and now a professor there: "Universities in the Marketplace: The Commercialization of Higher Education," where he explores the dangers as boundaries blur between corporate-academic worlds. Ms. Rimer, referring to Dr. Bok's book, states: "Drug companies pour billions of dollars into medical schools. Universities sell the rights to use their scientific discoveries to industry and faculty members occupy such industry endowed chairs as the 'Kmart Professor of Marketing.'"

"Prominent professors start their own venture capital companies, earn lucrative consulting fees and market their lectures through the Internet..... The virtues [of the academic life] and be rich at the same time." Commercialism "is now booming in medical schools and research labs." The Bayh-Dole Act made it much easier for universities to own and license patents for discoveries made through research financed by public funds. Industry's influence, however, does not began in higher academia, it starts in ordinary public school, inundated with commercial messages and Channel one commercials.

Recently, Merck & Co. and Pfizer, pharmaceutical companies, have come under scrutiny. [WSJ "Vioxx fallout spreads" Mark Gongloff 11/18/04] Dr. David Graham, associate director for science In the U. S. Food and Drug Administration's Office of Drug Safety, writing in The Lancet, January 24, 2005, writes that Merck & Co.'s arthritis drug Vioxx may have caused as many as 140,000 excess cases of serious coronary heart disease in the United States by the time it was withdrawn from the market in September, 2004. Dr. Graham's study analyzed the data from 1.4 million patients taking anti-inflammatory drugs in California from 1999 to 2004. People taking Vioxx had a 34% greater chance of coronary heart disease when compared with people who used other anti-inflammatory drugs.

[The Wall Street Journal,10/10/04 "FDA tried to tone down reports..." in an article by Jeanne Whalen,] reports a phone interview with Dr. Graham in which he states he had intended to publish this study last November, but withdrew the article at the last minute "under pressure from an FDA official." "Dr. Graham said that the official wrote him an email warning that there would be 'serious adverse consequences' for him if the article was published. Vioxx belongs to a group of drugs known as Cox-2 inhibitors. In addition, the consumer group Public Citizen asked the FDA to remove the two remaining drugs in the class, Pfizer's Bextra and Celebrex from the US market.

The New York Times, 9/2/09 "Pfizer agrees to pay 2.3 billion to settle marketing case" by Gardiner Harris; related to Celebrex, Bextra. Top federal drug regulators were accused of intending to suppress an important study. The FDA officials had forbidden Dr. David Graham to discuss before a panel convened to consider whether Celebrex and Bextra hurt the heart, a large study" of that very question according to Dr.Gurkirpal Singh of Stanford

University School of Medicine, Dr. Graham's co-author. "We have significant new information that will alter the thinking about these drugs,"Dr.Singh said. "I don't understand why they won't let us present this information."

The Wall Street Journal, February 7, 2005, "Merck documents shed light on Vioxx legal battles" by B. Martinez; reports that undisclosed company records, reviewed by The Wall Street Journal, "show that the external committee charged with monitoring the drug's safety in the clinical trial had early data suggesting that users could be at increased risk of certain heart problems after as little as four months. Notes from committee meetings show that members were watching the 'concerning nature of the trends' about Vioxx's possible effects on heart attacks and strokes from their very first meeting" (Merck spokesmen had maintained that the drug showed an increase in heart attacks and strokes only after 18 months). Later on, a government advisory panel concluded that the painkillers Vioxx, Bextra and Celebrex could all be safely marketed despite evidence of cardiac risk. The New York Times, in an editorial, points out that the decisive votes were cast by experts who had financial ties to the drugs' manufacturers. The Center for Science in the Public Interest, an advocacy group, found that at least 10 of the 32 panel members had consulted for or received research support from Pfizer and Merck. Had the votes of those 10 scientists been excluded, the panel would have favored withdrawing Bextra from the market and blocking the return of Vioxx. Only Celebrex would have been deemed safe to use. The FDA failed to announce the conflicts of interest at the time of the meeting.

Profits in child psychiatry for the drug companies

The pharmaceutical industry has not overlooked opportunities for profits in child and adolescent psychiatry. What had been a cornerstone of treatment that upheld the worth of human relationships, therapist/child and parent/child, is now replaced by a policy of mass dispensation of pills, even to two year-olds. The innocence of childhood becomes yet another fertile field for unbridled corporate profits – but not without consequences.

[The Wall Street Journal, January 25, 2005 reports: "Studies Linking Ritalin and Depression Highlight Risk of Over-diagnosing ADHD. By Tara Parker Pope] Dr. Eric Nestier, chairman of the psychiatry department at the University of Texas-Southwestern Medical Center in Dallas states: "Many kids are put on Ritalin when there is very weak evidence."

Dr. William Carlezon, a psychologist at Harvard co-authored a study on depressive symptoms that developed in adult rats exposed to Ritalin early in life. Researchers at the University of Texas-Southwestern have reported similar findings. It raises the question: what are the long-term effects of these drugs in humans?

Schools have tried to cope with overcrowded classrooms by pushing Ritalin. This same Wall Street Journal article reports that a recent McLean Hospital study showed that some teachers never rated any kids with ADHD while others singled out nearly all the boys as potentially ADHD. With both parents forced to work to make ends meet, it is highly likely that lack of parental supervision has more to do with ADHD then inborn brain dysfunction. The New York Times February 12, 2005 "Therapists question Canada/s action on hyperactivity drug" by Benedict Carey; reports that Canadian regulators had suspended the use of the commonly prescribed hyperactivity drug, Adderall XR indefinitely because the drug was linked to 20 deaths, 12 of those children. Adderall XR and its short-acting cousin Adderall, are amphetamines. More than 700,000 Americans take some form of Adderall manufactured by Shire Pharmaceuticals Group of Britain. These amphetamines, including Adderall and Dexedrine are far more potent than Ritalin. One doctor quoted in the article states that the 30 to 40% of his patients cannot manage their attention problems without amphetamines because Ritalin isn't strong enough. Prescriptions of the drugs have more than doubled during the 1990s, and children are now medicated daily, instead of only on school days, as they were once advised.

Psychiatric News (newspaper of the American Psychiatric Association), October 15, 2004, details the situation with the antidepressants known as serotonin reuptake inhibitors (SSRIs). On Friday, October 15, the FDA announced that all antidepressants marketed in the United States must carry a black-box warning about the increased risk of suicidal thoughts and behaviors, particularly when used in the treatment of pediatric patients. Officials of the US Food and Drug Administration first suspected an increase in suicidal thoughts and behaviors linked to antidepressant use in children and adolescents in March 1996. Yet no apparent action was taken by the agency until a pattern seemed to emerge in the first half of 2003. During a pair of hearings before the House Subcommittee on Investigations and Oversight, two committee members threatened to introduce legislation banning the prescribing of antidepressants to anyone under age 18 "if the FDA didn't act forcefully and swiftly to protect America's children." "Pharmaceutical company executives were grilled about their apparent selective disclosure and publication of clinical trial findings. Only four of the 15 trials of antidepressants in pediatric patients with depression have been published – all with favorable results."

A previously undisclosed letter from an FDA reviewer dated March 19, 1996, questioned Pfizer's data on the use of Zoloft (sertraline) for children because of a fivefold higher risk of suicidality when compared with those taking placebo. The subcommittee obtained the FDA's letter to Pfizer from the company, not from the agency. "On March 28, 1996, only a week after the letter asking for clarification and explanation, the FDA approved Pfizer's application for pediatric exclusivity without any apparent resolution of the medical reviewer's questions."

A report (2003) by FDA medical reviewer Andrew Mossholder, M.D., was the first to assert openly an increased risk of suicidal thoughts and behaviors associated with antidepressant use in children and adolescents. His report prompted an agency advisory committee hearing, but Dr. Mossholder was prevented from delivering his report at that meeting. An independent Columbia University analysis of Dr. Mossholder's conclusions verified that there is roughly a 1 1/2 to 2 fold higher risk of suicidal thoughts and behaviors in children and adolescents taking certain SSRIs.

The National Institutes of Health and the Office of Government Ethics [the New York Times February 1, 2005, "Agency scientists divided over ethics ban on consulting" by Gardiner Harris; contemplated a complete ban on private consulting arrangements between scientists at the institutes and pharmaceutical companies. A series of articles in the Los Angeles Times detailed conflicts of interest between N.I.H. scientist's public and private work. Studies show that researchers who except money from private companies are more likely to focus on commercially applicable ventures. Dr. Bryan Brewer Jr., for example, is chief of the National Heart, Lung and Blood Institute's molecular disease branch. In 2003, he wrote an article promoting the benefits of Crestor, a cholesterol-lowering medicine from AstraZeneca. "The article was published in a medical journal 'supplement' that was paid for by AstraZeneca and Dr. Brewer's NIH title was prominently displayed. The article failed to mention potentially serious safety problems with Crestor."

[Los Angeles Times 12/22/04 David Willman "508050 from Pfizer but no outside positions to note "]"Dr. P. Trey Sunderland, a senior researcher at the National Institutes of Mental Health, received more than $500,000 in consulting fees from Pfizer at the same time that he was collaborating with it in his government capacity of studying patients with Alzheimer's disease. Despite rules requiring that governmental scientists disclose their consulting arrangements to the health Institutes, [he] failed to make such a disclosure." These practices, rare until the 1980s, grew quickly after Dr. Harold Varmus, the Institutes director in the 1990s, decided to lift the limits on outside income and administrators loosened disclosure rules about these activities.

Bob Herbert, in his column for the New York Times, 1/14/05 "A gift for drug makers" writes: "But the administration is like an ardent lover in its zeal to shower the rich and powerful with every imaginable benefit. So tucked like a gleaming diamond in proposed legislation to curb malpractice lawsuits is a provision that would give an unconscionable degree of protection to firms responsible for drugs or medical devices that turned out to be harmful." The provision would prohibit punitive damages in cases in which the FDA had approved a drug or medical device. Mr. Herbert quotes Marcia Angell, the former editor in chief of the New England Journal of Medicine, from her book "The Truth about the Drug Companies": "...now primarily a marketing machine to sell drugs of dubious benefit, this industry uses its wealth and power to co-opt every institution that might stand in its way, including the US Congress, the Food and Drug Administration, academic medical centers, and the medical profession itself."

[NYT 6/8/2008] "Researchers Fail to Reveal Full Drug Pay" by Gardiner Harris. – A world – renowned Harvard child psychiatrist [Dr. Joseph Biederman – and Dr. Timothy Willins] whose work has helped fuel an explosion in the use of powerful antipsychotic medicines in children earned at least $1.6 million from drug makers from 2000 to 2007 but for years did not report much of this income to university officials Under pressure from Senator Charles Grassley, another colleague, Dr. Thomas Spencer, reported earning at least $ 1 million. Even these amended disclosures may understate outside income because of contradictions with payment information from drug makers. Dr. Biederman initially reported no income from Johnson & Johnson for 2001. Under scrutiny, he said he received $3,500. But Johnson& Johnson told Senator Grassley that it paid him $ 58,169. The Harvard groups arrangements with drug makers were already controversial because the researchers' promoted unapproved uses of psychiatric medicines in children. The Harvard group's federal grant money was administered by Massachusetts General Hospital, which in 2005 won $287 million in such grants. Dr. Biederman's work helped lead to a 40-fold increase from 1994 to 2003 in the diagnosis of pediatric bipolar disorder. It is far from clear that the medications improve children's lives over time, experts say. The drugs also contribute to the risk of weight gain and diabetes in children. In a subsequent NYT editorial, it was reported that Dr. Biederman's supporters claimed that he had "saved many lives." Critics complain, however, that the Harvard studies were too small, loosely designed and subject to biased interpretation through use of a subjective rating scale.

[NYT 11/25/08; "Research center tied to drug company" by Gardiner Harris] "Dr. Biederman pushed [Johnson & Johnson] to finance a research center at Massachusetts General Hospital…with a goal to 'move forward the commercial goals of J&J.'" Dr. Gahan Pandina, a J&J, executive, noted a problem with a study of children with disruptive behavior disorder that showed that both Risperdal and placebo were effective. An e-mail to Dr. Biederman states: "…please give some thoughts to how to handle this issue if it occurs." Dr. Pandina sent a draft abstract to Dr.Biederman of the study but it stated that only children receiving Risperdal improved "while those receiving placebo did not." Dr. Pandina asked Dr. Biederman to sign a form listing himself as author. It is not clear whether Dr. Biederman read only the draft abstract.

Comment: Thus, it is becoming increasingly clear why so many think they have "bipolar disorder" and that pills are magical solutions. But rearing children on drugs when they need parenting is inexcusable. Brainwashing by the drug industry plays a far greater role in the current belief system than the public realizes.

[NYT 12/3/2006, "Federal Alzheimer's researcher accused of conflict of interest" Associated Press] "U.S. Researcher Penalized for Drug Maker Ties." Pearson Sunderland a federal researcher in Alzheimer's who ran a geriatric research unit at The National Institute of Mental Health was ordered to forfeit $300,000 and perform 400 hours of community service for failing to disclose consulting work with the pharmaceutical giant Pfizer. He admitted to sharing thousands of the institutes much sought after tissue samples with Pfizer at the same time he was being paid as a private consultant. He told the federal judge: "I cannot tell you why except to say this is not part of my normal character." The institute identified at least 44 government researchers who were improperly paid for working on the side for biotechnology and drug companies.

Comment: He and the others are not the first to be corrupted by drug company money. [The New England Journal of Medicine; Erick Turner, M.D., Jan 17, 2008; 358:11761182]. The efficacy of antidepressants as reported in the medical literature is misrepresented because medical journals almost exclusively publish studies with positive results while negative results are suppressed. 94% of antidepressant clinical trials published in journals had data that showed significant drug efficacy compared to placebo. Yet, a more comprehensive FDA database showed only 51% of trials had positive results. "Medical journal readers only get the good news and none of the bad news," states Dr. Turner. Almost all (37 of 38) of the positive studies were published but only 3 of 36 studies that were judged negative reached publication. 11 of the latter were published in a way to make them appear positive. [WSJ 12/26/2006 "Medical journal spikes article on industry ties to kidney group" by David Armstrong] The New England Journal of Medicine warned that aggressive efforts to treat anemia in kidney disease patients with the drug erythropoietin (manufactured by Amgen), as recommended by The National Kidney Foundation, appear to increase the risk of heart failure and the need for dialysis. The medical journal, however, spiked an opinion piece by one of its senior writers critical of the foundation's reliance on multi-million dollar donations from companies that make such drugs. In 2006, the foundation received over half of its support from corporate partners, including $4.1 million from Amgen and $3.6 million from Johnson & Johnson. The foundations guidelines for such matters were criticized because of the 18 members who formulated the guidelines, two-thirds disclosed financial associations with Amgen or other related drug companies.

[NYT 4/16/2008 "Merck wrote studies for doctors" Stephanie Saul]] "The drug maker Merck drafted dozens of research studies for a best-selling drug, then lined up prestigious doctors to put their names on the reports before publication..." Dr. Joseph Ross of the Mount Sinai School of Medicine in New York and co-authors, writing in The Journal of the American Medical Association, said that an analysis showed that Merck had apparently manipulated dozens of publications to promote Vioxx. Dr. Ross states: "It almost calls into question all legitimate research that's been conducted by the pharmaceutical industry with the academic physician."

[NYT 1/24/2008 "Great drug but does it prolong life?" by T. Parker-Pope] "After a study ...showed Vytorin, an expensive combination of two drugs, worked no better than cheap Zocor alone in reducing artery plaque that can lead to heart attacks, The American

Heart Association came to the drug's defense." What the association did not reveal was that it receives nearly $2 million a year from Merck/Schering – Plough Pharmaceuticals... that market Vytorin.

It was also reported that the drug companies had planned to alter their statistical analysis of the above study (perhaps to come up with a more favorable outcome) but abandoned that plan because of mounting criticism.

[WSJ 6/14-15/2008 "FDA got left out on Paxil risk documents" Alicia Mundy] A study by Dr. J. Glenmullen at Harvard claimed that GlaxoSmithKline improperly counted patients taking placebos during clinical studies from 1989 through 1991 when it submitted information to the FDA for approval of the antidepressant Paxil. Glaxo said there was no difference in suicidality between those taking Paxil and those on placebo. However, Glaxo also counted patients taking placebo who had attempted suicide before the study started. The author concludes that the rate of suicidality for Paxil was actually 8x the risk for placebo.

[NYT 10/3/08 "Leading U.S.. psychiatrist failed to report drug income" by Gardiner Harris] Senator Charles Grassley is demanding that The American Psychiatric Association, "the voice of establishment psychiatry," give an accounting of its financing. He states: "I have come to understand that money from the pharmaceutical industry can shape the practice of nonprofit organizations that purport to be independent in their viewpoints and actions." In 2006, the latest year for which numbers are available, the drug industry accounted for 30% of the association's $62.5 million in financing. An analysis of Minnesota data by The NYT found that, on average, psychiatrists who received at least $5000 from makers of newer generation antipsychotics appear to have written 3 times as many prescriptions to children for the drugs as psychiatrists who received less money or none. A case in point: Dr. Melissa P. DelBello of the University of Cincinnati reported to the university that from 2005-2007, she worked for eight drug makers and received about $100,000. AstraZenica, the makers of the antipsychotic Seroquel, told the Senator that it paid her more than $238,000 in that period and sent some of the payments through MSZ Associates, an Ohio corporation Dr. DelBello established for "personal financial reasons."

Dr. Alan F. Schatzberg of Stanford, then president-elect of the American Psychiatric Association, has $4.8 million stock holdings in a drug development company.

[Archives of Gen Psychiatry; Tiihonen J., M.D. et al. Dec. 12, 2006; "Antidepressants and the Risk of Suicide, Attempted Suicide and Overall Mortality in a Nationwide Cohort"; Vol. 63 No. 12]. 15,390 patients without psychosis, hospitalized because of a suicide attempt from 1997 to 2003 in Finland were followed up for a mean of 3.4 years. Results indicated a 39% increase in suicide attempts among those who used antidepressants but also a 32% reduction in completed suicides. Dr. Tiihonen suggested that patients on antidepressants are more likely to overdose on them because they were available whereas those not on antidepressants used more violent methods such as shooting or hanging themselves [newer antidepressants, overall, tend to be less lethal after an over-dose than first generation antidepressants.]

[NYT 12/13/2006; 3/29/1990 "New antidepressant is acclaimed but not perfect" N. Angier] "Dr. Martin Teicher, a Harvard researcher, reported that six of his patients 'developed intense, violent, suicidal tendencies and preoccupations' after starting on Prozac." [I had a similar experience with one of my patients]. The article goes on to report that in late 2003, after reviewing previously unpublished data from drug company trials, British regulators effectively banned the use of most antidepressants in children and adolescents, citing a possible suicide risk..."

Comment: Establishment psychiatry, echoing drug company anger (antidepressant sales have slaked off), is feigning alarm that the FDA's black box warnings regarding the risks of antidepressant use in children and adolescents will cause diminished use of these pills and an increase in the suicide rate in that population (which is in fact occurring). Drawing that conclusion, however, conveniently overlooks the real reason for the rise in mental illness, namely, the complete destruction of intensive psychotherapy in office and hospital settings. The government – insurance – drug industry axis of evil has effectively dehumanized the care of children through bribery and propaganda, pretending that pills can substitute for parenting and proper psychiatric treatment. Young people who are seriously depressed need a relationship with a doctor. Furthermore, they often respond remarkably well in treatment and not infrequently exhibit more good sense than many of their parents. Intensity of treatment must be determined by the seriousness of the symptoms. Dailey sessions may be necessary for as long as is necessary. Treatment must be rendered by a professional who has had rigorous training. An untrained "psychotherapist" or a pill oriented psychiatrist are as oblivious of the real issues involved as an astrologer is of nuclear physics. The use of antidepressants: they are an adjunct to psychotherapy. The solution to the money problem must entail heavy taxation of the ultra-rich, 90% surcharges on golden parachutes etc. The money is there.

[Randomized Controlled Trial of the Effect on Quality of Life of Second vs First – Generation Antipsychotic Drugs in Schizophrenia; Peter B. Jones, M. D, Ph.D. et al. University of Cambridge, U.K., Arch Gen Psychiatry; Oct 2006, 63: 1079-1087]

Context: Second-generation (atypical) antipsychotics (SGAs) are more expensive than the older – line (typical) antipsychotics (FGAs) but are perceived to be more effective, with fewer adverse effects and preferable for patients. Most evidence comes from short term trials. This hypothesis was tested: 227 people aged 18 to 65 with a diagnosis of schizophrenia were assessed for medication review because of inadequate response or adverse effects. Results: "....there is no disadvantage across 1 year in terms of quality of life, symptoms, or associated costs of care in using FGAs rather than ... SGAs. (see article for details).

[Psychiatric News; published by the American Psychiatric Association; Vol 41, No. 23, Dec. 2006] An analysis from the National Institute of Mental Health in the CATIE trial found that treatment with FGAs compared to SGAs (see above) saved on average $300 to $600 per month. Moreover, there was no significant differences in measures of effectiveness, including symptom and quality of life ratings. The total treatment period covered 18 months [Neurocognitive Effects of Antipsychotic Medications in Patients With Chronchizophrenia in the CATIE Trial, Richard Keefe, PhD et al. National Institute of Mental Health; Arch Gen Psychiatry; June 2007, Vol. 64: 633-647] Patients treated with the older, cheaper, antipsychotic, perphenazine, in moderate dosage, after18 months, showed greater cognitive improvement than in patients treated with olanzapine or risperidone (representative newer antipsychotics).

Comment: Both the British and American studies question the validity of drug company studies that claim great advantages for their "newer," much more expensive antipsychotic drugs. A government study published online by The American Journal of Psychiatry, financed by the National Institute of Mental Health, Dr. L. Sikich, Dr. J. McClellen et al. found that the medicines most often prescribed for schizophrenia in children and adolescents are no more effective than older much less expensive drugs and more likely to cause harmful side effects. Two newer antipsychotics (the so-called atypicals), Zyprexa (Eli Lilly) and Risperdal (Jannsen) were compared with an older antipsychotic. After 8 weeks 34 % of the children taking Zyprexa, 46% of those on Risperdal and 50% on the older drug showed significant improvement. However, many gained too much weight on average: 9 pounds on Risperdal, 13 pounds on Zyprexa but only one pound on the older drug. The atypicals, in addition, showed changes in cholesterol and insulin levels which are risk factors for diabetes. Furthermore, the researchers found that 80% of prescriptions for atypical antipsychotics written for children are to treat something other than schizophrenia: 49% for disruptive behavior, 27% bipolar disorder, 14% depression, 13% anxiety. The suspicion exists that many anxious, upset children are given a diagnosis like ADD or bipolar disorder to justify prescribing these powerful, risky drugs that should be reserved for cases of true psychosis.

[www. fda.gov/cder/drug/infopage/ADHD/default.htm] The Food and Drug Administration expressed concern about cardiovascular risk after a review of reports of sudden unexplained death in patients taking usual doses of ADHD products. Concern about adverse psychiatric events, especially psychotic symptoms, followed another FDA review. [It is also a fact that stimulants stunt growth and cause weight loss in children and adolescents].

[NYT, 2/28/09] "Lexapro Maker Is Accused Of Fraud in Its Marketing:" by Barry Meier et al. "antidepressants were illegally promoted for children, U.S. says."

A recent television advertisement targeting consumers for Abilify, a drug hyped as just the thing for treating symptoms of "bipolar disorder" – and, of course, all the consumers out there understand the ins and outs of bipolar disorder. To the accompaniment of kitschy instrumental folk music, a gaunt youngish middle-eastern looking woman lolls her way along a poetic sea shore with windswept gray reeds, finally uniting with her rugged unshaven waspy boyfriend, and smiles were to be had by all. Then, a knowing voice says: "Ask your doctor if Abilify is right for you." Even more unconscionable is an Abilify television cartoon, as if drawn by an innocent child, that shows a little shy woman who stumbles upon the drug whereupon flowers pop up and her have-a-nice-day face is all happy again. Abilify can cost $1100 a month.

Then there are the ongoing shady television advertisements for drugs that supposedly dramatically improve memory replete with pseudo-neuroscience electron microscopy imagery.

[Psychiatric News, 4/3/09, newspaper of The American Psychiatric Association]: "The U.S. Department of Justice has accused Forest Laboratories of conducting a fraudulent scheme to market and promote unapproved indications for its antidepressants citalopram and escitalopram and paying kickbacks to induce physicians to prescribe those medications." The suit charges ...false and misleading information to doctors and the public about the safety and efficacy of Celexa and Lexapro in treating pediatric patients. A negative study showing that citalopram was no better than placebo was suppressed by the drug company according to the accusations.

[Psychiatric Times, "DSM-V Controversies"; Jan.2009; Vol. XXVI]: The American Psychiatric Association (APA) was criticized for "secrecy" surrounding the development of the upcoming DSM-V diagnostic manual. The manual helps to codify future trends in psychiatry and thus elicits keen interest from the pharmaceutical industry. Investigations by Cosgrove and others reveal that of the 170 panel members, 56% had one or more financial associations to pharmaceutical industry and in 6 of the 18 panels, more than 80% of the panel members had such financial ties.

Consider also the late night "infomercial" dramatizations anchored by oh-so-sincere sociopaths (they have perfected looking you straight in the eye.... but oftentimes are shaking their head "no") masquerading as scientific experts, and their "customers," aping wide eyed innocence (so eager to learn).Yet these crooks get away with stealing billions from the public all the while the networks cash in too. All manner of snake oil blares forth from television commercials assuring the public of sure-fire cures for memory loss, fatigue, obesity etc. highlighted by pseudo-scientific depictions of neurons and pretended research even though none of it has any proven worth.

The FDA's Eroding Independence

[AARP Bulletin July-August 2007] Fifteen years ago, faced with complaints that the FDA was taking too long to approve new drugs, Congress passed the Prescription Drug User Fee

Act, allowing drug companies to help fund the process. Susan Wood, a former FDA official and now a professor at George Washington University's School of Public Health, states: Over time, the FDA has "become more focused on the industry and less on what the science is telling us and what is in the best interest of public health."

In 2008, the drug industry will probably pay the FDA $ 400 million in user fees. "When you're getting paid directly from an industry you're supposed to be regulating, it takes quite a bit of edge out of the regulating, says Sidney Wolfe, M.D., director of health research for the consumer advocacy group Public Citizen, …" Risky drugs like Vioxx, Rezulin, Redux, Baycol etc. were approved and later withdrawn from the market. In addition, low cost generics whose approval depends on scarce federal funds, face a growing backlog while high cost brand names approval accelerates. The drug and health products industry directed $ 93 million to congressional and presidential candidates since 2000, according to the nonpartisan Center for Responsive Politics and the industry has spent over $ 1 billion since 1998 to influence the shape of drug legislation. From 1999 to 2018, $4.7 billion.

16

Media, and Mind Control. Psychiatry and the Fundamentals of Propaganda

An objective analysis of current economic realities in America compels us to conclude that there exists a state of unbridled capitalism, one that enriches a plutocracy at the expense of an increasingly disenfranchised, dehumanized public. As a consequence, basic American values that uphold the worth and rights of the individual are being subverted. An ethic of power and money is supplanting Judeo-Christian tenets, the bedrock of Western civilization. All aspects of our culture have been infected, including medicine, but especially psychiatry. One might rightfully wonder how an enlightened electorate could permit such a catastrophe to unfold, one so contrary to its own best interests? Of course, large segments of the public are not being enlightened. They are being manipulated by propaganda in the service of mind control, a necessary prerequisite to further distract the public from the real issue: The accelerating transfer of wealth from the middle class to a plutocracy. I define "propaganda" as the practice of telling partial truths, distortions and lies for a political end. Successful propaganda aims to control the organs of propaganda, the media and the dissemination of information. Let us briefly highlight propaganda in its historical perspective and then turn to its role in present-day psychiatry.

Earlier, we alluded to the fact that throughout recorded history, empires have sought self-enrichment through slave labor, cheap labor and the expropriation of wealth from an underclass. Republics and democracies devolved into plutocratic dictatorships as individual freedoms succumbed to the rule of an unprincipled gangster class bent upon control of societal resources. These totalitarian forces, whether fascist, communist or unbridled capitalistic, have similar ultimate goals. In time, the ruling class, regardless of ideological artifice (ideology is the cover-up that justifies dictatorship), unveils its true agenda, the pursuit of money and power. "The master race," "the dictatorship of the proletariat," the divine right of kings, Caesar anointed god, phony flag waving protestations of "free enterprise" were and are obfuscations to divert the people's awareness from the real issue: the flight of money to the oligarchy. Brainwashing insures the people's narcotized compliance. The control of money is contingent upon control of the media and the dissemination of propaganda. [www.pbs.org/

redfiles/prop/inv/prop inv ins.htm]: "Propaganda in the Propaganda State." The world's first modern propaganda state was created when the Bolshevik party came to power in Russia in the October 1917 revolution. The means of communication were seized as a matter of priority. Public opinion mattered; making sure rivals could not get their message out mattered more. The social order needed new kinds of glue: new myths, new gods and new beliefs. "New = good, old = bad." Alternative faiths like the church were prime targets. Slogans and sacred symbols of the new faith were created: Lenin was deified. "Indoctrination came in the guise of school age 'young pioneer' organizations.... sugary poems about [Lenin's] spirit and dedication to Communist revolution adorned classroom walls, community centers, even the toy stores." Generations of Soviet schoolchildren learned the story of little Pavlik who denounced his father, a rich peasant, to the secret police, and his father's subsequent disappearance into the GULAG. A climate of denunciation and terror took firm hold in Stalinist USSR. As Stalin signed the death warrants of thousands of his comrades and probably got rid of more people over all than Hitler, his own propaganda machine hailed him as the gentle, wise father-figure. His portrait and statues appeared everywhere, as the knowing, caring lover of Soviet children. Former friends, the old Bolsheviks, were suddenly listed as foreign spies and liquidated. The secret police were diligent in searching out fictitious "hidden enemies" of the state. Stalin was able to consolidate his power by picking off his rivals one by one while deluding the people into believing that he was rescuing them from deadly enemies. The source of any idea or mode of thinking that deviated from the party line earned an immediate death sentence. Independent thinking was abolished.

Hitler's propaganda minister Joseph Goebbels applied the same principles employed by the Soviet propaganda machine: create fictitious enemies (the Jews), control the media, consolidate political power by eliminating dissent, seize capital and the means of production, all the while distracting the public from what was going on by slogans, impressive public displays of solemn ritual and the fabrication of false issues that played upon the neediness of the German people by making fantastic promises. Just as Lenin was made sacred, so was Hitler. Just as the Reds had their minor deity, Pavlik, so did the Nazis, Horst Wessel, a manufactured martyr. Again, old was bad, new was good. The people were not supposed to have any other frame of reference but that authorized by the State. Die Neue Ordnung, the new order, was established. Terror was justified as necessary to subdue "enemies." Goebbels realized that brainwashing was indispensable. The repetition of lies over and over again convinced people that fabrication was fact. Goebbels states: "Je mehr es Luege gibt, glaubt man desto leichter ihr"... ".Man muss eine Luege nur oft genug wiederholen damit sie zur Wahrheit wird." (The more lies there are, the easier they are believed.... one has only to repeat a lie often enough for it to become true.) Hitler realized that the youth are especially impressionable, giving birth to "Die Hitler Jugend."

There are, of course, many examples of propagandistic systems. Elimination of rival ideologies or belief systems is a prerequisite for effective mind control. Such an agenda always entails the elimination of one's personal history as well as any form of independent thinking. Chairman Mao unleashed the Red Guard to destroy China's art, history, and pre-Mao culture so that the Chinese would have no other frame of reference beyond that defined by those in control. Currently, the Chinese government keeps Chinese students studying in American universities under surveillance ["Watchful Eye of Beijing Is Felt on Campuses Far From China"; NYT 5/5/17 Stephanie Saul]. Chinese students on leave from China to study in The United States bring vast sums to top American universities, paying more than twice what in-state Americans pay in tuition (at U.C. San Diego, over 10% of the under-graduates hail from China).All Chinese students know that what they say is under scrutiny by The Chinese Students and Scholars Association, an arm of the Chinese government. They are exhorted to increase their devotion to the Communist party and have been accused of harassing Chinese students who exercise free-speech (see article for details). The latter, knowing that Chinese tuition money has critical influence, organizes protests when universities invite speakers, like the Dalai Lama, who may question the Chinese government's political agenda. Stalin and Hitler liquidated Poland's intelligèntsia and Pol Pot of Cambodia murdered a million of his fellow countryman, anyone educated who could think.

Propaganda's blueprint for mind control

1. Control of the media, the organs of propaganda, eliminate dissent
2. Distract the public from the real issues by stirring up irrational fears, oftentimes by creating a fictitious enemy or exaggerating some threat
3. Convince the public that if they do not fall in line they are traitors (enemies of the state). Paranoia and mindless fanaticism are fostered
4. Sweep away a nation's history and culture, extinguish the individual's personal history, replace history with a "new order," promise an extravagantly rosy future
5. Suppress analytic thinking and introspection by encouraging frenetic activity, fill the air-space with unrelenting noise, saturate "entertainment" with bread and circuses, all to insure that the real agenda of transferring power to the oligarchy can proceed smoothly as an undercurrent.
6. Puppet-program the people by constant repetition of lies (brainwashing)
7. Obscure the real agenda of those in control by distracting the public with a false quasi-religious alternative faith replete with fabricated myths and self-righteous solemnity
8. Dehumanize the populace, devalue human relationships, and perfuse the whole of society with a value system based upon power, fooling the individual into thinking that, if they give up their humanity, they are honored heroes of the state. Above all, eliminate memory.

Unbridled capitalism in its race to cede control of the nation's resources to the billionaires has made extensive use of the principles inherent in a policy of mind control and propaganda. For example, a fictitious crisis is currently being created in regard to Social Security and Medicare solvency. The prior Bush administration repeated over and over again that these governmental programs will collapse due to lack of money. The solution it said is to dismantle Social Security and funnel the money to Wall Street brokerage houses under the guise of "private accounts," "empowering the individual" and creating an "ownership society." Administration propagandists feign moral outrage at any talk of raising taxes on the billionaires as if the average citizen was benefiting somehow from current tax policies that free the super-wealthy from taxation. We were warned that raising taxes would lead to economic Armageddon because the wealthy, "the job-creators," would stop spending. I have shown, however, how the billionaires and multimillionaires rake in trillions of dollars. These ill-gotten monies could be redistributed for the greater good of the vast majority of the population. The middle-class and the poor also spend when they have income to do so and it is the middle class that is the true engine of economic growth. What is the core value to the economy if a plutocrat purchases a $50,000 ladies handbag, buys another yacht or builds a 50,000 ft2 eyesore?

The Plutocrats and the Art of Propaganda: Past and Prologue

Frank Rich, The New York Times, March 20, 2005, reports on the "presidential roadshow" in which Mr. Bush had "conversations on Social Security" with "ordinary citizens" for the consumption of local and national newscasts: "As in the president's town meeting campaign appearances last year, the audiences are stacked with prescreened fans; any dissenters who somehow get in are quickly hustled away by security goons." "But, as the Washington Post reported last weekend, the preparations are even more elaborate than the finished product suggests; the seeming reality of the event is tweaked as elaborately as that of a television reality show. Not only are the panelists for these conversations recruited from administration supporters, but they are rehearsed the night before with a White House official playing Mr. Bush." "One participant told the Post, 'we ran through it five times before the president got there.'"

Mr. Rich also highlights the "faux reporter Karen Ryan" who "interviewed" administration officials hyping the Medicare prescription drug program. Armstrong Williams was paid $240,000 "for delivering faux-journalistic analysis of the No Child Left Behind Act." "The administration cycled the Ryan and Williams paychecks through the PR giant Ketchum Communications. Susan Molinari is another propagandist, according to Mr. Rich, and appears regularly on news shows: "As she bloviates from the right about Social Security to the fake newsman Jeff Gannon, she is invariably described as a former Republican congresswoman or a CNBC political analyst." Mr. Rich states that at present, she is CEO of the Washington Group, Ketchum's lobbying firm, and president of Ketchum Public Affairs. Other sources corroborate Mr. Rich's findings. Robert Pear, The New York Times, March 15, 2004 reports on materials produced by the Department of Health and Human Services which called them video news releases. Two such videos end with the voice of a woman who says, "in Washington, I'm Karen Ryan reporting." "But the production company, Home Front Communications, said it had hired her to read a script prepared by the government." In another segment a pharmacist talking to an elderly customer says that the new drug law "helps you better afford your medications." The customer says "it sounds like a good idea." The pharmacist replies: "a very good idea." In one script, the administration suggests that anchors use the following language: "In December, President Bush signed into law the first ever prescription drug benefit for people with Medicare. Since then, there have been a lot of questions about how the law will help older Americans and people with disabilities. Reporter Karen Ryan helps sort through the details."

On February 19, 2005, New York Times reporter Anne Kornblut reports: "The comptroller general has issued a blanket warning that reminds federal agencies they may not produce "newscasts" promoting administration policies without clearly stating that the government itself is the source. These "news releases" look indistinguishable from authentic newscasts and are often picked up by local news programs. Once again, Ketchum, the giant public relations firm is reported to be centrally involved. "Ketchum has received $97 million in government public relations contracts since 2001." American taxpayers fund these operations.

The latest wars are another example of unbridled capitalism's successful use of propaganda, not all that dissimilar to the methods Stalin and Hitler employed to justify preemptive invasions of other countries. The 9/11 tragedy was an opportunity to legitimize an invasion of Iraq. First, the American public was brainwashed into believing that Saddam Hussein planned the attack on the Twin Trade Towers even though all the evidence indicated that the Iraqi dictator and bin Laden hated one another. Second, the fictitious enemy was further burnished by inventing evidence that America was being threatened by weapons of mass destruction. Third, when no weapons of mass distraction were found, the war was justified because the United States was bringing freedom to the Middle East (Hitler and Stalin were also "liberating" invaded countries, as is Russia's Putin doing today in the Ukraine). It is not a policy of the military to estimate or disclose civilian casualties. By some estimates, however, 100,000 innocent Iraqi civilians have died. This "news" was hushed up along with pictures of the horribly maimed and scarred American soldiers, exploited by the only element in American society that really profits from this evil: Big Business ... Blood for oil. As of 2012, more than 6000 American youths have died in these evil wars "bringing democracy" to foreigners who hate us. 900 American young men have been horribly burned yet attempt to salvage what is left of themselves according to The New York Times, January 2012.

Nicholas D. Kristof, [NYT, "A Veteran's Death, the Nation's Shame," 4/15/12] alerted us to the fact that while an American soldier died every day and a half, on average, in Iraq or Afghanistan, veterans kill themselves at a rate of one every 80 minutes. "More than 6,500 veteran suicides are logged every year." Michael DeBow, in his 20's, was one of those suicides. After 9/11, he, followed by his younger brother Ryan, signed up for Iraq: 'I can't just sit back and do nothing.' When his Mother picked Michael up from the airport after he was discharged, she was staggered: '...it was like he was an empty shell...His body was shaking.' He bought the same kind of gun he had carried in Iraq. When Ryan returned home in 2007, he too began to show signs of severe strain and began abusing drugs. His Mother rushed him repeatedly to the V.A. emergency room but was told there was a six month waiting list for inpatient treatment. Ryan talked of suicide and, while waiting for treatment, killed himself. Three of his friends in the military also killed themselves on their return. Last year the United States Court of Appeals in San Francisco "excoriated the V.A. for 'unchecked incompetence' in dealing with veteran's mental health." A rock was lifted on V.A. corruption in 2014.

Cargo worker Tami Silicio took a photograph of flag draped coffins of fallen soldiers inside a plane at Kuwait International Airport. The Seattle Times published the picture. She and her husband were then fired by a military contractor, because the Pentagon prohibits photographs of caskets. Apparently, the American public has to be protected from the truth, otherwise they might think twice about unbridled capitalism's agenda.

The New York Times, "Rescued in Iraq" Associated Press, January 13, 2005, reports: "Mr. Bush did such a good job selling the weapons-hunting nostrum that 40% of Americans recently said the weapons were there." (Man muss eine Luege nur oft genug wiederholen damit sie zur Wahrheit wird....one must only repeat a lie often enough for it to be believed). Parallels also emerge with little Pavlic and Horst Wessel. Through no fault of her own, Jessica Lynch, a private in the US military, was exploited in a propaganda effort to make of her a sacred symbol, a gung ho war heroine who was captured by evil Iraqis and, in a blaze of gunfire, freed by her comrades. While a brave woman who was seriously injured in a Humvee accident, all the rest is fabrication.

Frank Rich [The New York Times, November 9, 2003] quotes Cher (one of those "Hollywood types") who visited the American wounded at Walter Reed hospital. She told of her experience talking with "a boy about 19 or 20 who had lost both his arms" and then asked: "why are none of Cheney, Wolfowitz, Bremer, the President,....why aren't they taking pictures with all these guys? Because I don't understand why these guys are so hidden and why there aren't pictures of them."

The plutocracy distracts the public from the real issues (where all the money is going) by dishing up diversionary fare. For the "right" it is prayer in schools for the so-called left, "sexual-harassment," gender rights, multiculturalism, etc.. Abortion (and even contraception) is decried yet there seems to be little interest in the well-being of the healthy child once it is born. An abortion of a fully formed fetus is morally questionable unless the survival of the mother is at stake but, as a psychiatrist, I have seen what happens to children who are brought into the world and are unwanted. Families grieving at the funeral of their sons who died in middle-east wars were systematically subjected to jeering taunts from a paranoid religious sect that relished these deaths as God's punishment for "homosexuality." What the rank and file of these dehumanized fanatics do not realize, however, is the extent to which they are being exploited and manipulated by politicians, the foot soldiers of the plutocrats. Social programs, medical care, education, Social Security and Medicare are under siege by the billionaire's minions who have provided a windfall for the billionaires and squandered the lives of American young men who, you can be sure, derive from the legions of the middle-class and poor.

Those in control have a double standard when it comes to "freedom of speech." Protesting against war is condemned as unpatriotic in spite of the fact that wars generally benefit only the military-industrial complex. It makes little sense for an individual to lose the only life they will ever have for the sake of politicians and big business profits. Even after 57,000 American young men died senselessly in the Vietnam War, right wing columnists for the Bush administration still planted articles about how that war could have been won. These are the people who have such reverence for the embryo. We recall Spiro Agnew, Nixon's vice president, who condemned the anti-Vietnam War protesters while he was taking bribes in the White House. His marble bust was unveiled in the Capital a few years ago. That the Bush administration was motivated by ideology is naïve. Their only ideology was one based on power and money, the prayer breakfasts notwithstanding.

The deterioration of humanistic values in American society has spawned two camps. At one end of the spectrum is the bread and circus camp. They ridicule and sneer at civilized standards of human decency. At the other end, is the so-called "religious right" who believe that only they own the truth. Ironically, both are unaware of the extent to which they are simple pawns of those who are really in control.

Control of the media is the blueprint for mind control. All powerful oligarchies have recognized this prerequisite and unbridled capitalism is no exception. In a series of investigative reports for public television in 1999, Bill Moyers addressed these issues in "Free Speech for Sale." The focus was the Telecommunications Act of 1996. The digital spectrum, it was explained, is a set of new channels over which it is possible to render a much better high-definition picture as well as limitless marketing opportunities, taking one existing channel and turning it into multiple channels, creating interactive TV to buy and sell products, watch movies, present programming, news and conduct business.

Mr. Moyers brought to light the tactics that broadcasters employed to influence congressman. Hundreds of lobbyists spread over Capitol Hill, working diligently prior to the vote. Millions were targeted for campaign contributions. Subtle intimidation was employed. Senator John McCain of Arizona stated: "When an issue comes up before Congress that affects the media, the station managers from the congressman's district sit down in a room with the Senator. Direct threats aren't necessary. They are the messengers who present the Senator to the public."

It was estimated that auctioning off the digital spectrum could have brought the public $70 billion but not one word on this issue was mentioned on any of the three major networks nor anywhere else on TV. Why? Because they were all going to make hundreds of billions of dollars by virtue of this giveaway. No auction was ever conducted and the airways were indeed handed over to media moguls, assets which, as Senator McCain pointed out, belonged to the public. President Clinton, congressman Gingrich and the owners of cable, phone, broadcasting and satellite companies were present for the signing ceremony. The media giants lobbied hard for this bill which would force consumers to buy new TV sets. It also lifted restraints on the number of stations the major networks could own while giving them free use of the digital spectrum. Fewer and fewer media giants were controlling more and more media outlets. Fox, Disney, CBS, GE, Cox Communications, Time Warner and AT&T, own cable, books, magazines, TV networks, and radio. They aren't going to present the news on any issue that affects them personally or their profits. The media giants have always claimed their First Amendment rights to "free speech" but, as Mr. Moyers points out, only they can afford to be heard.

Mr. Moyers also focused on the reaction of the tobacco industry to Senator McCain's attempt to legislate increased taxes on cigarettes and use the receipts to fund insurance and medical treatment for smokers harmed by cigarettes. Big tobacco reacted with a $40 million advertising propaganda campaign that depicted Senator McCain's bill as a measure foisted on "working people." Tobacco advertisements neglected to mention, however, what was being taxed, who was being taxed and how the receipts would be spent. Big tobacco orchestrated emotionally manipulated imagery of various proud minorities who were supposedly being pushed around by this anti-tobacco legislation. The McCain bill was defeated and probably in no small measure by Senator Mitch McConnell from Kentucky, an indefatigable foot soldier for big business and big tobacco (update: and the billionaire Communist China axis). Mr. Moyers reported that not a single major TV or cable network news program with the exception of a brief account on ABC covered the issue of the tobacco advertising blitz.

Mr. Moyers reported on the plight of other individuals targeted by big business propaganda who were smeared and their moral character questioned (former President Trump is a current example). Unflattering photographs accompany the smears.

William Safire, a voice that many would consider to be bona fide far right, had written extensively on the politics of the media. In The New York Times, June 16, 2003, Mr. Safire reported: "the Federal Communications Commission, in business to protect the public's interest in our nation's airways, has, by three to two vote, opened the floodgates to a wave of media mergers that will further crush local diversity and concentrate the power to mold public opinion in the hands of ever fewer giant corporations." He notes the risks of "homogenized news or a one size fits all entertainment forced down people's throats." Prior regulations allowed a single media giant to own TV stations reaching a third of Nations viewers. Proposed changes would up the percentage to 50% as well as no holds barred cross-ownership of newspapers, TV and radio stations. Mr. Safire attributes the proposed power grab to a "seemingly unstoppable lobby." Viacom (CBS, (UPN), Disney (ABC), and GE (NBC) etc.) intimidated the National Association of Broadcasters, who formerly supported its many independent members into caving in to, as Mr. Safire termed it, "giantism." He raised concerns as well about the fate of legitimate local mores since centralized mega business has never been prudish about exploiting the profit potential of sex, violence and pornography [AT&T profits handsomely on pornographic 911 calls]. Mr. Safire worries that the public airways will be turned into fiefs to undermine diversity of opinion, homogenizing our varied culture. Needless to say, CBS's60 minutes, NBC's dateline and ABC's 20/20 "found the rip-off of the public interest by their parent companies too hot to handle." (Homogenizing our culture is key to multinational corporations' globalization agenda.)

Bob Herbert's column in The New York Times, June 5, 2003, "Study finds the FCC took 2.8 million in industry paid trips" highlights the corruption within the supposedly independent FCC and the media giants it regulates. The Center for Public Integrity's study found that over the last eight years, commissioners and staff members of the FCC have taken 2500 trips costing $2.8 million "that were primarily paid for by members of the telecommunications and broadcast industry and that "many government agencies accept millions of dollars annually from industry and other special interests for trips to meetings, conferences, and retreats." The top destination was Las Vegas. Mr. Herbert states: "Control of the nation's airways which is the most direct and effective way of controlling how we think, feel, vote and spend our cash is one of the great prizes America has to offer."

A pusillanimous Congress is irate that drug companies give coffee mugs to doctors.

Does that mean that paying $10,000 for breakfast with your congressman is also off limits?

Paul Krugman writing in The New York Times March 25, 2003 "Channels of Influence" discussed the "Pro war rallies most of which have been organized by stations owned by Clear Channel Communications, the behemoth based in San Antonio that controls more than 1200 stations. He refers to a journalist who has written revelatory articles about Clear Channel and notes that the company is notorious and widely hated for its ironfisted centralized control. "Critics say it uses its power to squeeze recording companies and artists, contributing to the growing blandness of broadcast music." "The Telecommunications Act of 1996 nurtured this giant." Furthermore, "Clear Channel has a history with George W. Bush." The vice chairman of Clear Channel is Tom Hicks, Chairman of the University of Texas Investment Management Company, called Utimco and Clear Channel's Chairman, Lowry Mays, was on its board. Utimco had strong Bush family ties." In 1998, Mr. Hicks purchased the Texas Rangers in a deal that made Mr. Bush a multimillionaire." Mr.Krugman continues: "Scores of mid-level appointees.... now oversee industries for which they once worked."

You may recall the CD smashing rally organized by KRMD, part of Cumulus Media Radio chain, that banned the Dixie Chicks, a singing group, from playlists because they criticized President Bush and the second Iraq war. A 33,000 lb. tractor smashed Dixie Chick's CDs, tapes etc.. One could draw parallels to Nazi book burning bonfires but, on the other hand, the defenders of book burning counter that any criticism of the former Bush administration and its policies is also rooted in Naziism. Saying makes it so. After all, Hitler had his struggles too as exemplified in "Mein Kampf."

Brent Staples writing in The New York Times 2/20/03 "The day protest music died" observes: "...but independent radio stations that once would have played edgy, political music have been gobbled up by corporations that control hundreds of stations and have no wish to rock the boat. Corporate ownership has changed what gets played and who plays it. With a few exceptions, disc jockeys who once existed to discover provocative new music have long since been put out to pasture. The new generation operates from playlists dictated by corporate central..... wallpaper music." "The point of these sterile playlists is to continually repeat songs that challenge nothing and no one, blending in large blocks of commercials, 30 minutes or more per hour during morning drive time." Independent radio where "unknown bands might once have come knocking at the door no longer even have doors." [The only alternative to nothing-music is violent dehumanizing rap].

The big city newspaper is also moribund, The New York Times and others are losing circulation. After 146 years of publishing, The Seattle Post-Intelligencer will survive only in a much smaller online version. The San Francisco Chronicle may also close along with Chicago and Detroit papers. The public is less literate and thinks less. The same one liner sound-bites that masquerades as news is mind-numbingly rehashed over and over again on so-called newscasts. AOL that had presented introductory news coverage now substitutes Hollywood gossip, as if for a mentally retarded public. Free speech is also under attack around the world. An Afghan journalist received a death sentence commuted to a 20-year jail term for blasphemy. He wrote something about the role of women in Islam. Newspaper closings in The United States will lead to further dumbing-down of the public and the repression of dissent through the plutocracy's agenda of conformist brainwashing.

The Orwellian Plutocrats Refashion Education To Better Serve Their Interests

For years, corporate advertising (brainwashing) has infiltrated the public school system [The New York Times January 5, 1997 "Corporate classrooms and commercialism" Deborah Stead]. School hallways are adorned with corporate logos and billboards. 40% of secondary schools have home rooms that start the day with news and commercials transmitted by "Channel One." Classroom packets promote Hershey's chocolate or Kellog's Rice Krispies or third graders practice math by counting Tootsie Rolls. Young children learn to read with software using corporate logos like Kmart, Coke and Pepsi or Prozac representatives give a talk at a high school assembly on National Depression Screening Day. A Hershey Foods Corp. video's shows four young people learning how chocolate is made along with some math and science lesson. One teenage actor states: "I didn't know they used real whole milk in chocolate." "Mr. Hershey did," another replies, "His company still does today" [have you ever had the courage to taste a Hershey Bar?]. Campbell Soup Company sponsors the Prego thickness experiment. The kit contains a slotted spoon and a Prego poster "explaining the scientific methods students could use to prove that Prego was thicker than Ragu." Calvin Klein donated free textbook covers to a Staten Island school featuring young models dressed in Calvin Klein clothing and free tattoos with initials CK for Calvin Klein.

Corrupt the young and make money. That was 1997. Have things changed? Hardly. We are well on our way to "1984" and "Brave New World".

Bill Gates and fellow billionaires to overhaul the nation's education policies

[NYT 5/22/2011 "Behind Grass-Roots School Advocacy, Bill Gates" Sam Dillon] The New York Times [Indianapolis] reports that "a handful of outspoken teachers helped to persuade state lawmakers this spring to eliminate seniority-based layoff policies. They testified before the legislature, wrote briefing papers and published an op-ed article in The Indianapolis Star. They described themselves simply as local teachers who favored school reform – one sympathetic representative, Mary Ann Sullivan, said 'they seemed like genuine, real people versus the teachers' union lobbyists.' They were, but they were also recruited in a national organization, Teach Plus, financed significantly by the Bill and Melinda Gates Foundation." Bill Gate's new strategy is the overhauling of the nation's education policies. Tactics include creating new advocacy groups, paying Harvard-trained data specialists to work inside school districts, "bankrolling many of the Washington analysts who interpret education issues for journalists and giving grants to some media organizations [Education Week and public radio and television stations that cover education policies]." "We've learned that school level investments aren't enough to drive systemic changes, said Allen C. Golston, the president of the foundation's United States program."

The foundation spent $373 million on "education" in 2009 but will pour in $3.5 billion more over the next several years. Few policy makers, reporters, or the public who encounter advocates like Teach Plus or its pundits realize that they are underwritten by the foundation. Bruce Fuller, an education professor at the University of California, states: "It's Orwellian in the sense that through this vast funding they start to control even how we tacitly think about the problems facing public education.

Frederick M. Hess of the American Enterprise Institute received $500,000 from the Gates foundation in 2009 "to influence the national education debates." He added: "There can be an exquisite carefulness about how we're going to say anything about the foundation." "Everybody's implicated," he added.

Harvard got $3.5 million to place "strategic data fellows" who could act as "entrepreneurial change agents" in Boston, Los Angeles etc. school districts.

The foundation's latest annual report highlights its role "in the development and promotion of the common core academic standards that 45 states have adopted." "The National Governor's Association and the Council of Chief State School Officers, which developed the standards, and Achieve Inc., which coordinated the writing of tests aligned with the standards, have each received millions of dollars."

Fordham's president praised the standards after their 2010 release. He was quoted in scores of newspapers but the Gates connection was not noted. The Fordham Institute received $959,000 from the foundation in 2009.

The Center on Education Policy, which calls itself "a national independent advocate," was given $1 million to track which states adopted the standards.

"The New Teacher Project," a Gate's financed group, issued an influential report cited repeatedly by Arne Duncan, the Obama Secretary of Education, who wrote it into the rules for the federal "Race to the Top."

Mr. Gates spent $2 million on a campaign supporting the film "Waiting for Superman" "which demonized Randi Weingarten," the president of the second biggest teacher's union. The foundation created an advocacy group as part of a $290 million program designed to "establish strong ties to local journalists" and "should go toe to toe with union officials." The document said the group should "maintain a low profile."

In Chicago, union activists have accused Teach Plus of being an "Astroturf grass roots organization."

There are "bad teachers" but also bad principals, delinquent kids, and irresponsible enabling parents whose children are impossible to teach absent discipline in the classroom. Poverty is deadly and teachers are not its root cause. Why the call to arms against senior teachers? It appears to be another Big Business union busting agenda. At a deeper level, the aim is the remolding of education to fit the priorities of the billionaires: suppress individuality, eliminate a liberal arts education that promotes critical thinking and churn out more cogs for business profits. Is the Chinese ant-colony-model really the best for Americans? Could American innovative creativity suffer in more ways than one? Will America end up with a computer literacy but illiteracy in thinking?

[NYT 4/26/14; "A Walmart Fortune, Spreading Charter Schools – Foundation Finances a Conservative Tack on Education" M.Rich]. Since 2000, the foundation has awarded more than $1billion in grants nationally to educational efforts. In Washington D.C., the Walton foundation has subsidized an entire charter school system in the nation's capital, including teachers who are alumni of Teach for America, whose largest private donor is the Walton foundation. While the D.C. charter students are mostly poor and black and far outperform neighborhood public schools, charter schools can pick and choose who can attend, receive taxpayer's dollars but are privately operated (the teachers are also non –union). Even the local board that regulates charter schools receives funding from Walton. The foundation also ear-marks grants to business think tanks like the Thomas B. Fordham Institute and the American Institute for Public Policy Research.

The public school system, on the other hand, must accept all students. The public school system is at the foundation of America democracy and is being undermined by billionaires who want to mold the young as they see fit. Their motivation is not just altruistic. "Silicon valley billionaires remaking America's schools" Natasha Singer [NYT 6/7/17].

Tech companies have been taking over programs in public schools. Megan Tomkins-Stange, assistant professor of public policy at the University of Michigan, states: "They have the power to change policy, but no corresponding check on that power.....It does subvert the democratic process." And it directly benefits the tech industry (companies need more programmers). The pitch is made directly to students (starting in pre-kindergarten) and teachers, bypassing school boards. Campaigns are financed to alter policy and subsidize teacher training alongside a push to sell computers and software to schools. DreamBox Learning develops algorithms to instruct children on goals, while devaluing the role of teachers. The article points out that there is little evidence that DreamBox improved learning.

[The Washington Examiner "Facebook's Mark Zuckerberg is focusing on personalized education" 11/7/15 by Jason Russell], promoting the idea that children the world over should teach themselves ("a personalized education"): Students cluster together with laptops, while teachers become "helpmates" rather than leaders. Children select their own assignments and work at their own pace with software provided by Facebook (software that will help children to think the right way). In 2015, Urban Promise Academy, a public school, experimented with Mr.Zuckerberg's approach but Claire Fisher, the school principle, and one of the voices of dissent, stated: ".....students...did not know how to pace themselves.... Kids were self-pacing to failure." Inculcating the need for Mr. Zuckerberg's software in the classroom and ultimately eliminating the teaching human is a perfect vehicle for brainwashing. First take over the politicians, then the minds of children.

["How Goggle Conquered The American Classroom"; NYT 5/14/17, Natasha Singer]. Google is leaving no stone unturned to de-emphasize the teaching of traditional academic knowledge in favor of training children in skills like teamwork and problem solving (group think).The long term end result: turn out skilled workers rather than knowledgeable citizens. Jonathan Rochelle, director of Google's education apps group, states: "And I don't know why they can't ask Google for the answer if the answer is right there." Google makes lots of money by selling management services to schools "but by habituating students to its offerings at a young age, Google obtains something much more valuable." Students graduating high school are shepherded into uploading their school Google account into a personal Google account along with all their school Gmail, Docs and other files. Google derives most of its revenue from online advertising. Personal Gmail accounts can serve ads – "much of it targeted through sophisticated use of people's data." Building and fashioning a specific profile of each individual into maturity becomes a powerful marketing tool for selling that information to Big Business. Google lawyers have fought privacy restraints.

William J. Broad, in an article for The New York Times, 3/16/14, writes: "Billionaires With Big Ideas Are Privatizing American Science." They are filling the vacuum created by the cutbacks in public funding of the basic sciences. Steven A. Edwards, a policy analyst at the American Association for the Advancement of Science, states: the practice of science in the 21st century is becoming shaped less by peer-review groups and more by the particular preferences of individuals with huge amounts of money." Their agenda will aim toward a society of puppets.

[NYT "'Tom Sawyer' and Court Opinions: A New Mix in English Class"; 6/20/15 Kate Taylor] The Common Core requires increased use of non-fiction texts in English classes. "Tom Sawyer" is to be understood in the context of current teenage unemployment and Salinger's Holden Caulfield clarified by research on bipolar disorder.

Comment:

"Non-fiction" is not necessarily factual. It is corrupted by political propaganda. Who is selecting the "non-fiction?" Children will be inculcated with propaganda rather than being allowed to critically think for themselves about the eternal truths. The human ties are the royal road to maturity and independence, not the physical sciences. Holden Caulfield is written off as "bipolar disorder" [he is genetically mentally ill] because he is white (read one of the white supremacists) and consequently undeserving of sympathy that is reserved for non-white downtrodden. In realty, the billionaire fascist manipulators are aiming to destroy American history and culture to institute globalization. They lie about their concern for minorities and the whites are the only remaining power block that stands in their way.

Psychiatry and Propaganda

Current news reports lead one to believe that psychiatric "disorders" are the results of gene interplay, viruses or some as yet undetected physical causation. From official journal articles to the popular media, this attitude is promulgated as if it were a mathematical or Scriptural certainty. It is, however, propaganda, not information. Of course, genes may exert influence, but, as I have pointed out: man's success in the animal kingdom is the result of his ability to adapt to diverse environmental cues and conditions (whether positive or negative). Our genetic makeup allows for this adaptability. Take note of the fact that, regarding schizophrenia, for instance, recent adoption studies throw doubt on the dogmatic assertion that schizophrenia is unalterably inborn. Tienari's Finnish adoption studies show the environment to be the final determining factor of whether or not the child becomes schizophrenic. Adopted away children whose biologic mothers are schizophrenic clearly tend not become schizophrenic if the adoptive family is emotionally healthy. (The issue of genetics will be discussed in much greater detail in another book/.

A thinking person, in touch with reality, and possessing common sense, might wonder what is behind the relentless gene drum-beat. Most people are aware that we react keenly to loss, stress, aggression and rejection. Such adverse experiences can leave searing emotional wounds that are not easily forgotten, as a patient of mine who lost a fine 31 year old son to a hit and run driver knows all too well. Some genetic studies indicate that individuals with a particular gene configuration are more susceptible to depression (although more recent studies fail to corroborate these claims). Intrinsic to the findings, however, is the fact that a worsening depressive outcome is contingent upon an accumulation of environmental set-backs and stress. In any case, serious depression does not come out of the blue. People that grow up in a crazy, economically and emotionally impoverished environment become very troubled adults.

Incredibly, it seems one has to point out some obvious realities. The arts, for example, in literature, poetry, the plastic arts, music and the theater give testimony to the pain of tragedy, and our yearning for love, acceptance, harmony and truth. Those artistic expressions that have enduring value reaffirm our being and humanity in the face of the catastrophic adversity that threatens our emotional integrity. To read the psychiatric journals, however, one would think that the environment didn't exist. If one mentions the parent, especially the mother, as having anything to do with the causation of emotional problems, the reaction is angry and irrational. And yet any child who loses their mother is devastated. Later Reviewing the research literature shows how profoundly the brain interfaces with and reacts to environmental stimuli. One apparently needs to remind the organicists (defined as one who views human behavior as more or less exclusively inborn) that, for the small child, the parents are the environment. The skewed journal "research" that systematically leaves out the effect of parenting on child development is a clue of the degree to which current views of human behavior are distortions.

Propagandistic distortions are evident when psychotherapy and clinical evidence are assessed. "Studies" of large populations that employ statistical techniques are supposed to disclose "facts," while thousands of in-depth studies of individual psychotherapy cases are dismissed as unscientific or just "anecdotal," no matter that these in-depth psychoanalytic and psychodynamic studies repeatedly corroborate the same fundamental findings. How can a grossly superficial set of questions administered by people with no training, and orchestrated by biased investigators, be deemed "objective"? How can it stand up to the findings forthcoming from an investigative treatment that has dug into the deepest recesses of another person's mind over a period of years? A psychoanalytically oriented clinician who has made a serious effort to understand his or her own emotional conflicts is a more objective and worthy investigator then someone tainted by grant money from big business or big government who has never taken the step to investigate themselves (there is no proof that parachutes save lives because this issue has not been verified by randomized controlled trials).

Preconceived bias invalidates even the most impressive sounding statistical analysis. Statistically significant is not equivalent to scientifically significant. Garbage in, garbage out. Furthermore, no research money is available from corporate sources, the drug companies etc., unless it promotes the "born that way agenda." "Research" currently marches to the tune of big business priorities. Politicians need to justify slashing expenditures for the poor and middle class as "cost effective" and "scientific." Unbridled capitalism and those who hold the reins of power have a vested interest in eliminating psychoanalytic/psychodynamic treatment, downgrading human relationships, and creating born-that-way-puppets. The principles of mind control are at play here: abolish independent thinking, eliminate memory and an individual's personal history and marginalize human relationships so that the only frame of reference is the one created by those in control: Big Brother. Propaganda is an indispensable tool to achieve dehumanization. "Man muss eine luege nur oft genug wiederholen…."

Part II

Dehumanization of the Individual

17

The Plutocrat Puppet-Master's Agenda

"My opinion is that, in the world of knowledge, the idea of good appears last of all and is seen only with an effort and when seen, is….." [Plato, "The Republic", book 7]

History books glorify Alexander the Great, Caesar, Napoleon, Frederick the Great, Peter the Great, the empire builders, particularly if they fit certain cultural and racial criteria ("us", not "them" not Tamerlane, or at least we see "them" more clearly). Little noted is the fact that for all these "giants" the individual was expendable. They achieved what they did by bringing millions to their deaths. La gloire de la France, Napoleon, willingly offered up the lives of his 500,000 men liquidated in the invasion of Russia. Frederick the Great, lauded in the encyclopedias as a military genius for his innovative blitzkrieg tactics, inaugurated a 23 year war that eventually cost 500,000 Prussians their lives. His relentless political machinations and the ensuing destruction did not prevent him from composing music and writing poetry in idyllic San Souci, his palace "without cares." It is not surprising that the gilded spider-web was a recurring decorative theme in Potsdam palaces. Yes, the powerful are admired in spite of the innocent victims sacrificed in their frenzy for domination.

Judeo – Christianity, however, teaches a quite different ethic, namely that each individual has intrinsic worth. That concept is embodied in both The Torah and the New Testament as The Golden Rule. One day, that message spreading like a conflagration, shook a mighty empire to its foundations. We remember also that the bedrock of Western ideals is the worth of the individual, born in ancient Greece, imperfect as their nascent attempts at Democracy may have been. That belief in the potential equality of all human beings lived on even in ancient Rome and was embraced, incredibly enough, by a Roman Emperor, Marcus Aurelius Antoninus, a stoic, philosopher-king who withstood, as many lesser men could not, power's corrupting influence. One might even point out that the ancient philosophers espoused the Golden Rule long before the Judeo-Christian code came on the scene. Even today, humanism as a value system based on the worth of the individual and the value of human relationships is not without adherents.

The pursuit of power that excludes mutually caring human relationships, ends in personal unhappiness, emotional fragmentation and a failed life. What some may dismiss as romanticism, rests on both psychological and biologic truths. For example, the brain will not develop normally, or at all, without the foundation of a healthy mother – child bond.

As for empires, they cannot come to pass without restricting the individual's freedom to think independently of "the national interest." "Threats to our country" are all too often propaganda to consolidate control by the powerful and suppress individual dissent. Those persons who do not prioritize their own best interests will become victims. Sadly, not many lose sleep over the senseless deaths of soldiers and civilians in the course of various wars, except perhaps the families of the dead or the still suffering maimed and disfigured. For these reasons, this book primarily addresses the health needs of the individual. They are not necessarily synonymous with what the politicians call "the greater good."

Self-assertion and having the right to control one's life are essential to personal survival. Money is not in itself evil and if one has to suffer, better with it than without it. The pursuit of power and money becomes pathologic when it becomes a value system that substitutes for human relationships. Why one elevates power over intimacy with others is a fundamental issue in life. In the course of these discussions, there will be many references to the classics in literature, music and the arts because, as flawed as their authors may have been, their works have endured the test of time by virtue of the enduring truths they manifest.

Why do we turn to Power and reject our human core?

Richard Wagner's stupendous Ring cycle, Der Ring des Nibelungen, is instructive in this regard. In Das Rheingold's debut, the first opera of the cycle, the dwarf Alberich, from the underworld, espies the three lovely Rhein maidens who guard the Rheingold in the river's depths. He falls madly in love, first with one, then another [Die schlanken arme schlinge um mich dass ich den Nacken dir neckend betaste mit schmeichelnden Brunst an die schwellende Brust mich dir Schmiege ....The lithe arms embrace me and I become one with their naked enticing, burning on the swelling breast]. Unfortunately for him, alternately, after playing with his emotions, they taunt and spurn him: "Deine Kroetengestalt.... deiner Stmmme Gekraechz." ....Your lizard-like form....your hoarse voice. It is then, in his impotent rage and burning shame, that he catches a glimpse of the gold's radiance [Power]: einem blendend hell strahlenden Goldglanze entzuendet; ein zauberisch goldenes Licht bricht von hier durch das Wasser" ....burning blinding rays of gold; a magical golden light breaks forth through the water. The lesson is: rejection precedes the lure of power.

Commanding unbridled power, one controls others and creates an illusion of invulnerability that is immune to loss and rejection. One has turned the tables on fate. The problem, however, is not a simple one for those who sacrifice everything in that all-consuming quest. As the Ring cycle unfolds, the competing forces for the Ring (absolute power) sacrifice the real treasure: their own virtue, integrity, love and happiness. Treachery, manipulation and dishonesty beget corruption and, ultimately, the destruction of the gods themselves. These are the consequences of the unbridled quest for power and control: dehumanization, emotional sickness and the death of the spirit.

The bonding of human relationships is intrinsic to the highest expression of what it means to be human, beginning with that of the mother and child.

Through its control of the political process, the Nation's resources and the media, unbridled capitalism, whose only interest is profit and power, has extended its influence over every facet of American society, fashioning a culture that is itself increasingly obsessed with power in all of its manifestations, an environment that begets personal dehumanization, frantic competition, and cruelty. Historically, the transformation of a republic to empire follows this pattern and a greedy controlling oligarchy is always at the heart of the process, the worm in the apple. Ancient Rome is a case in point.

The Billionaires Foster Dehumanization in the Arts as They Efface Personal Identity

The Renaissance means rebirth, referring to the rediscovery of the face and form of man kindled by Greece and Rome and lost in the Dark Ages. The Renaissance resurrected the beauty of the human face and form in all its art, rejoiced in children and the enlightenment of the human spirit.

Unbridled capitalism aims for cookie-cutter, comatose, dumbed-down consumerist machines oblivious of truth and beauty, unthinking cogs they can control. Totalitarian forces have always found the arts and entertainment industry to be an effective and essential brainwashing tool and modern-day plutocrats are no exception. Brainwashing aims to blur individuality and devalue human relationships. A critically thinking opposition poses problems for the oligarchy. If you thought that Western Culture was so great, the plutocracy thinks you need to be re-educated. In the era of globalization, cheap labor, and overall homogenization, all cultures are equal and no art is superior to any other art, or so goes the refrain. The plutocrats pretend great concern for minorities. Their treatment of minorities, however, belies their hypocritical propaganda. Their real goal is to dismantle the humanistic heritage of Western Culture, wipe the past from our memories, eradicate our personal history and with it our unique identity as individuals.Only the super-rich will have the luxury of an identity.

With that in mind, we shall continue our investigation of present day culture, the matrix in which psychiatry finds itself. Psychiatry is, of course, profoundly shaped by societal values (for example, Soviet psychiatry was primarily interested in eliminating dissent). Our own dehumanized culture has not left psychiatry unscathed.

The arts are a reliable gauge of societal trends and values, reflecting as they do, a culture's soul. What do they say about our society? In our present era, remarkable technological advances aside, enduring creativity, at least as it exists in the official realms of the art establishment, is dead. The art sections of newspapers, the media, art exhibitions, bombard us with preposterous examples of so-called artistic innovation, but pretensions of creativity that lack substance aren't very convincing. To highlight one recent absurd example, The New York Times ["Heads, Yes, Tails, No, at a Dinner Starring Rats"; 7/27/2012 author not listed] devotes a full page coverage in its arts section to a New York art gallery that served its guests Rat Braise – replete with recipe – for the jaded guests. The gracious hostess was dressed in a vintage gown decorated with rat skins. One of the guests, an artist, ate with gusto and the gallery owner, also an artist, states: "…skinning and eating rats represents the survivalist instincts she likes to explore in her work." One may evoke head shaking for failing to give a joke its due. The only problem is that, as one peruses the art sections, it's one joke after another.

There are, of course, exceptions. Many a young artist, self-trained, or lucky enough to have found a true teacher, haven't forgotten the beauty inherent in the human form and face. They are not, however, given a forum except as the occasional lonesome examples in art shows. One won't find them represented amidst all the junk in contemporary art museums. As Karl Marx might have said: You may think this display of art is garbage but my money will make you say it is fantastic. After all, who dares point out that the emperor has no clothes? Ridiculously pretentious critiques cannot disguise the fact that, in the politically motivated official art world, real creativity is extinct. Where, for example, are the tunes to equal those of Carousel or even one contemporary song that is worth remembering, if one could remember it? Art is yet another victim of the vast trend of dehumanization engulfing contemporary society.

It is silly to blame, as some do, "The Rise of the Machines" for this state of affairs. Rather blame those who control the machines, the media leviathans and their billionaire friends. Fantasizing that a master computer will someday eclipse human intelligence is science fiction. Faster and faster computing is not intelligence and it is the human mind that created the computer. The danger lies in the increasing effectiveness of computers in the hands of those who control society to police behavior and manipulate thinking, altering the perception of reality. Movies like "The Matrix," "Dark City," and "Revenge of the Sith," reflect an awareness that the "aliens" in our midst, who hold the reins of control, seek to program every facet of our existence and exchange individual creativity and spontaneity with bread and circuses in the new coliseum of technology. The movie "The Invasion of the Body Snatchers" is not so much science fiction as it is an allegory of our own society in which the thinking person is targeted as Enemy of the State. Virtual reality is reality for a legion of programmed puppets. There is scant trace of the human face in our society, the symmetry and harmony of the human form, or a human voice able to rise above the chaotic din. The arts reflect better than my words the state of dehumanization in our culture. It is the puppeteers of the plutocracy who are the real aliens in our midst.

Abstraction in the arts, at the beginning of the 20th century was, at least in part, a rebellion against reigning conventions, supposedly. Classical form and harmony of the established order gave way to disharmony. Mahler's music anticipates the coming perturbation when his bittersweet refrains abruptly plummet, collapsing into dark foreboding surges as if the bottom had suddenly dropped out of reality. Leonard Bernstein, in his radio talks to young listeners, highlighted the significant portent of Wagner's melodic line in "Tristan und Isolde" that ends without harmonic resolution. Perhaps one is justified in making the claim that disharmony reveals forces and realities that lie below the surface of amiable appearances. Nevertheless, abstraction also fragments form and feeling. In pruning details and foregoing reality's depths, abstract art stylizes and simplifies but, in the process, also dehumanizes. Yes, one abstracted aspect or fragment may evoke a special intensity, but reality is many faceted, its depths fathomless as is the totality of every unique human being. It is not my experience, subjective as it may be, that abstraction can bring one face-to-face with the reality of one's own being, those immortal moments when time itself is arrested, so intensely compelling is the beauty and truth of a work of art experienced (Donatello's bronzes for example). Abstraction and its cousin, minimalism (emptiness), by definition reflect the part but not the whole.

The ruling mafia in the art establishment claim that new art is always greeted with hostility but people must accept the new because, well, because it's new. Regarding contemporary music, an elderly gentleman who sat next to me at the symphony recently commented on a "newly commissioned work" which had little redeeming value. Clearly, he was more than a little bewildered by its frank unpleasantness but affirmed in a small depleted voice that we have a responsibility to support new music. Of course, had this terrible work been placed last on the program he would have left early along with most of the audience. The wonderful new works are strategically placed in the middle of the program thus averting the likelihood of the audience coming late or leaving early. There is a music critic of The New York Times who seems to find all abstract musical works "remarkable" and "fantastic", such "giants" as Ligeti and Schoenberg. He blames symphony subscribers because the stunning, incredible, remarkable new American composers aren't being heard much. What's wrong with the public? Why can't they get it? Perhaps it's because they still remember beauty and they take ugly noise at face value. As for the "young" flocking to Disney Hall for modern fare, they won't sustain orchestras. Most just want to be seen, like wearing a baseball cap backwards, or rubbing their parent's nose in the latest fad. And yet two adolescents at a performance of Mahler's second symphony were transported by the uplifting beauty of the last movement. The young could be educated in the classics had they some exposure to these truths in school, but corporate profit priorities have shoved the humanities out of the schools. They want cogs and puppets for their mills not educated well rounded, discerning adults. "Math and science" are important but should we follow the script of the Chinese dictators who fashion their society on the model of an ant colony?

As for the contention that new art is always poorly accepted, the Italian Renaissance generated intense enthusiasm. Even that citadel of reaction, the papacy, was swept up in the esthetic fever that every newly discovered classical fragment generated. A boulverse-ment of all preceding conventions in the arts ensued. Or, consider Athens, in the space of 50 years and with no help from technology, whose alchemistic fires transformed Egyptian archaism into the golden age of classicism that mesmerized Rome and had enough reserve fuel a thousand years later to rekindle the Renaissance.... and we still remember its truth and beauty. In 15th century Florence, far from rejecting the new art, even the simple trades-men of the guilds commissioned works that beautified the Gothic church of Orsanmichele with innovative sculpture: the foreign wool merchants, St. John the Baptist by Ghiberti; the guild of the butchers, St. Peter by Donatello; the tanners, St. Philip by Nanni di Banco; the guild of linen dealers and old clothes men: St. Mark by Donatello; the tribunal of the merchants: the incredulity of St. Thomas's by Verrocchio.

By contrast, what have our times to offer? For the general public, contemporary arts remain as incomprehensibly sterile as ever. Schoenberg codified his 12 tone scale in 1921 to be exact. Almost 100 years later, most people still find it alien. In contrast, a revolu-tionary Beethoven was exalted by the public in his own lifetime. Bernard Holland, the insightful former music critic of The New York Times wrote, referring to a performance of Berlioz by the Orchestre de Paris at Carnegie hall: "...perhaps audiences and perform-ers starved for innovation that has substance, don't mind going back 150 years to find it" [Mr. Holland was offered and accepted a buyout from the paper. Could it be that the Times wasn't friendly anymore to his critiques of "modern" music? It has been pandering to the latest fads ever since – and losing subscribers]. The pathetic excuse of contemporary music dogmatists is that music had run out of ideas and there was no place else to go. Thus, ca-cophony and lyrical frigidity approaching absolute zero Celsius, better heard on some far away asteroid, was the only answer.

Curiously enough, the average person, including probably most music critics, never seem to tire of physically attractive people whom we continue to admire, secretly or oth-erwise, because of their visible harmonious beauty. If we have learned anything in life, we realize that a person's inner beauty is immeasurably more important than their surface attri-butes. Be that as it may, harmony and beauty, at whatever level, have never become passé.

The arts dehumanized, a history

Even Grand Opera has fallen into the hands of charlatans, directors who must be laughing up their sleeve as they tarnish great music with corrupt productions that are neither grand nor have anything to do with the music or the intentions of the composer. Gerard Mortier, formerly director of the Salzburg Music Festival and, later, the Paris Opera, had been graced with the honorary title of "provocateur" for his "daring" productions that jarred the sensibilities of the public. He carried on in this manner for years dishing up repulsive fare to the public owing to the support of government politicians and shallow business sponsors bent upon putting their power brand on the art scene. Apparently, according to the press, immersing the ethereal operas of Mozart and Donizetti in degrading productions is a great achievement. This may fool the ignorant and the abrutis but the purpose of attending opera is to experience the message of the composer not that of some "look-at-me-I hate-the establishment" manipulator pretending to be a provocateur. Mon. Mortier and the others like him cannot create so they rely on shock. The trivializing, pseudo-creative politics of "updating" is no substitute for true creativity. Western culture gave birth to humanism and the worth of the individual and it is no wonder that totalitarian forces hate its heritage.

Jeremy Eichler [NYT 7/21/04 "Berlin Tarts Up Opera With Sex and Violence"] Describes Philipp Himmelmann's production of "Don Carlo" and the brutality of the second act where five bound infidels lie naked in front of the king's table. Executioners duct tape their mouths, douse them with gasoline, string them up by their ankles and, as the executioner's spark their lighters, the curtain falls. "Why this flight into such sadistic realism… or perhaps he knew such a stunt would draw press attention." Mr. Bieito, the Catalan director, serves up worse fare for Mozart's "The Abduction From the Seraglio." Instead of a Turkish harem, the opera takes place in a modern day Berlin brothel. Pasha Salim drags the heroine Konstanze around on a leash. Osmin slits the throat and cuts off the nipples of a prostitute. There is rape, masturbation, drugs, suicide, and the drinking of urine. Of course, all this may capture the spirit of our times but makes it impossible to pay attention to the music.

Alex Ross, writing in The New Yorker ["Nausea"; August 9&16, 2004] describes his nauseating experience at the Bayreuth Festival in Christoph Schlingensief's premier production of "Parsifal." Schlingensief dispenses with Wagner's stage directions for the maximally transcendent final moments of the opera: "A ray of light; the Grail is fully radiant. A dove floats down from the dome above." Instead, the director substitutes two dead rabbits, the rotting of their bodies on a screen. A sped-up film shows accelerating decomposition, to the final frothy maggot-laden end stage. When Endrik Wottrich, the tenor who sang Parsifal criticized the transplant of the action to Africa and Nambia, the director accused him of racist slurs. Singers were done up in blackface. When the curtain fell, the audience roared with boos. Audience disapproval was not registered in the press, however. Interviews with the Minister-President of Bavaria found the production to his liking "because it presented an entirely new point of view." Jose′ Manual Barroso, the President of the European Commission found it only logical that it had been transplanted from Germany to Africa.

Mr. Cross points out that it's all politics, of course. Because German opera houses are heavily supported by state and local governments, the audience's opinion is irrelevant. These contemporary updates fit the spirit of the classic works they sully no more than would a cockroach crawling across a Rembrandt painting.

Here in The U.S., Peter Gelb, the general manager of the Metropolitan Opera responds to critics who question the artistic merit of the 50 new productions he brought to the Met since 2006 [The New York Times Magazine, 3/24/13]: "I think there is a lack of understanding about our efforts to make these productions appealing to an audience that may or may not know much about opera." Again, his solution is to educate the public by updating Wagner and Gounod and hiring movie and theatre professionals (who know a lot about opera?). "Opera News," published by the Metropolitan Opera Guild, posted a column by feature's editor, Brain Kellow, as follows: "We are in the midst of a very bad period… The public is becoming more dispirited each season by the pretentious and woefully misguided, misdirected productions foisted upon them." Mr. Gelb, apparently enraged, pressured "Opera News" (a step he later reversed) to desist from writing reviews of Met productions. He also telephoned the president of WQXR, the classical music station, to complain about a critical blog on their website which the radio station then removed. The Met's current production "Faust" drew boos and empty seats. Clearly, the harebrained updating is contributing to declining membership. The public rightfully questions the politics or the need to distort the classics. Does the Parthenon need updating?, Titian?, Renoir? Of course, the fact is that few see the creative merit of ugly, fragmented new music. The updating masquerades as creative but few beyond the establishment of music critics (who would lose their jobs if they didn't nod their approval) are fooled by the emperor's new clothes. Due to falling attendance, The Metropolitan announced it will reduce ticket prices by 10% this coming season.

Music critics like Anthony Tommasini of The New York Times all too often write as if they were the arbiters of culture and public taste. The cultured public who appreciates harmony and lyrical beauty needs to be educated, or so it goes. As of yet, the public still doesn't understand that "musical trailblazers" like Carter (who is already 100) and Ligeti are mind-blowingly brilliant. We are told that opera directors should mount contemporary music productions because college students, who are already hip rock and rap fans, will dig it (they always dig what's new and have little to learn from the past because they are manipulated into believing that they already know everything. Plus they have to get get along with their administrators or they won't get a good grade). The ultimate manipulation: give them a snappy uniform and make of them cannon fodder. After all, here is music to warm-up the dust swirls on distant planetoids. All that and contemporary too! Newly appointed opera directors, of course, will have to pass the reviewing board of politicians and banal business men so that all the "important" people have a go at the branding iron that will put their stamp on the "new generation" of automatons.

To Mr. Tommasini's credit, even he fails to see the merit of the, at the time, new $ 32 million Los Angeles production of "the Ring," conceived by Achim Freyer [NYT 4/9/09]. Mr. Tommasini writes of "Walkuere": "...but much of Mr.Freyer's magical imagery is not so much strangely alluring as just strange." The warrior maidens ride atop wire-rim horses, part bicycle and part sewing machine. Woton's skull capped head is enclosed in a wire helmet that looks like a protective device for a giant industrial light bulb. Of Siegmund and Sieglinde, he notes: "...these characters after all are half mortal and achingly vulnerable" [yet depicted like outer space aliens]. "I badly missed a human dimension."

Such "human dimensions" haven't seemed, up to now, to trouble Zachary Woolfe another New York Time's critic ["Opera's Sad Goodbye? How About, 'Good Riddance'?" 12/31/13]. Mr.Woolf finds the 1969 glittering, sumptuous, "pseudo-Vienna" production of "Der Rosenkavalier," sets by Robert O'Hearn, "vaguely pernicious: a symbol of the deep-seated resistance to change." Peter Gelb, the Met's general manager, is replacing the production because it has run nearly 200 times. The new production will take place in the past but not the 18th century. Mr. Woolf takes us through a forced march of what he considers to be the public's typical whining protestations when it comes to ugly updating of the classics so that he can note and then dismiss them. According to Mr.Woolfe the Merrill and O'Hearn production, having been left lying out in the sun too long, becomes "faded," "stale" and even had it retained some semblance of vibrancy, that is no excuse to stand in the way change. He likes a Madrid production of "Cosi Fan Tutti" because it is "savage," introduces the politics of gender norm confusions and the current global financial crisis. It must be a head-scratching mystery for this critic that people are still putting up with Rembrandt.

Mr.Woolfe chooses not to address a number of facts, however. Appealing to constant change as his guiding artistic principal, he overlooks the principal reason why the cultured public remains unimpressed by current faddish updating of the classics. Whether from the theatre houses of Broadway to grand opera itself, creativity is dead. Were it not for what we have inherited from the past there would be little worth attending. Of course, my observations, if they are given a forum at all, will probably not sway the art establishment mafia, but the fact remains that most new operas by living composers are ugly freaks that are shelved after one hyped up staging. Updating is not creativity. The reason that the classics endure is that they communicate an enduring message, the antithesis of the drumbeat for constant change. The composer's instructions and ideas should be inseparable from his music. The classics don't need politically correct adulterations. Whatever political message they communicate (and they are concerned with ethics and values) is intrinsic to the work and sufficient in and of itself. Otherwise, the work would have been forgotten. If a work is set in the 21st century, let's have new works that have the truth and beauty to remind us that our souls have not been extinguished.

Even Mr. Woolfe fell off his wave-length with the hip up-daters in his review of The Los Angeles Philharmonic's Disney Hall production of Mozart's "Cosi Fan Tutte." Mozart's glorious music, that celebrates the human, finds itself staged in a vast abstract white sand-dune, the characters outfitted bizarrely by prominent fashion designers. Mr.Woolfe finds the whole not quite legible [NYT 5/26/14 "Spotted in a chic sand dune"]. Equally empty and depressing for Mr. Woolfe is the current Munich production of Wagner's Parsifal. By contrast, however, A.J. Goldmann, also an art critic for The New York Times, finds the same production "stunning," graced as it is with huge blow-ups of black and white skeletal blobs by the German painter Georg Baselitz. Mr. Baselitz's original set would have been "a black box, nothing else." Mr. Woolfe might be treading on thin ice with The Times if he continues to deviate from the party line.

The unremitting parade of sadism with a public-be-damned attitude was featured at the Aix-en-Provence Festival's production of Mozart's "Die Entfuerung aus dem Serail" 2004 NYT author not listed.].The opera is reset in the 1920s with much talk of beheadings and a rewritten dialogue full of obscenities and "inexplicably alternating between German and English." The charlatan that conceived this production filled the scenes with brutal images including, at the very end, bloody clothing thrown at the pasha's feet (originally, but deleted, it was to have been four severed heads). Mozart's joyous ending and his celebration of marriage had fallen by the wayside. The audience booed long and hard. Opera is being delivered into the hands people who hate the family, traditional male-female relationships, and humanistic values.

Trying to breath excitement into current opera updates and underline the plutocrat's phony concern for the downtrodden (globalization's agenda), politics is center stage. Thus the Metropolitan Opera's current production of Humperdinck's Hansel and Gretel forces the guilty audience to contemplate world hunger. Of course, relating the witch to certain types of mothers would be a real "no-no."

The high priests of the contemporary music mafia ecstatically pontificate about the great abstract works being offered the public. The only problem is that this dehumanized fare is leading to falling attendance and risks the shutting down of major American orchestras and opera houses that do not have the luxury of state subsidization as is the case in Europe. Amusingly, no criticism in the art sections of the major newspapers of this reality is allowed. Hoping to reverse this erosion of public interest, the politicians imagine that the answer lies in attracting the young, whose eager hormones, they hope, will fire-up enthusiasm for innovative newness. In 2014, The Seattle Symphony commissioned the grandson of Serge Prokofiev to write "Dial 1-900-MixA-Lot." After its performance, the stage was joined with Sir Mix-A-Lot, a black rap artist, backed by the orchestra. But the young, with their frantic attention span, are ignorant of the classics which have been eliminated from education. They can't see the depths of a Rembrandt beyond the paint.

Bernard Holland, the former music critic of The New York Times wrote: "I hope it is not unreasonable to suggest that composers, not listeners, are the servants here, and that every new opera or orchestral piece they write should be brought in on a tray with hopes that it has something substantial to say that we can like."

Charlatans have a grip on classic theatre. Vincent Canby [NYT, 6/14/1998 "A cock-eyed view of Elsinore"] exposed the senseless trivializing of Shakespeare's ageless plays under the pretext of "updating" (the charlatans answer to creativity). The R.S.C.'s production of "Hamlet" is a case in point. It begins with home movies of Hamlet as a small boy and then jumps to the present: what looks to be a madcap Long Island party, complete with a swing band, on the occasion of the marriage of Claudius and Gertrude. "Pay no attention to the dialogue, which still contains references to kings and queens….". "Claudius could be the new head of his late brother's brokerage firm, Gertrude, a bored, middle-aged socialite who winters in Barbados, Hamlet a Yale student who drinks too much." "As with so many attempts to update and find contemporary associations to the classics, this concept has no place to go once it is established. It simply gets in the way….makes the governing passions seem petty and renders the violence more wanton then inevitable." "The language is all but lost amid these bizarre images….This is a "Hamlet" in which the gravedigger sings "September Song"… Every now and then, when you [recognize] familiar speech, it seems to be a mistake, as if the soundtrack from another movie were butting in."

Unfortunately, in allowing directors like this leverage, we risk losing the heritage of great works of art in the process. Behind it all lurks the shadow of the Roman Colosseum: serve up sadistic shock, beckon inexperienced youth with a good freak show and frantically offer competition with the latest demented video game. But such ugly trends in the long run can only accelerate the problem of falling attendance. Most people who attend the opera and symphony hope to be uplifted by the experience, one that affirms our personal worth in spite of the tragedy that life can suffer upon us. Tragedy visits everyone but only human relationships heal. We need to revisit Mozart and the reasons why his music has endured. Mozart, who ended his operas joyously in a marriage, the triumph and healing powers of friendship.

How did dehumanized art forms succeed in suffocating humanistic art?

So why have the arts become so ugly, cold and fragmented and why is there a public be damned attitude on the part of those that commission new works? The artists are not to blame. If they don't say Heil Hitler they will have no forum to show or perform their works. It is banal businessmen, politicians, smug university professors, administrator bureaucrats sitting on boards, and manipulating shock-artists who hate normal people, that promote these trends. They dictate and the public should stop complaining, just accept, and be "educated."

Recently, I was talking with a gifted young soprano who sang the title role in Berg's "Lulu." Although the opera was composed in the 1920's, she extolled a production that had been "updated" so that the public could "get it" better (as you know, the public must be pretty stupid). I mentioned that Botticelli, Da Vinci, and Donatello don't seem to require updating to maintain their esthetic impact and I wondered if certain current directors of opera hope to hide their meager creative talents through egocentric gimmickry. She found my question difficult to answer. The fact is that banal business men and politicians with little aesthetic sense commission works that they think will put their Lilliputian ego, look-at-me-stamp on posterity. Money talks and artists have to eat. Score another round for unbridled capitalism. The dead hand of government subsidies are another sure way to scotch creativity. Bernard Holland pointed out that once Sibelius received support from the Finnish government, his creativity faded. The compositions that followed his gorgeous second symphony were increasingly emotionally remote.

Why the classics and classicism?

It is unfortunate that most Americans have had little exposure to classicism, the Renaissance or the Great Masters. Their historical context is of interest but these works stand on their own independent merit and can be appreciated as such. What followed the Impressionists and German expressionists makes little sense, however, except through explanations of their historical context. Or again in music, Schoenberg's 12 tone scale was a calculated rejection of harmony but otherwise, in and of itself, has no real reason for existing. I had a conversation with someone about contemporary music following an address by conductor and composer Pierre Boulez. For her, (and I paraphrase), Maestro Boulez's compositions were a direct and natural evolution of Berlioz and Strauss. Her initial aversion to atonal music, through diligent study, became enthusiastic acceptance and she saw it as a thoroughly natural consequence of the music that had preceded it. She continued: the reason that not even 100 years has sufficed for the public to accept Schoenberg lies in the public's unwillingness to devote study to what is different and new. The artistic tradition of Europe (she was Austrian born) is only "one small part of the artistic production of the world" and in no way the measure for all of art. Plus, there are many forms of modern music, Greece and Rome were horrendous examples of civilization (One could have mentioned that Greece was the birthplace of western democracy) and music that seemed to invoke imagery of outer space affirmed our unity with the cosmos. The apology for modern music rests upon an understanding of its historical\evolution, much the same argument that is made for embracing abstraction in the visual arts. Be that as it may, the dinner companion did finally admit that perhaps there is some intrinsic natural essence to which we humans respond that modern music may lack.

As the human form is physically harmonious, even more essential is the yearning and need for inner harmony through the resolution of conflict, fragmentation, and discord. Richard Strauss challenged the far boundaries of harmonic's but ultimately sought resolution, a higher goal that unifies and reveals beauty's potential within us, as grieving Ariadine in her state of oblivion and despair is rescued by Dionysus and carried into Paradise. Like Hans Castorp in Thomas Mann's "The Magic Mountain" (Der Zauberberg), personal growth, life against death, is in battle against the forces of the Antihuman, the inorganic, Das Absolute – The Absolute.

Early on, I was quite captivated by contemporary abstraction in all of the arts but a temporary interlude in Europe and elsewhere that grew into a four and a half-year quest allowed me to look into the matter more deeply. Time allowed for spontaneous discoveries, and a passion for the Renaissance and for those favorable temporal conditions that allowed a humanistic art to flourish: usually small city states, ancient Greece, the Amaravati culture of India, and Quattrocento Italy, eras in time that allowed the un-fragmented self to arise like a Phoenix out of darkness, revealing the beauty of the human form and mind, the whole person.

In fifth century B.C. Greece, a miraculous transformation took place. The mind's eye saw man for the first time in history, whole, unabstracted. The archaic wide-eyed specters of Egypt and the Cyclades were transfigured into images of incomparable beauty. No doubt the freedom to think, restricted as it may have been, was essential to bringing about this metamorphosis. In the dark centuries that followed the collapse of the Roman Empire, abstraction again reigned until man was reborn anew in Florence, Venice and Rome itself, the resource of classical antiquity. Witness the collection from Epidauros at the National Museum of Athens where crystalline stone is transformed into a radiant smiling youth, his beautiful face alive with friendly human warmth. In the same collection, the Nereid on horseback, emerging from the sea, her sheer tunic rippling across her breasts and thigh, surging energy, stone become flesh and airy light. But there is a deeper beauty here, sensing from crystals of inorganic marble, thoughts and feelings of the artist who departed this space and time millennia ago.

There is the tiresome dogma that the ugly and alien foisted upon us by those who have a stranglehold on the art scene – the new establishment – must be accepted because it's art for our age and its "new," when, in fact, abstraction is very, very old, as old as the Neanderthals and clearly preceded figurative art [The New York Times, "New Portrait Emerges of Europe's Cave Artists", 6/15/12, John Wilford]. Of course, not that we just copy masterpieces from the past (although Ancient Rome got away with it for centuries). When, in some future point in time, we experience another Renaissance, it will be because we have gotten back in touch with ourselves and it will reflect man unfragmented and whole. The classics embrace and reveal the whole person. That is why they eternally, timelessly, endure.

Fragmentation in architecture

Regarding architecture, few are the voices that dare criticize the "Giants" of our time, Frank Gehry, Rem Koolhas, Daniel Liebeskind, Lord Richard Rogers and Sir Norman Foster, "the most powerful architects of the land." One wonders, however, if their buildings have true enduring value. The giants of the past, Bramante, Palladio, Wren, embodied unifying concepts that complemented the cities for which they built. They were gems in a setting not preposterous ego trips. Like alien tumorous swellings on an otherwise healthy host, Mr. Gehry's architecture, for example, betrays its neighborhood environs. He had a big laugh regarding his $300 million Stata Center at M.I.T.: it "looks like a party of drunken robots got together to celebrate" (he is being sued by M.I.T. for the building's impracticalities). Frantic gimmickry may set these architects apart. What they do share in common is grandiose emptiness.

Paul Goldberger writing in The New Yorker 4/30/09 "Prince Charles's long war on modern…" takes Prince Charles to task for "an error in judgment" because, from the outset, he [Charles] cast the issue of Britain's architecture in moral terms… between the inhuman and the human. But doesn't architecture and all the arts for that matter reflect values and priorities? Visit the Medici chapels in Florence's and walk from Michelangelo's new sacristy 1520 to the tombs of the princes 1620. Note the contrasting values apparent in these vastly different connected realms. Michelangelo's timeless space employs classical forms of Greece and Rome but adapted to his own age. The room and sculpture that grace it are exquisitely noble and evoke the mystery of the human condition, the courage to face life fully although we know our vulnerability to death and loss. The tombs of the princes by contrast were built after the Medici became the Grand Dukes of Tuscany under the shadow of the Austrian Empire. That chapel is grotesquely grandiose, fragmented in mismatched colored marbles and clearly intended to radiate power first and foremost. The human scale is obliterated.

Stalinist and Nazi architecture hardly evoke humanistic warmth. The uninformed associate Nazi architecture with classicism. To the contrary, Nazi art was in spirit abstract like all totalitarian political art. It was not a celebration of the person but cold, dead, and devoid of the qualities intrinsic to the Renaissance, nor did it burn with the timeless nobility of Greek or Roman art at its best. Mussolini's Vittorio Emanuel Monument and the Stalinist vision for East Berlin are good examples of the emptiness of totalitarian architecture.

Even subjectively, one cannot and should not dismiss all contemporary art as "degenerate" but much of it does appear to reflect the values of a power driven society in which the individual is being eliminated. Mr. Goldberger, quoting architect Rogers states that Britain and Tony Blair are saying we have to be seen as a creative society while Prince Charles is "vicious" and "questionably democratic." Charles's crime apparently is that he spoke the truth, that the edifices going up in Britain are ugly, like a carbuncle on the face of a friend.

Yet, shouldn't one be upset by vandals that destroy an irreplaceable heritage? As for democratic pedigrees, we can trace those of Lord Rogers to corporate financial interests. His strange $1.4 billion millennium Dome resembling as it does a highly magnified AIDS virus, grappling hooks and all, is a colossal flop and shunned by the British public. Les Halles in Paris, a wondrous cathedral of soaring glass canopies, light, and elegantly wrought iron decorative elements was bulldozed by George Pompidou despite international outcry to make room for, of course, The Pompidou Center, a hideous sore on the face of Paris. One of the two architects by the way was none other than Richard Rogers.

Dennis Smith, "Memorials Without a Memory" [NYT, November 26, 2003] wonders "Why no heroes in the Trade Center designs?" After four months of secret meetings (as of 2003), eight designs for the Sept. 11, 2001 tragedy reached the finalist stage. Mr. Smith writes: "The universal elements – air, water, earth and light-are celebrated. Nowhere is there a representation of a human being." "None of the designs conveys the strength and spirit of the American personality, as represented by the kind of men and women who not only know how to suffer but who, when times are tough, will step up and say, "Follow me." Not here is represented in the jury of bureaucrats and administrators any of the police and firemen, the more than 400 brave souls who chose to go into those buildings to help people who desperately needed them. "Where are the images of people who will inspire the generations to come…?" "Think of the Parthenon, Trajan's Column, the Arc de Triomphe, and what those images tell us." Instead we are left with eight designs that look more like trendy hotel lobbies than awe inspiring monuments. (Mr. Smith is a former firefighter).

The public needs to remind the art establishment mafia that beauty need not go the way of the dinosaurs. Anyone who has had the good fortune to see the Hôtel Soubise, les chambres de la Princess, in Paris, knows that beauty on a human scale is eternal.

The psychology of contemporary Art: the human vs. the anti-human

In contrast to egocentric gimmickry and the dogma of minimalism, some of us who have had the good fortune to see it are persuaded by a Renaissance view of art and architecture, one that allows for decorative elements, the human face and form, where mathematics serves beauty and harmony. In Venice we are reminded as the vaporetto carries us down the Grand Canal, the classical masks on the façades of palazzi in the crystalline Mediterranean light of Venice, as if in a timeless dream; or the Temple of Apollo at Side, Turkey, whose carved faces, reflecting the gamut of human emotion, search the horizons of time beyond an eternal sea. Art critics of current trends say they are well acquainted with the "what is art" debate, they have "heard it all before." Be that as it may, one may still ask the question: what do these trends signify psychologically? Painters of our time, like Rothko, Kline, Pollack, DeKooning and Bacon found their own signature style and they repeat this over and over again. Contemporary art expos exhibit such poverty of ideas and unapologetic ugliness that one has to wonder what separates these works from what might otherwise be classified as junk? A photo in an investment magazine shows a smug, apparently nouveau riche couple and the work they purchased that appeared to be a half carcass of a dog with a looping floor duster like tail and the caption: "we get worried when too many people begin to like it."

Contemporary art critics routinely write raving affirmations about some work, yet their words seem a total disconnect from the thing being described. Michael Kimmelman in a New York Time's article, June 2005, is transported by "A Dramatic Turn for Abstract Sculpture," namely, eight massive twisting steel sculptures by Richard Serra at the Guggenheim Museum in Bilbao. Supposedly, this work is "deeply humane." The snake like twistings "press on from one to another, how the spaces inside the sculptures, which are private, psychological and tight, yields to the ones outside, which are public, social and open, and vice-versa." "The sculptures are catalysts for memory." "What sticks in the mind are the general sensations they provoke, that one is claustrophobic, that one, mazelike." "Now enshrined here, it becomes a benchmark for the young century.".... Yet, one sees from the picture in the newspaper oppressive hulks that tower over the little human forms meandering through mazes that lead nowhere. It is scary enough to be a fitting setting for "1984." Mr. Kimmelman does admit that Mr. Serra's previous sculpture, then installed in Foley Square in downtown Manhattan, was carted off to a dump in 1989, because it was regarded as "menacing."

If the art critic really wants to experience mind blowing space, he should once again step inside the Pantheon in Rome, perhaps the most successful and extraordinary space in the world of architecture, an interior that dissolves all barriers, it's peach and rose gold Corinthian columns supporting the Dome of the world, its oculus eye opening to the eternal heavens and the universe beyond. It is no wonder that it has stood for two millennia. No pope, king, barbarian or miserable bureaucrat could bring it down.

Diana Jean Schemo writing in The New York Times highlights "The Jabberwocky of Art Criticism": "younger artists like [so & so] have also begun to investigate the possibilities of painting in a post – Kantian context, without giving up their work's traditional epistemological character in favor of a verbal mode of production" (International Flash Art).

The message of contemporary art trends is threefold and interrelated. Firstly, it reflects society's emptiness, a cold, increasingly dehumanized culture where the individual is systematically fragmented and reduced to machine computer equivalents. Secondly, so-called contemporary expressionism mirrors an increasingly abrasive, cruel and sadistic value system that celebrates power over the individual. A deadened frantic society substitutes shock in lieu of creativity. Thirdly, one sees what happens to beauty when money becomes the measure of everything. As Karl Marx might say: you say it is ugly? But my money will make you say it is beautiful. The unworthy becomes worthy, the lie, truth, ugliness beautiful, the inhuman, wonderful.

Corporate money counts on a big pay back for troubling itself with the arts. Unbridled capitalism hopes that the public, subjected to repetitive brainwashing, will suspend critical judgment and accept advertising masquerading as art. Chanel, the fashion brand, hired a "renowned London architect" to design a 7,500-square foot spacecraft structure to house "15 hot contemporary artists" each of whom was to create a work inspired by Chanel's 2.55 chain handbag, first issued in February 1955 [NYT 7/24/08 "A 7500 square foot ad for Chanel with an artistic mission" by C. Vogel]. The New York Times [5/13/16 "Piercings and eye popping tattoos" by La Perla] in their "Styles" section informs us of "the latest": "Fashion labels, celebrities and street-style stars are helping to usher once transgressive body modifications like allover tattoos and unusual piercings into upscale quarters." Barney's, a department store, takes pride in displaying window-dummies as such. A New York lady had the independence of mind to note it was "beyond disgusting." Of course, the foregoing are symptoms of a degenerate culture.

Contemporary "chick-lit" novels find the fashion world fascinating, swooning over the fashion world – the clothes, the famous brand names, the big shot characterizations.

Ugliness is wonderful say the plutocrat's minions

One might also highlight additional examples. For instance, the much hyped show "Sensation" (read Shock) which originated at the Royal Academy of Arts in Britain and ended up at The Brooklyn Museum of Art a few years ago. [New York Times. "Art, money and control"; 12/6/99, by David Barstow] The exhibits included a huge portrait of the convicted mass murderer of children, Myrna Hindley, made from the tiny handprints of children (were the feelings of the parents of the murdered children taken into consideration by the bureaucrat administrator of the Royal Academy?). Also on display was a glass box with a rotting cow's head complete with flies and live maggots. The journalist, another laughing hyena in The New York Times, sees a similarity between these works and Phidias's Athena in the Parthenon because Phidias was arrested after he carved an image of himself and his sponsor Pericles onto the goddess Athena's shield. He finds the Sensation's offerings shatter "our preconceptions and widen our perspective so that when a great work of art comes along we're ready." Of course, that writer probably figures if this freak show can make money why couldn't he cash in on it too? (after all, he got published in a prestigious paper… maybe a book will follow).

One might also point out as a psychiatrist that sophistry is oftentimes the stock and trade of a good psychopath There are, after all, strong psychopathic trends in our society: for example, the current view that people are just objects to be manipulated.

Other exhibits included a frozen cast of the artists own head made with 8 pts. of his own blood, whole sharks and pigs floating in formaldehyde etc.. The show was the private collection of Charles Saatchi, "the most powerful collector in British contemporary art."

Damian Hirst, the Ripley's-Believe-It-Or -Not self-promoter who created the floating shark in formaldehyde (a symbolic nod to unbridled capitalism), sold his stockpile at auction in September 2008, 223 works all made by Mr. Hirst within the last two years, for $127.2 million. The selections included dead animals submerged in formaldehyde, cigarette butts, and diamond skulls. Very, very good timing for "art" that would otherwise, except for the diamonds, fit the definition of garbage. Of course, other times promoted freak shows, typically at U.S. state fairs, but they weren't the main attraction of museums and their true merit was widely recognized. Following the money, as usual, reveals the motivation for touting shows like this: [NYT "Dealer's Money Nudges Museums"; 11/18/07 by Jori Finkel] "... it's hard to remember another season when so many dealers were writing checks to museums for solo shows devoted to their artists, and being credited publicly for it."

Another heralded art event was The Turner Prize exhibition in Britain's Tate Gallery. [NYT "A symbol of renewal in south London" 5/1/2000, Alan Riding] Candidates for the prize included a pornographic movie, a film of a building under construction and a large suspended ceiling of colored panels. A government minister in the culture department commented: "the attempts at conceptualization are particularly pathetic." The Tate Modern was described by a writer in The New York Times, May 2000, as "a bright star," "a Temple of Modern Art in a space that has kept its industrial soul." The soul of this "bright star" was a gargantuan prison-like void that could have served as headquarters for the secret police. Illustrative photos of the art included a pile of rocks.

A show at the Atlantis Gallery in London began touring in Japan in 1996. Around the world, 8.5 million visitors had seen it. The art objects are real former human beings whose bodies have been flayed and dissected, then subjected to "plastination." They are posed in various activities such as running, fencing, playing chess, smiling etc.. One suspects that the titillation this show generated has more in common with what took place in the Roman Colosseum than any sincere interest in education or gross anatomy.

Jeff Koons "the American superstar artist" made it to Versailles [NYT,9/11/08 by E.

Sciolino

[NYT "An invasion of American art at Versailles" by Elain Sciolino]. His artistry of 17 sculptures in the halls of Versailles include an aluminum red lobster hanging from the ceiling in the room dedicated to Mars, a plexiglass-encased display of vacuum cleaners and floor polishers etc. Mr. Koons also placed a marble portrait of himself in the same room as portraits of Louis XIV and Louis XVI. The lobster, Mr. Koons states "goes back to medieval type times." Each of his works is a dialogue with the setting, he said. "It comes from just thinking what it would be like, I mean, what Louis would kind of have the fantasy to see when he would wake up in the morning…" A "little known right-wing group" expressed dismay about the exhibition (only right-wingers criticize great artists like Mr. Koons). Le monde revealed, however, that six of the works on display came from the private collection of Francois Pinault, France's wealthiest art collector, whose business empire includes GucMet ci etc." The newspaper contended that the showing of the works at the palace would raise their value." Jean-Jacque Aillagon, the chairman of Versailles and a former French cultural minister, once ran a private art foundation of Mr. Pinault.

One might refrain from including the paintings of Jasper Johns with the aforementioned nightmares and junk, but what is it about his paintings that warrants high excitement by the critics and commanded such fantastic prices (actually modest prices by today's standards).[NYT "Met buys its first painting from Jasper Johns by Carol Vogel] In 19/291998, The Metropolitan Museum of Art in New York purchased its first John's painting from the artist himself, a painting whose' estimated value according to the experts was $20 million. Entitled "White Flag," it is a monochrome depiction of the American flag in gradations of white. Individual brush strokes are highlighted. In 1999, another painting by this artist held by The Lincoln Center for the Performing Arts was suggested as a possible candidate for sale in hopes of raising $15 million. A writer in The New York Times describes this "Number 1964" as "monumental," "imposing" and notes that it has graced the lobby of The New York State Theater for 35 years. A picture of the painting shows a motif employing numbers fashioned out of sculpmetal bolted onto squares of a grid. The measure for the grid is derived from the foot length of the choreographer Merce Cunningham. From the photo, the color appears to be a metallic beige. Mr. Johns and some others decried its possible sale.

Then there are the drippings of Jackson Pollock, the puzzling scratches and smears of Cy Twombly etc.. Incredibly these pathetic posturings commanded tens of millions of dollars at recent auctions. A hedge fund billionaire "scooped up" a de Kooning, "Woman," for $137.5 million "adding to the prestige of a personal collection that is fast becoming one of the world's greatest" [NYT 11/16/2006 "Landmark De Kooning crowns auction…" C.Vogel]. Some Russian gentleman bought a portrait by Francis Bacon with its sadistic slashes of paint for some sixty million dollars. Other Bacon paintings sold for $27.4 million, $34.4 million, $86.3 million. Six other works brought over $25 million apiece. In 2012, a Rothko's watery blobs sold for $87 million. Aside from critiquing the value of this art as art, how is it that the culturally illiterate ultra-rich have more billions than they can spend and at a time when the middle class is being obliterated? In 2013, Mr.Cohen, of SAC Capital, bought a Picasso from another billionaire for $155 million shortly after he recently agreed to settle a civil insider trading case with the Federal government for close to $700 million. And then there is the Bacon triptych of "Lucien Freud" that sold at Christie's in November, 2013, for $142 million. It could just as well have been titled "Butcher-shop Trimmings." The New York Times, 3/16/14, devotes a full page to a young artist whose family comes from Columbia. While one is sympathetic to struggling young artists, it is difficult to understand how one could ascribe any value, artistic or otherwise, to a canvas of crazy scrawls and scribbles from someone who apparently can neither paint nor draw. In the write-up, a Manhattan "art adviser" is quoted thusly: "This is a market hungry for the players of the future." The sagging contemporary art market was propped up recently by Christie's sale of a Jean-Marie Basquiat canvas, untitled, for $57.3 million to a Japanese patron who deems it "a masterpiece" [NYT 5/17/17 "Why spend $110 million…? By M.Rich]. Various paints vertically run down the work along with a devil's face. It's too big to fit in an average-sized trashcan. A subsequent nightmare by the same artist sold for $110.5 million to the Japanese admirer. Another collector of his graffiti states: "The dimensions Basquiat is more apparent in the world today – his impact on music, lyrics, dress – even hair – is totally integrated and embedded in our culture." "[He] is now connected to the greats of art history" [NYT 5/18/17].

Andy Warhol's pop art has sold for tens of millions. One might be surprised to learn that in his own home, he surrounded himself with antiques and period furniture.

[NYT 6/20/14 "At Art Basel works with a museum presence" Carol Vogel] The Art Basel Fair featured up and coming trendy young players. One such produces works on ink-jet printers. Protesting the enormous price tag for one of his paintings at auction, he made copies and posted them on Instagram (one brought in nearly $6 million). He then gave one of each to five dealers he works with for display at the Art Basal, accompanied by philosophical musings: they should be shown all at the same height "so each time you walk up to one, you would have a similar physical encounter." Black paintings, all the same size, they all sold for $350,000 apiece.

[NYT 7/3/14 "Tracy Emins 'My Bed' headed to the Tate" author not given] Then again, no need to study drawing, painting, or sculpting at all. A "door buster" at Christie's in London sold for $4.3 million. The art work entitled "My Bed" was the artist's bed presented with crumpled sheets, cigarette butts, dirty underwear, and condoms strewn around. It's a shame that some of the homeless weren't welcomed at Christie's with an invitation to put their shopping bags and lice-ridden linens up for the exclusive sale.

One reads that the super-rich are rushing to sew up purchases of contemporary art destined for the auction block even before it gets to the Christie's and Sotheby's show rooms by guaranteeing a reserve price in advance. With money to burn, they hope to flip faddish works at an enormous profit before the music stops. They will have to pay attention, however, since the typical modern/contemporary work is not exactly painstakingly created nor does it involve the investment of time that the great masters devoted to their creations nor do the in-demand contemporary artists have the training to draw and paint properly (hence they rely on shock and the abnormal). As a result, the contemporary art market is flooded with fakes. There never was a more perfect vindication of Marx's prediction that in a soulless culture dominated exclusively by a plutocratic profit-motive, money becomes the measure and substitute for the intrinsic value of everything.

Most of today's super rich lack schooling in the humanities and therefore equate money with value. They rely on the greater fool theory that they practice so artfully in the manipulated casinos of Wall Street and elsewhere. People who value Truth and Beauty are ignored because the human dimension has no forum in a culture that is obsessed with Power. As for the sycophantic minions of the powerful, not a one has the courage to say that the emperor has no clothes. An unintentional affirmation of the latter comes to mind on seeing a full page spread in The New York Times [1/15/12] of an installation at the Guggenheim in Bilbao: just white light, no more, no less. The columnist raved over it. A more organic class act is a Dutch museum exhibition of four towering giant turds [NYT 6/7/18 "In this exposition you walk through excrement," N. Segal]. We are being educated.

Deborah Solomon writes in The New York Times January 9, 2000 that the Met might be "phobic about contemporary art." Philippe de Montebello, the museum's former director, apparently singled out a sculpture by Kiki Smith (1992) on view at The Whitney Museum of Modern Art: "a crouching female figure excreting a trail of dark matter, as "disgusting and devoid of any craft or aesthetic merit." He also "dismissed the Sensation show as unredeemed rubbish." Ms. Solomon considers Mr. de Montebello "phobic" but misunderstands the meaning of the word. Phobias are imaginary fears whereas Mr. de Montebello has proven himself in good touch with reality. Hawking sideshow freaks to bolster failing museum attendance degrades both art and the public. A better solution would be to reintroduce the humanities in the public school system, but, then again, the humanities don't serve corporate profits.

[NYT "Art/Architecture for the moment (but only for the moment") 8/1/99]. Michael Kimmelman, The New York Times art critic, commenting in 1999 on the Venice Biennale said: "We now have a new species of art geared specifically to the circus environment of the big international survey show and video is a part of it.... to encapsulate the spirit of the moment. Artists have caught on to the nature of these extravaganzas. Their strategy is to accept rather than fight against the short attention span and impatient gaze of people meandering among hundreds of disparate works. What we get are the visual equivalent of sound bites, quickly digestible and user-friendly."

Mr.Kimmelman subsequently reviewed the 2009 Venice Biennale [NYT June 11, 2009 "Small world crammed on Biennale's grand stage]. Germany charitably turned over its pavilion to a British artist. The latter's artistic brain storm was an installation of bare pine kitchen cabinets. In reading Mr. Kimmelman's critique, it occurred to me that the show could have served as a pretty good pictorial clinical survey of schizophrenic illness.

Movies, photos and video are also a must in current opera productions. They project flatly on the set, a disconnected irrelevance of two dimensional banality jumping around that adds nothing and to which no one pays any attention. There were, however, examples of creative lighting that actually comprised an integral part of the production. At the Stockholm Opera's production of "Medea" by Cherubini, rippling waves of light flowed across the whole set, reflecting Medea's lapse into psychosis and "A Winters Tale" at Stratford on Avon in which the characters and action were frozen in blue light that heralded the King's paranoid jealousy of his friend and his wife. Those productions were years ago. The 2016 Chicago production of "Les Troyens" also showed what magical effects videos are capable of.

The establishment in the name of "progress" considers abstraction a sacrosanct art form. Current dogma decries comparing the art of our times with art of other epochs. One suspects that the reason for this lies in the fact that abstraction does not stand up well to the comparison. Of course, my critique is also based on a value judgment because I do hold higher, art from other eras that neither abstracted reality nor excluded man's image, that neither exalted cruelty nor degraded the person. For example, Rembrandt's "The Man with a Magnifying Glass" and "A Woman with a Pink," "these mysterious and poetic portraits" are (states the Met's caption), among the deepest paintings in the world. Words alone cannot suffice to do justice to the profound beauty of these paintings. As Schubert's trios must be heard, so must these paintings be seen. In the former, his eyes express an ineffable existential sadness, yet, they acknowledge us and express compassion for fellow travelers in a world often blind to our vulnerability and hopes. The man and woman portrayed have endured adversity and persevered – that would not have been possible without the human bond, evoked anew between artist and viewer.

Another compelling and enigmatic painting is Rembrandt's "The Polish Rider" at The Frick Museum of Art. Astride his phantom mount, he rides alone through a dusky hermetic landscape, his face, turned toward the viewer, framed in a golden light from an unseen source, his quiver of arrows ready to meet fate come what may. Rembrandt is a painter who reveals eternal truths. Inorganic paint plumbs the mystery of existence, our own life's journey that hopefully will carry us from darkness into light. Can one compare Ruben's (after Titian) "The Bacchanal of the Andrians" and Boucher's "The Birth of Venus" both at The National Museum in Stockholm or Titian's "Bacchus and Ariadne" in The National Gallery, London, with Jasper Johns or Jackson Pollock? Of course one can. And, in architecture, the great buildings that have withstood the test of time, that remember the human spirit above and beyond geometry or computer graphics: Thomas Jefferson's Monticello and the University of Virginia, Palladio's Il Redentore on the Guidecca, Bramante's and Laurana's cloister of Santa Maria della Pace in Rome, La Chambre de la Princess in the Hôtel Soubise, Paris. An inspiration in modern architecture is James Stewart Polshek's spectacular Rose Center for Earth and Space in New York, worthy of admiration and awe. Mr. Polshek seems to be a different breed of architect, one who maintains: "Architecture should serve people instead of egos."

Art forms can be instructive of underlying cultural values. An ethic of power sterilizes art and dehumanizes artistic representation. Looking across the Roman forum from behind Michelangelo's glorious Campadoglio one compares the arch of Titus at the far end, the inner reliefs of which are sculpted with revitalizing energy, quality and beauty, with a much larger and later arch of Septimius Severus whose little stick figures crawl in a confused jumble over its surface. It was during Severus's reign that the Roman Empire took a turn toward a military dictatorship and the Emperor assumed absolute despotic powers, replacing the Roman Senate with military henchmen.

18

The Dehumanized Arts The Bread and Circuses

Panem et Circenses

The people that had once bestowed commands, counsulships, legions and all else.... now longs eagerly for just two things, bread and circus games. [Juvenal:Satires X.lxxviii]

Contemporary entertainment for the masses reflects more than any other measure the intent of materialistic forces to dumb down the public and suppress critical thinking. These corporate forces aim for programmable brainwashed automatons who are addicted to immediate gratification, humanoid-machines who will look no further than their basest appetites, as Aldous Huxley so presciently foresaw in "Brave New World." Consider the technique of the hypnotist in the induction of a hypnotic state. A few simple steps are employed. The more mental steps involved, the less effective the induction. The more analytical a person, the less susceptible they are to hypnotic suggestion and brainwashing. An unthinking public will believe what the authorities want it to believe. Mephistopheles encourages Faust to relinquish thinking and act out in accordance with the Devil's agenda, to enslave him. Canny Mephistopheles knows that the thinking person is not so easily manipulated. Ideal targets for the Prince of Darkness are those isolated souls in dire need.

Depression and the defense against depression, psychopathic acting out and paranoia, are the product of dehumanizing social forces. Individuals who have fulfilling interpersonal relationships, who have freed themselves from their childhood, do not succumb to the ravages of mental illness. If personal growth falters and meaningful human relationships are eclipsed, behavior may become increasingly frantic as the isolated person attempts to forestall a collapse into depression. The brainwashed and exploited are aware unconsciously that their identity has been sacrificed. Bread and circuses can only divert them from the terrible truth of what they have lost.

A few preliminary remarks about depressive and sociopathic (psychopathic) disorders. These mental disorders are an increasingly prevalent by-product of our progressively dehumanized society. We might think of depression as the ultimate dead-end. It underlies both the mania of manic depression (bipolar disorder) as well as the sociopath's aggressive pursuit of power over others. Depression, has its nascent roots in parental, especially maternal, rejection/loss. The pseudo-euphoria of manic-depression, is a defense against acknowledging that loss ("I'm not depressed, I'm wildly happy"). On the flip side of the coin, the sociopath experienced not only rejection but also exploitation. Never having experienced real love from either father or mother, the psychopath, in turn, sees others as objects to be manipulated, just as they themselves were manipulated in childhood. Psychopaths are made, not born.

Mania, psychopathy and paranoia can also describe whole societies. In Iraq in the early seventies and practically everyone I met said they were with the police. The entire country was shrouded in paranoia. As for the controlling plutocrats of unbridled capitalism, they, as a group, clearly meet the diagnostic criteria for "psychopath" ("sociopath"): 1) lack of conscience 2) manipulation and exploitation of others without regard to consequences 3) prioritizing power without regard for human relationships (For example, they are eager to send young people off to their deaths if there is a financial profit to be made or if they, as politicians, can win an election). As I have pointed out, this faction aims at absolute control of society. Dissent is frowned upon as "hate talk." Some say that the way to get ahead in corporate America and in society in general is through sycophancy and shallow cocktail chatter. Lewis Lapham, author of "Lapham's Rules of Influence," explains the technique of cultivating friendship with the powerful: "Practice with inanimate objects. Look at a balloon for 90 minutes with an expression of close attention and profound respect; talk to a box of Cheerios about Martha's Vineyard and Monica Lewinsky."

Unbridled capitalism exploits entertainment to debase the individual
The pattern in recent history: dumbing-down the public

A survey of current programming in the media and entertainment industry is instructive in two regards:1) it shows the extent to which a value system obsessed with power has debased the individual and 2) it reveals the hidden agenda of those who control the money, to eliminate an upward aspiring thinking public through the vehicles of bread and circuses.

Let us review the data:

Current "reality based television" reveals such programs as "World's Scariest Police Shootouts" and "When Stunts Go Bad." Apparently tragic footage of people actually losing their lives is titillating enough to dramatically increase viewer ratings. Marx would have pointed out that money, when it becomes the ultimate measure of everything corrupts and debases a culture.

TV networks foster cruelty and dehumanization in their programming, debasing the impressionable young in order to ensure high ratings and an unobstructed flow of dollars regardless of consequences to the individuals they harm. Money and power becomes THE standard. As reported in New York Times Magazine December 6, 1998, by Tom Vanderbilt, television executives review such footage as a passenger consumed by flames struggling to escape a burning car, or put the finishing touches on "When Animals Attack."

Tuning in on a supposed "documentary," an anguished woman in churning waters pleads for help as a huge shark undulates around her in a feeding frenzy. In a country that considers itself humanitarian, witness a "talk show" in which an adolescent boy is subjected to the disgraceful confession of his mother, a professional prostitute. The cameras zoom in on him as he breaks down sobbing, pleading with her to stop, his life broken. Canada and Norway do not allow such an assault on children but in the United States, big money calls the shots. Humiliation and cruelty are the consequences. Movies dehumanize and degrade children. That's the kind of country we live in.

The producers of the "Jennie Jones Show" thought it would be amusing to shock a young man with the homosexual interests of another male and put it on film for viewer enjoyment: "Did you think Donna had a crush on you?, Jenny Jones asked. "Well, it's Scott." She also played back a tape of the other male's sexual fantasy that involved whipped cream and the talk show guest being tied up in a hammock. The result was a murder and subsequent imprisonment of the talk show guest. Did anyone stop to think what the emotional impact of such a humiliating experience would be on a troubled individual? Why weren't the producers who masterminded this tragedy indicted? Meanwhile, the show, of course, was still being aired because there were more profits to rake in, $50-$60,000,000 a year to be exact. Another case in point is "Scare Tactics" on the sci-fi Channel where two employees find body parts in plastic bags in the freezer. The funny high point arrives when someone announces "you're on Scare Tactics, afraid you're going to vomit?"

Young people are juicy exploitable fodder for sadomasochistic scenarios, a discovery that has made enormous profits for big money's MTV network. Their show "Kidnapped" depicts four friends competing in each episode. One plays the hostage while the other three try to guess how the former answered such questions about the latter as who would be most likely to push an old lady in front of a bus to save himself? Caryn James, writing for The New York Times, February 4, 2002, highlights several shows of this genre such as family oriented NBC's "Fear Factor": contestants bobbing for chicken feet under a pile of live worms etc.. Her ridiculous psycho-blabber claims these "torture games" tap into and defuse an undercurrent of anger in the country "related to a wartime society." For her, these programs, because they are so "silly," "disarm our genuine fears." Her posturing sophistry aside, understanding this kind of entertainment is far simpler: greed for money. Were there no laws against outright murder you can be sure they would waste no time rebuilding the Colosseum, if they have not already.

[NYT 1/3/09 – Television Review: "Humiliation For Sale, At New Low Prices" Ginia Bellafante

An FTC study deplored the pervasive and aggressive marketing of violent entertainment to children, the New York Times September 12, 2000: "The vast majority of the best-selling restricted movies, music and video games were deliberately marketed to children as young as 12." A movie studio's internal memorandum regarding its R-rated movies said its "goal was to find the elusive teen target audience and make sure everyone between the ages of 12 and 18 was exposed to the film." Another memorandum about an R-rated movie described how it would be distributed in Kansas City to organizations like the campfire boys and girls (R-rated films require an adult to accompany children younger than 17).

Bob Herbert writing in The New York Times March 1, 1996 highlights "Daytime TV's Child Porn" and rancid topics such as "My Daughter is a Tramp," "Teen Sex Better in the House Than in the Back of the Car," "Mom, I am a Teen Prostitute," all hosted by Sally Jessy Raphael; "Deadly Erotic Teen Games" and "Poor Black Teen Buries Her Baby Alive" (Jerry Springer) etc. plus "Teen Girls Who Have One Night Affairs." Young girls are often dressed provocatively in miniskirts with lots of makeup. Mr. Herbert continues: "like pornographers and pimps the talk show hosts and their producers found a gold mine in the sexuality of troubled children." 12-year-olds are humiliated while subjected to boos and curses and youngsters "left weeping and bewildered." Ms. Raphael hosted a 12-year-old who slept with 25 guys all the while the host "wore a cloak of sanctimony throughout." "With all due respect, "Ms. Raphael sniffed, I don't think they need understanding. They need to be told it isn't right."

Other examples of American culture's obsession with power in a manner reminiscent of Ancient Rome at its point of decline is evident in the changing standards for male and female physical beauty. The frenzied culture of anabolic steroids and testosterone taken to induce massively inflated musculature in athletes and young men (and now geezers too) has been spurred on by a culture that makes power its number one priority, a culture where grotesque muscular hypertrophy accompanied by vapid smiles of supposed superiority is the idealized standard for the average younger man. Ridiculous magazines like "Men's Health" preach to the gullible of six-pack abs and inflated pectorals, articles which promise brain dead males a good lay with an air head of the opposite sex. Nowhere is there mention of a relationship between a man and a woman built on trust and love, only posing and posturing. Admiring physical beauty is one of life's pleasures but cartoon-like caricatures of the masculine ideal reflect the celebration of power for power's sake. More recently, the masculinization of women is being promoted as psychologically liberating. A 2012 editorial in the ever modernizing New York Times, thinks women are being discriminated against in combat and deserve the opportunity to fight on the front lines along-side the men. Women are made to feel ashamed of themselves if they find raising children fulfilling.

Corporate advertising depicts macho-women frantically body-build on television. Some women have been sold a bill of goods that men have caused all their problems (divide and rule is the plutocratic template) and determinedly march down the sidewalk in the currently fashionable high black leather boots. As for the latter, some men already passed through that phase as members of S.S. Division Adolf Hitler. Of course, women and men should have equal opportunities but is breaking the "glass ceiling" the ultimate goal of every strong woman? Those at the helm of giant corporations are all too often despots regardless of their sex.

Strong women and men think for themselves regardless of politically inspired propaganda. Amy Wolf (NYT, 4/8/2013) reports on a Vanderbilt study that finds that female graduates of elite colleges (with superior earning potential) are working much fewer hours than their counterparts from less selective colleges. Joni Hersch, a professor at Vanderbilt states that the presence of children strongly influences how much a women works.

Louise Story, a journalist for the New York Times writes "Many Women at Elite Colleges Set Career Path to Motherhood"; 9/20/2005. "What seems to be changing is that while many women in college two or three decades ago expected to have full-time careers, their daughters, while still in college, say they have already decided to suspend or end their careers when they have children."

"At the height of the women's movement and shortly thereafter, women were much more firm in their expectation that they could somehow combine full-time work with child rearing," said Cynthia E. Russett, a professor of American history who has taught at Yale since 1967. "The women today are, in effect, turning realistic."

Dr. Russett is among more than a dozen faculty members and administrators at the most exclusive institutions who have been on campus for decades and who said in interviews that they had noticed the changing attitude.

Shannon Flynn, an 18-year-old from Guilford, Conn., who is a freshman at Harvard, says many of her girlfriends do not want to work full time. She plans to work part time after having children, though she is torn because she has worked so hard in school. "Men really aren't put in that position," she said.

Uzezi Abugo, a freshman at the University of Pennsylvania who hopes to become a lawyer, says she, too, wants to be home with her children at least until they are in school. "I've seen the difference between kids who did have their mother stay at home and kids who didn't, and it's kind of like an obvious difference when you look at it..."

The journalist states that the shift emerges repeatedly in interviews with Ivy League students, including 138 freshman and senior females at Yale who replied to e-mail questions sent to members of two residential colleges over the last school year. The interviews found that 85 of the students, or roughly 60 percent, said that when they had children, they planned to cut back on work or stop working entirely. About half of those women said they planned to work part time, and about half wanted to stop work for at least a few years. The fact that only 20% of the work force in Silicon Valley are women is not necessarily proof of discrimination.

Michael Oriard writing in The New York Times December 23, 2001, "King Football" former player for the Kansas City Chiefs and presently Professor of English at Oregon

State University writes about how the sport of big-time college has changed. The 225 lb. weight he reached in his senior year of college at Notre Dame and 242 lbs. in the NFL compares with the 300 lb. frame bred for today's college teams. During his day, the purpose of college was still to achieve an education in preparation for a viable career perhaps in Engineering or English. Afternoon classes were not blocked out for fear of conflicting with football. Today, Division I sports require full-time commitment and recruited football players attend coaches summer camp from the ninth grade on and work in year-round training. The vast majority of these young men are never picked by the NFL and have no career development to fall back on. His six-foot 6 in. basketball playing son was passed over by Division I programs because he was not 6-foot 10 in.. Universities and big money in media are exploiting these young people. The pervading message is clear: Force counts. Sportsmanship is for losers. I am reminded of the Roman mosaics of gladiators on the floor of the rotunda of the Vatican Museum, heavily muscled brutes in a savage blood sport of life and death.

Again, the master puppeteer behind this corruption of college sports is the plutocracy. Big money is high-jacking the citadels of higher learning and the pursuit of excellence in education is falling by the wayside: ["College Football's Biggest Player? ESPN – Spending and Reaping Billions, Network Rules Schedule"; NYT 8/25/13 Andrew Miller et al.].The journalists write that 2012's national champions, the Alabama Crimson Tide, who would battle Virginia Tech in the Chick-fil-A Kickoff Classic, Oklahoma State that would play Mississippi State in the Texas Kickoff Classic and Louisiana State and Texas Christian that were to face off in the Cowboy Classic were games not just to be televised by ESPN but creations of ESPN, "…the chief impresario of college football." The network infused the sport with $10 billion in the prior 5 years to pay for television rights. "ESPN has become both puppet-master and kingmaker, arranging games, setting schedules and bestowing the gift of nationwide exposure on its chosen universities, players and coaches." Professionalized sport's empires are being created in the midst of academic institutions, state the journalist investigators. The millions of dollars that flow to athletic departments go to athletics not academics. Lavish facilities are financed by rich donors and corporate sponsors.

Tamar Lewin, writing for The New York Times in 2014: "Colleges Increasing Spending on Sports Faster Than on Academics, Report Finds," highlights the findings of the American Association of University Professors regarding the rapid increase of spending on sports while spending on classroom learning stayed flat. The organization states: "Increasingly, institutions of higher education have lost their focus on the academic activities at the core of their mission." Division I athletics was not the only focus. From 2004 to 2011, instruction spending at division II and III schools declined while athletic spending per athlete increased 35 %. The ranks of administrators and their salaries are growing far more rapidly than that of tenured professors. Coaches at big-gun colleges are commanding multi-million dollar salaries.

Finland, Poland, and South Korea, by contrast, have catapulted to top world academic rankings by virtue of a rigorous curriculum where academics is the priority. Nowhere in Europe would anyone imagine that the goal of a university was football.

Academics teaches critical thinking. Athletics can degenerate into diversionary entertainment for the masses, not an insignificant agenda for the plutocracy.

Children's toys are reflecting these trends. Compare G.I. Joe figures from 1964, 1982, 1992 and the mid-nineties. The earlier models are on a human scale but become progressively distorted. In the mid-to late nineties the figures show outrageous muscularity with the grimaces of rage sported by professional wrestling clowns. Hasbro made a nice profit off of children. As reported by Jim Rutenberg, The New York Times January 28, 2001, violence also makes its way to these shores in cartoons imported from Japan and aired by the Cartoon Network on cable: examples include "pug nosed thug kicked in an elderly storekeeper's face. Then he punches a young heroine… and cracks herin the small of the back with a heavy barstool. Her limp frame collapses to the ground as he stands over her with his gun drawn and pointed at her head." "Two young boys are in a fistfight on a moving boxcar. A friend tries to intervene. But an older and very respected boy advises: let the fight continue. Sometimes, he says, friends need to bare fists." (Nazi propaganda posters fostered just this kind of ideal). "Network executives who show the new style cartoons say no extra scrutiny is necessary."

Bob Herbert's column, The New York Times, December 28, 2002,"The Gift of Mayhem", describes "Forward Command Post" being marketed by Toys "R" Us and JC Penney and recommended for children five and up which features a bombed out dollhouse with smashed furniture and bullet holes in the walls. Accessories include a machine gun, magazine belt and explosives. Also being sold is a videogame rated appropriate for six year-olds is "Burnout 2: Point of Impact" featuring car crashes. An ad shows a man's head smashing through a windshield: "the last thing to go through your mind," the ad says, "will be your [behind]." The biggest selling videogame in recent years has been a PlayStation 2 game called Grand Theft Auto 3. This is an interactive game in which you shoot whom you want, beat women to death with a baseball bat, have sex with prostitutes and then kill them. At $50 each, millions of copies are sold annually to teens. Rockstar Games, maker of the Grand Theft series also makes State of Emergency which promotes rioting, looting and extreme sadism. The player can kill and maim at will. Mr. Herbert concludes: "the building blocks of violent behavior are dehumanization and desensitization. The lessons begin at a very early age." The "Art Section" of The New York Times regularly critiques updated versions of "Grand Theft Auto." The journalist-writer describes the game in rapturous language reminiscent of Mussolini's son's poetic rendering of the exploding bombs he dropped over Ethiopia ...like unfolding Lotus blossoms. The games also make a lot of money. [NYT, 9/19/13 "Grand Theft Auto v muscles its way to sales record" Nick Wingfield] Grand Theft Auto V, the latest version, "generated more than $800 million in sales Tuesday on its first day on store shelves."

Dehumanization is mirrored as well in wildly sadistic hazing rituals not only on a college-level but also in high school. Andrew Jacobs's reporting in The New York Times, March 5, 2000, quotes Gary Powell, a hazing expert in Cincinnati, who writes a legal newsletter for schools and fraternities: "hazing has changed from the goofy high jinx of the fifties and sixties to something that is remarkably brutal and vicious": beatings, forcing bloody fistfights, sexual penetration, and humiliation and cruelty reminiscent of Nazi Jugend boot camps.

Breaking down individual identity assures unquestioning subjugation to the group and ultimately to those who hold the reins of power. The individual, both male and female, is being primed for their role in the Empire as an obedient slave.

Boxing has given way to "Ultimate Fighting," a brutally sadistic "sport" that has a ubiquitous presence nowadays on television and a mass following of fans excited by the prospect of seeing someone beaten to a bloody pulp, no holds barred. There is a local tavern. In the past, they showed slides of great master paintings to the accompaniment of classical music and good hamburgers. All had been updated, however. Gone were the paintings and music. In their place were a series of flat screen T.V.s all showing the blood-sport. It was packed with young people from a nearby university. The young men were roaring with approval as one fighter was being kicked into submission. Times have changed. The shadow of the Roman Colosseum is lengthening over America.

Television and movies imitate the overall relentless obsession with power. Human relationships that engender mutual caring are in plutocracy's cross-hairs and systematically expunged from American cinema, with few exceptions. These days, Hollywood stars, like roman candles, have little staying power. The great screen personalities of a bygone era are history. Dispensing with flesh and blood human beings obviates the need for an intelligible story. Pseudo human characters are fabricated that have no personal history and no past. They share accolades with computer generated virtual humans who let nothing stand in their way and view with unbridled contempt the weak. It's the race to be #1. Power dictates, spawning power's offspring: violence and mindless frantic activity. Innovative sadism garners rave four-star movie reviews. Typical programming pits the criminal element against intrepidly cute policewomen-starlets who know just how to show serial killers whose boss. The latter, however, have their day before their comeuppance as fans are treated to graphic anatomical dismemberment that makes the drama in the surgical suite seem like an old-fashioned Disney movie (not current Disney movies). One television series, "Breaking Bad," served up nauseating sadism and was rewarded with an Emmy. Its finale goodbye:

“Even bad things have to end.” The Plutocracy achieves dehumanizing mind control by eliminating values based on human relationships that could offer an alternative to Big Brother’s agenda.

[NYT 5/3/14 “Rising Unease Over Rape’s Recurring Role” Dave Itzkoff]; Not to be trumped in the citadels of sadism, the HBO series “Game of Thrones” enjoys its fourth season of explosive growth, averaging 14 million viewers nightly and HBO’s most watched programming. It takes place in medieval times and is based on a book series that has over 31 million copies in print. According to the front page of The Times, the novels depict such scenes as a warrior king who claims his child bride on their wedding night and the gang rape of a young women “by half a hundred shouting men behind a tanner’s shop.” In the space of three minutes, two different women are raped, an infanticide, an old man being tortured by a gang with knives, and a young man being beaten. Michael Lombardo, the president for programming at HBO, said: “We fully support the vision and artistry of [the creative team Dan and David’s exceptional work and we feel that this work speaks for itself.” It seems clear that this content reflects not so much medieval times as it does the times we live in.

Desperate to avert being dismissed as behind the curve, The New York Times enlists journalist, G. Bellafante, to thoughtfully review a sequel on “The Real Housewives of Orange County.” A 19 year old comes home with a few friends to find his mother in a bikini entertaining her 40ish friends in a hot tub drinking wine. The fashionable liberal, Ms. Bellafante, finds this experience far from discomfiting: “But what it conveys instead is a not entirely unwelcome consequence of feminist ambitions: the breakdown of obstructive Freudian barriers between mothers and sons, a triumph over the once-prevailing notion that a women in midlife must downgrade her sexual valuation.” (who cares about the feelings of the son anyway? Is a book in the offing?).

A night at the theater offers us the opportunity to experience the plays of Thomas Bradshaw, who according to The New York Times “is fast becoming the American theater’s most distinctively provocative playwright.” His play “Intimacy” is captioned in the article:[NYT 1/29/14 “Sure, Son I’ll Help you Make A Skin Flick With Neighbors.” By Ben Brantley]. “Eventually, even James, Mathew’s dad, is able to banish his religious scruples to join in.” The Times reporter notes that disgusted theater-goers routinely walk out of Mr. Bradshaw’s plays. He philosophically parallels the mainstream reviewer’s reactions to the same kind of outrage “that greeted Ibsen’s ghosts more than a century ago.” [The nauseated public is not sufficiently open to deep modern insights]. Sex, we are informed, “in all its varieties, becomes as routine as moving the bowels. And yes, that, too, is a highly visible part of life here.”

The depreciation if not trashing of human relationships as mandated by a controlling, autocratic, unbridled capitalist state has ominous consequences for community, family and individual. The Golden Rule is a thorn in the side of a system that only recognizes good in corporate profits, a system that aims for an underclass of clueless automatons. Expunging the human bond between us destroys the only real security we have in an otherwise hostile universe. Mindless activity, frantic empty competitiveness and the diversions of bread and circuses becomes psychologic heroin. It creates the false euphoria that masks the depression of an increasingly vacant, fragmented society. A simplistic dehumanized category is instituted for everyone, men, women, children, young and old. Big Brother seduces the unthinking and punishes independence.

Hollywood movies command ever bigger budgets where every second exhilarates in perfected mayhem and digitally generated catastrophes on a scale of exploding supernovas that render us punch-drunk. But It isn't the "walking dead," brain eating viruses, vampires, zombies, or oncoming asteroids that threaten the American public, it is the totalitarian plutocratic goal to render obsolete the critically thinking mind, the bedrock of Western civilization.

19

Don't Think – Obey! "1984" Refined for the 21st Century

The self-appointed gurus of technology, fluent in mumbo-jumbo, try to sound cool and prescient when they explain how technology changes everything now that we are all connected and ten year olds shall lead the way to a bright new future. Virtual relationships are to replace real relationships and thousands of virtual friends will replace the need for that old-fashioned concept of a best friend. But even extended chatting online is a threat to the technology billionaires: enter censorship and mind control. The young, abandoned by their parents, desperately need to feel connected and accepted.

Harry Hurt III reviews "Grown Up Digital: How the Net Generation Is Changing Your World," by Don Tapscott [NYT 12/21/08]: "But what really makes Net Geners different, Mr.Tapscott says, is their lifelong experience in using the internet." Their parents were a television generation (22.4 hours a week) but Net Geners watch T.V. "only" 17.4 hours a week on average, but spend up to 33 hours on the internet, "a collaborative medium…all over the world." Facebook and Myspace helped elect Mr. Obama while Hillary Clinton lost because she relied on old fashioned media. (I suspect, however, that everybody tired of the Clintons and wanted "change you can believe in"). Mr. Tapscott identifies eight norms of the Net Generation including: "they prize freedom"; "they scrutinize everything"; "they insist on integrity in institutions and corporations"; "they want to have fun even at school or work"; "they believe that speed in technology and all else is normal"; "constant innovation." He contends that brain-imaging studies show "that Internet use by Net Geners has fundamentally changed – and improved – the way their brains are wired.": I.Q. scores have been rising three points a decade since World War II across all boundaries (if indeed the statistic is true, it's hard to imagine how the Internet could be responsible since it only recently became operative) Video game players "notice more" and have highly developed spatial skills, "useful for architects, engineers and surgeons." "They care strongly about justice." "The Net Geners are smarter, quicker and more tolerant of diversity than their predecessors."

Mr. Tapscott makes a lot of claims that he touts as facts. What used to be "I saw it on television so it must be true," is now echoed by "I went online so it must be true." His statement that the Internet has improved brain wiring is junk-science. What does "improved" mean? If young people can no longer read or write, what does that do to their "wiring"? Wiring must be likewise affected, but adversely so. That Net Geners are "smarter" isn't born out by test results. If they can't read or write, how can they become surgeons? And if their math skills are among the poorest among industrialized nations, how can they graduate as engineers? If Net Geners are so socially conscious, why are unbridled capitalism's plutocrats getting away with murder? Where are the protests and marches that take place in Europe or Asia? (hopefully there were some beginning stirrings with the "Occupy Wall Street" movement). Many American teenagers are comatose addicted zombies glued to their video games, smart phones, and a virtual reality, neglected by their wonderful parents and distracted from the vital events that are destroying the American middle class. Obsessive wheel spinning should not be confused with creativity (if indeed there is much creativity taking place beyond consumption-driven advertising for the latest technology gizmos). I also notice that Mr. Tapscott's work is being financed as part of a $ 4 million grant from "large corporations." Quelle surprise.

Sara Konrath, a researcher at the University of Michigan Institute for social research, presented a study at the annual meeting of the Association for Psychological Science that analyzed the data on empathy among 14,000 college students over the past 30 years. "We found the biggest drop in empathy after the year 2000. "College kids today are about 40 % lower in empathy than their counterparts 20 or 30 ago, as measured by standard tests of this personality trait." In this meta-analysis, 72 different studies of American college students between 1979 and 2009 were combined.

Jennifer Schuessler [NYT 6/21/09; "Get a Life, Holden"] talks about the contemporary teenager's view of the Holden Caulfield character in J.D Salinger's "The Catcher In The Rye." "Holden may be losing his grip on the kids," she states. He strikes many as "weird," "whiney" and "immature." She quotes a high school teacher: "Holden's passivity is especially galling and perplexing to many present-day students....In general they do not have much sympathy for alienated anti-heroes; they are more focused on distinguishing themselves in society as it is presently than in trying to change it." Ms. Schuessler continues: "These days teenagers are more concerned with getting into Harvard....[and] with their compulsive text messaging and hyperactive pop culture metabolism, are more enchanted by wide-eyed, quidditch-playing Harry Potter of Hogwarts..." "Today's pop culture heroes, it seems, are the nerds who conquer the world – like Harry – not the beautiful losers who reject it." She thinks Holden would have felt more at home in today's multibillion-dollar cultural-entertainment complex catering to the taste of teenage boys. Stephane Savage, allied with "Gossip Girl" television series, thinks that in Holden's world you could go to the carousal in Central Park or have a prostitute come up to your room but there's "really not that sense of teen culture that there is now."

One suspects, however, that few of today's teenagers will be getting into Harvard or conquering the world. The real world for many young people has in great measure been usurped by a phony virtual matrix-world, the creation of corporate forces bent on mind control to homogenize individuality, suppress dissent and control money. Technology is an extraordinarily useful tool to manipulate people. Our billionaire bosses intuitively know (it doesn't have to take place in a smoke filled room) that human relationships are a fundamental antidote to the addiction of bread and circuses and the false lure of the Sirens that preach power. The current teen culture is a puppet culture and there are many a lonely Holden Caulfield, many more than before, who have no forum for expression.

The frantic texting of today's teens masks anxiety and depression. It is a frantic attempt to make contact with someone real in an increasingly dehumanized world where teenagers and even children are put on pills because they have no one to talk to. "Texting May Be Taking a Toll on Teenagers" reports The New York Times by Katie Hafner [5/26/2009].

Holden's favorite word "phony" isn't heard much these days because the brain washing is nearing completion. Pathetically, false prophets are now showcased who hope to usher in "the post-human" (and, of course, they will be its new priests and maybe even publish a best seller). Be not mistaken, while youth is tragically impressionable, it is not bereft of its God-given creative imaginative energy. For now, the young are trapped in a crass power oriented culture that has suppressed and narcotized their individuality, but they will always be a potent threat to the establishment when and if they revolt. As for Harry Potter, he resorts to magic because he is impotent.

Mark Bauerline's book "The Dumbest Generation," critiqued by David Robinson [NYT, 5/13/08], writes that among young people, TV viewing is constant, the time spent on the Internet notwithstanding. Moreover, the Internet is not making "kids" smarter. The National Assessment of Educational Progress concludes that 46% of 12th-graders are below the basic level of proficiency in science. Between 1992 and 2005, the NAEP reported that reading skills "dropped dramatically" and "only 24% of 12th-graders are 'capable of composing organized, coherent prose in clear language with correct spelling and grammar.'" The "blind celebration of youth" is a source of frustration for Mr. Bauerline. Of course, all movements bent on totalitarian control aim to control the minds of the young. They are more easily brainwashed and can be exploited to spearhead favorable changes, favorable to the billionaire puppet-masters who pull the marionette strings.

Some of our elders have actually learned something from their life experiences. They could get in the way of current political agendas. All the more reason for the plutocracy to suppress their voice and create youth-hype. During the Third Reich, you would have had to pay careful deference to the Hitler Jugend when they boarded the streetcar. The Red Guard is a more recent and perhaps even worse example of how the young can be manipulated. As for the contention that the young are addicted to their own world of peers, what does one expect when the family disintegrates, adults have abandoned their young and the pages of once mighty newspapers are devoted to "Style" and the latest botox treatment.

Kevin Kelly writing in The New York Times Magazine [11/23/08] enlightens us as follows: "The past is a rush of data streams cut and rearranged into a new mashup, while truth is something you assemble yourself on your own screen as you jump from link to link. We are now in the middle of a second Gutenberg shift – from book fluency to screen fluency, from literacy to visuality."

Mr. Kelly's analysis of these issues is short-sighted (the pun is intentional). To be sure, not all books are profound or even worth reading but books have stood the test of time and some are, as they say, "classics." Language also holds a worthwhile place in the lives of most people. The capacity for language elevates homo-sapiens over the apes. It is doubtful that "the truth" will be grasped by jumping around from link to link or that it is just something that you assemble yourself on a video screen. Books and information on a screen can be altered by the delete button and posted false information can masquerade as truth. A book on the shelf, written by someone a hundred or two thousand years ago, is still in existence because it has withstood the cleansing purge of time.

Rearranging the past to suit yourself may not be the independent, objective endeavor you think it is. The past is carved in stone, not ephemeral electrons. It may be hidden but skimming along the surface of seeming reality will not call it forth. We cannot shed light on the past, alone, in a vacuum. Replacing myriad-minded Shakespearean English with illiterate computer-talk impoverishes the human spirit and creates an underclass of mindless marionettes. It is through the fullness of language that real humans, face to face, enrich one another, learn and grow. Virtual internet friends are electronic figments that give the illusion of sharing without incurring the uncertainty of true intimacy. Needless to say, the rewards of closeness with another are never realized. From the beginning of time, a true teacher has been a real person, someone a student could look up to as a role model and a guide. A computer generated electronic image is not in any sense a teacher. Were that not the case there would be no need for families or parenting. Mr. Kelly's vistas are two dimensional. What he thinks he "sees" is, to borrow Mr. Kimmelman's wording, "the visual equivalent of sound bites," evanescent, momentary, desultory. The visuality of experiencing a Rembrandt painting, in person, is not the visuality of an electronic screen. What Mr. Kelly is extolling is virtuality not visuality. Illiteracy is illiteracy. Reality is in four dimensions, the fourth of which is time. Memories render us real.

Video-games and electronic entertainment:

The stairway to higher intelligence?

David Deming, at the University of Oklahoma, writes "What I Learned From a Brainiac"

[WSJ, Jan. 2012]. In the 1960's, he notes, children were expected to rise up and meet standards set by adults. He and his brother assembled their own computers from construction kits. They also read books to build their vocabulary, science fiction, "Doctor Doolittle" etc. (a series I fondly remember). Chess enhanced analytical skills. Television back then tended to be instructional, not vulgar or degrading. Both brothers, encouraged at home, went on to become scientists, the writer, a geophysicist and his brother, one of the world's leading astrophysicists. Deming reserves a harsh indictment for the computer entertainment industry: "Video-games have no educational value whatsoever. They are degrading, addictive and stultifying. The promise of the high technology developed by previous generations has largely been squandered." He states the obvious when he points out that books, by contrast, increase the command of language and thought. Education begins at home and teachers can do little with children "who have been indulged and entertained with an array of electronic devices." [it is no wonder that all of them are on Ritalin]. Computer access should be discretely supervised by parents. "If you set high standards, your children will rise to them."

[WSJ 1/17-18/2015; "Skills Gap Found in College Students" Douglass Belkin] Four in 10 U.S. college students graduate without the complex reasoning skills to manage whitecollar work, according to the results of a test of nearly 32,000 students administered by the Council for Aid to Education. 40% of the graduates were unable to distinguish the quality of evidence in building an argument or express the appropriate level of conviction in their conclusions. [NYT 11/10/2013 "Warned of a data deluge" by William Yardley] Over 25 years, Clifford Nass, a Stanford professor, pioneered research into how humans interact with technology until his untimely death at 55. Dr. Nass majored in math at Princeton and later became a professor of communication at Stanford. At Intel, he helped develop the 286 processing chip. His research found that "the increasingly screen saturated, multitasking modern world was not nurturing the ability to concentrate, analyze or feel empathy." A 2009 study revealed that "multitaskers are terrible at every aspect of multitasking. They're terrible at ignoring irrelevant information, they are terrible at keeping information in their head nicely and neatly organized; and they're terrible at switching from one task to another (notwithstanding the fact that they think they are great at it). He showed that heavy multitasking shortened attention span and the ability to concentrate. He argued that increasing use of media and social media eroded social and emotional development.

Comment: Regarding computers, television and new media, Dr.Nass showed that far from just being tools, "...these things talk, they have relationships with you, and they make you feel good or bad." That makes them an ideal vehicle for brainwashing.

Dr. Vincent Mathews of Indiana University, speaking at the 2012 annual meeting of the Radiological Society of North America, presented evidence from functional magnetic resonance imaging that showed that one week of violent video game play produced significant changes in brain function in a study of men aged 18-28 compared to controls [Clinical Psychiatry News January 2012]. Active role playing in violent video games may make them more harmful than violent television or movies. Behavioral studies show detrimental effects including desensitization to violence and the encoding of aggressive behavior as appropriate. Recent research with adolescents by Dr. Mathews revealed decreased activity in the area of the brain involved in inhibition after 30 minutes of game time. In the current research, the game group showed decreased activation of the dorsolateral prefrontal cortex (associated with inhibition) and the anterior cingulate cortex (involved in attention).

Holden Caulfield vs. "What should I think?" "Tell me what I want."

"The Catcher In the Rye" was written in an era where the critically thinking individual could still find a forum for self-expression in American society. That was a time when a dynamic America respected an individual's God-given right to feel lonely and hold accountable the phony, posturing movers and shakers that strove to expunge all traces of individuality from our culture and eliminate potentially dangerous criticism in the process. Back then, palpable emotions could touch a stranger and miraculously find a friend. Friendships were sacred bonds between two individuals, an inexplicable mystery born out of a hostile universe.

America's energy is the hermetic creation of its unique individuals but, today, an individual like Holden Caulfield would be dismissed as weird and hopelessly dated. Too bad he didn't have the advantage of verifying what he should think and like with Facebook, the giant internet company that connects you instantaneously with everyone else on the planet, "your friends," so that in "sharing" everything you do and think, you will be able to feel the security of knowing that you are the exact cookie-cutter replica of everyone else. What a breakthrough for the plutocracy and the government!! The young will come to enjoy being programmed and brainwashed and the powerful will wield unprecedented control over everything and everyone. No need for the puppet-masters to worry about messy revolutions because everyone who counts will be happily compliant, like Pavlovian dogs. Besides, there is no need to hide your thoughts from the established power brokers or the State. They just want to help you share. It's all for you!

Evgeny Morozov writes [NYT, 2/5/12, "The Death of the Cyberflâneur"]: "Through clever partnerships with companies like Spotify and Netflix, Facebook will create powerful (but latent) incentives that would make users eagerly embrace the tyranny of the "social," to the point of pursuing any of those activities on their own would be impossible." And, of course, everything that we do and think will be easily sold to advertisers.

Rush! Live in the instant, you may miss something!

Instagram (recently bought by Facebook) realizes INSTANT photo sharing with friends and is entirely mobile (computers are so yesterday!). Foursquare lets users share their instant location with everybody and has 15 million members. Everyme analyzes a user's contacts and generates miniature social networks around people it thinks belong together ("Me" is so yesterday!).

[NYT 3/11/14] In "Wired Well," "The Monitored Man," Albert Sun. The Times reports on increasingly popular activity trackers that wire up our privacy in addition to our social life. Sleeping, eating, meditation, exercise, in fact our every movement, whether asleep or awake, as well as such physiologic responses as heart rate, perspiration etc. are recorded. These devices could help the police state in their efforts to establish careful profiles on every citizen. Not only can we be assured of strict rules for healthy living but potential enemies of the state could be monitored in advance should they eventually show their true colors by deviating from the norm.

[NYT 8/11/13] Stories "I Flirt and Tweet. Follow Me at #Socialbot." by Ian Urbina. Robotic programs are proving cleverly successful at passing themselves off as human. Chatbots greet users when they enter online chat rooms. Spambots hawk "miracle stocks," and Nigerian bank accounts while Bimbots deploy photos of seductive women to sell get-rich-work-from home job ploys. Socialbots keep up-to-date databases as well as their own Facebook sites so that they can piece together a real person image as they lure in real people and amass "friends." The goal is to influence elections, the stock market, lure the lonely to pornography sites and ensnare susceptible non-robots for mercenary purposes. Bots can be designed to self-activate when key words are detected whereupon an adversary is inundated with a barrage of fabricated propaganda. University computer specialists in Brazil revealed that "Carina Santos, a much followed journalist on Twitter, was actually not a real person, but a bot…." Her ratings ranked Ms. Santos as having more online influence than Oprah Winfrey." Politicians use bots to undermine the opposition both in this country and abroad. The article states that of the 500 million Twitter accounts, some estimate that only 35% of the average user's followers are real people. Christian Rudder, co-founder of OkCupid, redesigned the dating site and noticed a drop not only in the bots but a 15% drop in use of the site by real people. He attributes the decline to the decrease in falsely intimate bots that affected the site: "Love was in the air," Mr.Rudder said. "Robot love."

The puppeteers who control our society goad the citizenry into increasingly frantic activity to divert the public's attention from the real issues, such as where all the money is going. Inducing such an environment of constant change creates insecurity and is a fundamental principle of brainwashing. Without moorings or the familiar signposts of one's identity, the ensuing identity-vacuum is exploited by those who wield the power in our society, the billionaires who promote globalization. The underpinnings of a humanistic culture are broken down and fragmented so that the only point of reference is crowd-think, dictated by the corporations. Everything must be new. Appreciating the classics is reactionary. Entertainment, increasingly bizarre and crass, is excused as creative and innovative, extreme sports become ever more extreme with scant attention paid to its forgotten quadriplegics and the citadels of art contort themselves to attract a public whose schooling aborted the humanities that teach critical discernment.

Judith H. Dobrzynski, [NYT 8/11/13, "High Culture Goes Hands-On"] writes about the museum culture that promotes public participation to offset falling attendance such as the New Museum of Contemporary Art that gives visitors an opportunity to slide down a corkscrew from the fourth floor to the second and was described by the New York Times as "an art world amusement park" that drew lines around the block in 2011. Marion Abramovic's "The Artist Is Present" in 2010 had New Yorkers queuing up for hours to sit opposite the artist who simply stared back. The Metropolitan Museum installed a summer roof-top bamboo walk (2010) and a walk through a mirrored modular habitat, "Cloud City" in 2012. Other additions in some museums include interactive games in painting galleries, asking visitors to vote for which paintings should be sold, which altered paintings should be restored as well as parties and sleepovers. Ms. Dobrzynski quotes Glenn D. Lowry, director of the Museum of Modern Art,: Museums have to make a "shift away from passive experiences to interactive and participatory experiences, from art that hangs on the wall to art that invites people to become part of it." And, he said, they should shed the idea of being a repository and become social spaces. She also had a conversation with Alexander Bortolot, the "curatorial content strategist" at the Minneapolis Institute of Arts who told her that younger people want museums to connect them to the creative economy. They don't want to listen to some art historian flown in from New York; they'd rather network with members of the local arts community and take part in a conversation. She added the thoughts of Thomas P. Campbell, the Metropolitan's director, who, after the terrorist attack in Boston, offered the Museum of Fine Arts three paintings dealing with contemplation. Mr.Campbell said: "Great museums are places of solace and inspiration particularly when tragedy strikes a community." Ms.Dobrzynski suggests that visitor engagement changes the very nature of museums and places their very identity at risk.

One might add to her observations that the individual's identity is also at risk. Seducing the young through frantic crowd-think and technology fads is the contemporary version of bread and circuses. The sinister time-tested goal of those at the helm of power is always the same: brainwash the malleable young, create a cadre of dehumanized puppets, eliminate our multidimensional identity, eliminate introspection, contemplation, and critical thinking. The art in Museums should speak to us of the depth of our humanity and reminds us that adversity and suffering have not extinguished our soul.

The young and old do not realize how seamlessly the plutocracy is exploiting and dehumanizing them.

A Blueprint for Brain Manipulation. Mind Control Will Be Camouflaged as Progress. [NYT "Big Leaps in Linking Computers and Brains" 8/5/13" by Nick Bilton]: "Scientists haven't yet found a way to mend a broken heart but they're edging closer to manipulating memory and downloading instructions from a computer right into a brain." Researchers from the Riken-M.I.T. Center for Neural Circuit Genetics said they were able to create a false memory in a mouse. The scientists reported in the journal Science that they caused the mouse to remember being shocked in one location when in reality the mouse was shocked in a completely different location. They took a neutral memory and artificially changed it to a negative memory. Steve Ramirez, an M.I.T. neuroscientist, said that one day such procedures could lead to computer-manipulation of the mind for treatment of such things as post-traumatic stress disorder. Technologists are already working on brain-computer interfaces to allow us to interact with our smartphones and computers simply by using our minds. Technology already exists that can read our thoughts to control games etc..

In 2011, scientists at Boston University and A.T.R. Computational Neuroscience Laboratories in Japan described a process called Decoded Neurofeedback which sends signals to the brain from an M.R.I. machine that can alter a person's brain activity pattern. Thus, writing to the brain could, they say, teach us to learn how to play a musical instrument in our sleep, or learn a language, or allow us to interact with our computer or other human beings "just by thinking about it." [or someday allow the state to control our minds].

[NYT "Monkey's thoughts propel robot…" 1/15/08, by Sandra Blakeslee. Miguel Nicolelis, a neuroscientist at Duke, successfully connected the brains of two rats over the internet so that when one pressed a lever the other did as well even though they were in different countries and monkeys were each given half of a piece of information which they would have to share through the brain to move a robotic arm. At Harvard Medical School, scientists created a brain to brain interface that allows a human to move a rat's tail just by thinking about it. Dr. Nicolelis predicts that techniques will be developed to allow humans to read one another's thoughts.

[NYT 3/16/14 Gary Markus and Christof Koch; "The Plug-and-Play Brain"]. "How soon can we expect to see brain implants for perfect memory, enhanced vision, hypernormal focus or an expert golf swing? We are closer than you think." The writers inform us about some of the technical problems yet to be overcome in interfacing the brain but are confident that sooner or later neural implants will be able to enhance the performance of "normal people" as opposed to merely reparative usefulness as in paralysis or blindness. "They will be used to improve memory, mental focus (Ritalin without the side effects) perception and mood (bye, bye Prozac)." "The augmented among us – those who are willing to avail themselves of the benefits of brain prosthetics and to live with the attendant risks – will outperform others in the everyday contest for jobs and mates, in science, on the athletic field and in armed combat. [The rubbish in print is amazing. Brave New World anyone?]

Comment:

These three articles in the lay press share certain characteristics. Firstly, there is no mention of human relationships in this grand scheme being outlined for all of us. Eliminating interpersonal relationships from a discussion of human behavior is a dead giveaway for a dehumanized power-oriented value system. The last article in particular hyped naked power as if that was what life was all about, including prowess in every domain, jobs, athletics, the "right mate" etc. Of course, this brings to mind "Brave New World" with its cast of top-dogs, the alphas, and then the lesser breeds, the betas and on down the line (by the way, would one really want to invest in a mate who valued power above intimacy in a marriage –. These noisy and dull mouthpieces for the current cultural obsession with power are not even scientifically grounded even if the word "science" is continuously parroted.

Overwhelming evidence proves that human relationships are foremost in determining both psychological and brain development. These self-appointed "brain experts" might pay some deference to the billions of years of evolution that gave rise to the neo-cortex in Nature's own grand scheme to advance man to the apex of the animal kingdom, a pinnacle whose foundation rests on mutually trusting human relationships. If no one cares about us we are nothing. The thrust of these article is underwritten by a plutocracy. If perfected, such technological advances would give the state and those who control the state, a tool to eliminate our independence once and for all and refashion our memories and identities in accordance with the priorities of the plutocracy. The movie "Dark City" was an allegory dealing with these issues. As for a method to treat post-traumatic stress disorder or mood disorders, while medication helps, only another human being can heal emotional wounds. Manipulating the brain will only deepen trauma as it communicates indifference to our suffering.

Corporate Profits and Priorities Decree Personal Privacy Is Out. Torture may be Necessary

Like all ultimately totalitarian systems, unbridled capitalism realizes the value of complete control of the individual, knowing his/her whereabouts, vulnerabilities and predilections. Why safeguard the constitutional right of privacy when privacy interferes with potentially windfall corporate profits? Abrogating privacy can also come in handy for smearing those who would defy the plutocracy. The super-rich are, after all, insulated from law suits as a consequence of the discriminatory system of justice in the United States that makes it financially impossible for the average person to defend themselves against corporate lawyers or the government, or levy law suits against plutocratic titans.

The Supreme Court itself has become a tool of the billionaires. The Court's term ending in June, 2008, was exceptionally good for the U.S. Chamber of Commerce and American business: "The chamber's litigation center filed briefs in 15 cases and its side won in 13 of them." [Jeffrey Rosen,The New York Times Magazine; "Court Inc."; 3/16/08].The politicians, of course, as unbridled capitalism's willing lackeys, always lend a helping hand to their corporate masters who finance their campaigns and find lucrative jobs for them after they leave congress. As for the public, they are distracted by bread and circuses (what little bread they still get).

The public docilely accepts systematic spying on Internet users. Technology companies (like Facebook) and Internet service providers track and compile a record of every Website visited, ads clicked, every word entered in search engines, all without telling you or asking permission and they then sell this information. Facebook gathers your personal information even if you don't have a Facebook account. They can target those who seek specific medical treatment, buy medications online, seek out meetings for Alcoholics Anonymous (anonymous no more), visit adult Websites, or Websites that might raise the suspicions of Big Brother. The information can be sold to sociopaths, employers or insurance companies. Corporate profits and furthering a police state agenda are thusly well served.

An individual's detailed history, "criminal record" (including traffic violations) is now readily accessible on various websites for free with no guarantees as to accuracy. Unlisted telephone numbers and the owner of a particular license plate are also available online for a small fee. Spying satellites and Google Earth's mapping software, will soon be capable of following a single person's peregrinations and reading their license plate numbers. Cellphones track a cellphone user's whereabouts through satellite systems. "Friends" will be able to keep tabs on you. Forced DNA testing at the dictate of the police is now common practice for anyone charged with an offence even before a trial and conviction, including misdemeanors.

Electronic medical records are touted as patient friendly because private medical information can be forwarded quickly and efficiently with the touch of a computer key. Yet confidential data, including details on psychotherapy, has fallen into the hands of hostile third parties who have in turn made disclosures to insurance companies. The latter have used confidential information to deny claims, in spite of federal laws that are supposed to safeguard confidential medical information. Many thousands of complaints have been lodged with the Department of Health and Human Resources but the agency has failed to act on any of them. Peter Swire, a law professor at Ohio State University who helped write the regulations states: "It sends the signal that the health system can ignore this issue" [WSJ 11/27/12 "Privacy professor to try to break do not track logjam" S. Shankland]. Secretly spying on our privacy, corporate interests collect data on our website visits and enjoy free license to do so.

Spying on us: "1984" refined for the 21st century
The Billionaire/Politician Totalitarian Axis

Somini Sengupta [The New York Times; "Should Personal Data Be Personal?"; 2/5/12] explores the threat to our independence posed by a plutocracy bent on mind-control. Selling our independence to the corporate agenda and the government spying apparatus will insure that those in control will stay in control and profit thereby:

Max Schrems, a 24 year old law student from Salzburg, Austria, wanted to know what Facebook knew: "He requested his own Facebook file. What he got turned to be a virtual [B]ildungsroman, 1222 pages long. It contained wall posts he had deleted, old messages that revealed a friend's troubled state of mind, even information that he didn't enter himself about his physical whereabouts." "Why was it there at all, he wondered, when he had deleted it?" "We in Europe are oftentimes frightened of what might happen someday."

Ms. Sengupta wonders how the laws of various nations manage the multinational companies that control our digital lives. All the data that we share is used by companies to target advertising based on the personal opinions and desires posted online. She adds that companies spend $2 billion a year to collect that information. German newspapers published instructions on how to retrieve personal data files from Facebook, and German authorities have scrutinized facial recognition technology. The European Commission will empower a citizen of Europe to demand the deletion of his or her personal data. By contrast, the United States has no law that controls how online data is used. In China, 200 million facial recognition surveillance cameras are in place everywhere and authorities are working on refining the technology to capture all of its people on a vast police database called "Skynet." While the system is still a work in progress, a Chinese narrator states: "No matter which corner you escape to, we'll bring you to justice." Chinese police have also upgraded Google-type glasses that now have facial recognition ability.

Ms. Sengupta continues:

Stewart A. Baker, a former assistant secretary at the Department of Homeland Security sees "enormous benefits for private companies and government agencies alike." He feels that to fight these trends on privacy grounds is "futile": "You can't have really a property interest in data." [The totalitarians wouldn't approve].

Lori Andrews, a lawyer, writes "Facebook Is Using You" [The New York Times, 2/5/12]. Cookies and other tracking mechanisms are used to sell your personal information to companies that in turn target you with custom tailored advertising. If you did a Google search for stress, expect ads for medications etc.. "The bits and bytes about your life can easily be used against you. Whether you can obtain a job, credit or insurance can be based on your digital doppelgänger." A company called Spokeo gathers online data for employers and anyone else who wants it. Women are asked for their boyfriend's e-mail for an analysis of their online photos and activities. Ms. Andrews makes the case for a do-not-track-law similar to the do-not-call one.

Never Forgetting a Face

[NYT 5/18/14 "Never forgetting a face" Natasha Singer]. Joseph Atick, a pioneer in the technology of face recognition now fears that if face-matching is taken too far, it could allow mass surveillance, "basically robbing everyone of their anonymity." "Online we are all tracked. But to Dr.Atick, the street remains a haven, and he frets that he may have abetted a technology that could upend the social order." Once companies amass consumer's facial data, government could gain access to it too.

The advancements of biometrics are such that your face becomes your code, accompanying you everywhere. Dr.Atick noted that an app called NameTag, according to a news release, was available in an early form to users of Google Glass. Name Tag users, in a glance, could instantly identify a stranger's name, occupation, and Facebook profile. Owing to complaints, Google said it would not approve the app for Google Glass. However, several tech giants have bought up face-recognition start-ups. In 2011, Google bought Pittsburgh Pattern Recognition, a computer vision business developed by researchers at Carnegie Mellon University and, in 2012, Facebook bought Face.com, an Israeli start-up.

Face recognition can be used at a distance without the person's knowledge and then linked to pictures they have put online. Both Google and Facebook have technology to identify faces on videos.

Software converts each face into a mathematical code called a "faceprint." Once faceprinted, they can be identified by photographs or after walking in front of a video camera. In 2018 [NYT 7/10/18 "Facebook's push for facial recognition software raises privacy alarms" by Natasha Singer], Facebook re-launched its facial recognition software. It can scan your unnamed photos or videos and then match the code of their facial patterns to the data base of named people. This tool and other patented Facebook facial recognition software can be used in stores to track shopper's purchases, whereabouts etc. Critics fear that these tools could serve to promote a police state. (the software was later shut down.)

Police departments already employ face recognition systems. In 2001, a company supplied the Tampa police with a Face-recognition system that was used to scan tens of thousands of fans at the Super Bowl XXXV. No one was arrested.

["For Marketers, TVs Act as Priceless Sets of Eyes"; NYT 2/26/17, by S. Maheshwari] "While Ellen Milzand her family were watching the Olympics last summer, their TV was watching them." TVision Insights, a marketing company using Microsoft technology, installs a device on the TV that analyzes the viewer's eye movements and facial expressions in response to advertisements. The information is of keen interest to advertisers. This and other related companies plan to launch such technology across multiple platforms. Vizio, one of the biggest makers of internet-connected TVs said it would pay $2.2million to settle charges that it was collecting and selling data from millions of smart TVs without the viewer's knowledge. Samba Interactive TV [NYT 2018] teams up with a number of TV manufacturers and, if consumers who bought newly purchased smart TVs opt in, everything they are watching is being read and fed to advertisers, including which political programs they favor.

[NYT "The Bright-Eyed Talking Doll That Just Might Be a Spy" 2/18/17 by K.FreytasTamura]. Germany pulls a U.S.-made toy manufactured by Genesis Toys that records children's conversations and transmits the voice prints of children to Nuance Communications.

[NYT "Documents said to Reveal Hacking Secrets of C.I.A." 3/8/17 by Scott Shane et al.]. WikiLeaks released thousands of pages describing sophisticated software tools and procedures used by the agency to break into smartphones, computers and internetconnected televisions (to turn selected televisions into secret microphones), and even commercial antivirus programs used by millions of people. Audio and message traffic can be intercepted and collected before encryption can be applied (see article for details). "There is no evidence that the C.I.A. hacking tools have been used against Americans." (But….). In 2015, Samsung included in its fine print the warning for its smart TVs: "Please be aware that if your spoken words include personal or other sensitive information, that information will be among the data captured and transmitted to a third party through your use of Voice Recognition."

The government arbitrarily suspends civil liberties

Well on the way to an Orwellian state, the military-industrial complex, as part of the Bush – Cheney administration's "war on terror," methodically dismantled America's constitutionally safe-guarded civil liberties. Captured enemy combatants or simply "detainees," who were never charged with a crime, as reported by the Red Cross and Physicians for Human Rights, were subjected to torture, including near suffocation by drowning, confinement that recalled Viet Cong tiger cages, humiliation, bombardment with intolerable constant noise, beatings and electric shock, burns, military dogs, extreme cold or heat injury, torture ("enhanced", "special" methods) that one would expect to have taken place at the hands of some South American dictator. These practices were considered justified and legal at the Office of Legal Council, under John C. Yoo, then a pentagon lawyer and now a law professor at the University of California, Berkley campus. The Bush administration outsourced interrogation of war detainees to mercenary private contractors like CACI and Titan, both of whom were linked to torture of prisoners [NYT 9/11/09, "Torture case against Iraqi contractors is dismissed" Reuters (they have immunity)..

Ali Soufan, an F.B.I supervisory special agent from 1997-2005, writes how the F.B.I. fought terrorism without using torture [NYT 4/29/09 "CIA uncensors memoir of former FBI agent" Charlie Savage et al.]. Mr. Soufan interrogated high-ranking terrorists like Abu Zubaydah and elicited important intelligence but objected to "the harsh techniques" that shortly thereafter were instituted and forced upon C.I.A. agents. "My C.I.A. colleagues who baulked at the techniques, on the other hand, were instructed to continue." Pat D'Amuro, an F.B.I. assistant director affirmed that "we don't do that." From the recently released memos, "It seems clear that it was [private] contractors, not C.I.A. officers, who requested the use of these techniques." The C.I.A. destroyed hundreds of hours of interrogation tapes. Suspicious deaths were reported. [NYT 12/7/07]

In 2005, Steven Bradbury, then acting head of the Justice Department's Office of Legal Council in a memo notes: "Torture is abhorrent." He then painstakingly defines in legalize the meanings of "severe" and "physical pain and suffering" to justify the conclusion that what the CIA did was not torture. Near drowning, slapping, "walling," were among the ten "approved" techniques as well as the use of insects. Methods were tailored to a detainee's primary fear as, for example, a fear of insects. Interrogators placed one detainee in a box with an insect and told him it was a stinging insect when it really wasn't. [WSJ 4/17/09 "Bush officials defend physical abuse as revealed in memos" by Ewen MacAskill]. (Of course, the use of psychological terror and precisely such methods as these appear to be directly lifted from the pages of Orwell's "1984").

Jose Padilla, an American whom the Bush administration accused of being an enemy combatant has been held prisoner for years without ever being charged with a crime. He was allowed outside of solitary confinement to see a dentist. His feet were shackled, fitted with blacked-out goggles, hands manacled, noise-blocking head phones over his ears, "his expressionless eyes briefly met the camera before he lowered his head…" [NYT 11/3/06, "Why is the NYT covering up the torture of Jose Padilla?" David Walsh] What is to prevent any of us from being labeled "an enemy of the state," illegally imprisoned without ever filing charges and then subjected to torture? What has happened to the constitution?

Former President Bush succeeded in his efforts to win congressional approval for his "massive warrantless wiretapping and surveillance" program, enlisting the secret cooperation of the telephone companies and the approval of President Obama for domestic spying. The National Security Agency, once confined to foreign surveillance, sweeps up data on American civilians including e-mails, internet site visits, cellphone numbers, phone numbers, financial records and airline information. "Scale of U.S. Wiretapping Exceeded Law, Officials Say" [NYT 4/16/09 by Eric Lichtblau].. Military Data Reveal Tips on Antiwar Activities.

Paper mail is also watched. The Mail Isolation Control and Tracking program, through the Postal Service computers photographs the exterior of every piece of paper mail processed in the United States – about 160 billion pieces a year, according to The New York Times.

[NYT 4/16/09 "Wiretapover collection at the NSA" Jennifer Devries] monitoring can also track your whereabouts through your mobile phone. Records from cellphone networks include an ID number of the nearest cell tower and often say which direction that tower is in, states Matt Blaze, a computer science professor at the University of Pennsylvania. The New York Times also reports that stores are tracking shopper's movements through their cell phones.

[NYT 8/30/13 "Facial scanning is making gains in surveillance" by Charlie Savage] Ginger McCall, a lawyer and privacy advocate, is the founder of Advocates for Accountable Democracy. She obtained documents under the Freedom of Information Act and learned that the Department of Homeland Security is making progress on a tool called the Biometric Optical Surveillance System that will use video cameras to scan people's faces in public etc. and then identify them. At present there is little or no legal oversight of such technologies. But let us continue……

The Edward Snowden affair

[NYT 6/4/15 "The world says no to surveillance" by Edward Snowden] Edward J. Snowden, an ex-contractor for the National Security Agency, who most recently was part of a Booz Allen team that worked directly with the N.S.A., leaked secret N.S.A documents to the British newspaper, The Guardian, and the American newspaper, The Washington Post, concerning the existence of a top secret court order allowing the N.S.A to monitor millions of telephone logs of American citizens. Booz Allen is an independent defense contractor. Mr. Snowden forwarded the information to Glenn Greenwald, a lawyer who previously worked for a high-powered New York law firm and who now writes for The Guardian. The Guardian exposed the detailed nature of this spy program, called Prism. For the past six years, Prism has secretly collected information on foreigners overseas from the nation's largest Internet companies like Google, Facebook, and Apple and, for the past seven years, N.S.A. has swept up all the telephone records of every American in the nation. The Internet surveillance program collects data from online providers, including e-mail, chat rooms, videos, photos, stored data, file transfers, video conferences and logins, according to classified documents.

"It cannot be used to intentionally target any U.S. citizen…." states James R. Clapper Jr., the former director of national intelligence. However, this is the same Mr. Clapper who seemingly lied in testimony to the Senate in March, 2013, when he stated that the N.S.A. was not gathering data on millions of Americans.

Rajesh De, the N.S.A.'s general counsel, sought to debunk what he called "false myths" about the agency, including the idea that "N.S.A. is spying on Americans at home and abroad with questionable or no legal bases." [NYT 6/12/13 "Earlier denials put cyber ['chief in awkward position" by Scott Shane]. U.S. lawmakers who support the program say it is only "metadata" like logs of calls sent and received and not invasive listening. Not so reassuring is the fact that Americans' e-mails who communicate with someone overseas can be swept up without an individualized court order. N.S.A. obtains direct access to companies' servers. Section 215 of The Patriot Act allows the government to obtain a secret order for business records if it is deemed relevant to a national security administration. Representative Mike Rogers of Michigan claimed that the program averted a terrorist attack in the last few years….no details were given. Nor is it explained why this wholesale spying on non-terrorist Americans didn't ferret out real terrorists like those responsible for the Boston Marathon bombings, even though the Russian government gave the U.S. advance warning concerning the perpetrators identities. Could it be that the real basic premise for such unbridled spying on one's own citizens rests on the historical precedents that underlie all totalitarian agendas? Pursuing "enemies of the state" is always the excuse used to justify an evolving police state. Mr. Snowden said that he released only what he found to be the greatest abuses of a surveillance state that he came to view as reckless: "If you realize that that's the world you helped create and it is going to get worse with the next generation and the next generation and extend the capabilities of this architecture of oppression, you realize that you might be willing to accept any risks and it doesn't matter what the outcome is."

[NYT 6/9/13 "Leaks are literally gut-wrenching" by Aaron Blake] it was also revealed that the Justice Department had secretly obtained phone logs for reporters at The Associated Press and Fox News. Mr. Clapper warned that these revelations were "gut wrenching" "because of the huge, grave, damage it does to our intelligence capabilities." Mike McConnell, A former head of the N.S.A. who later was made vice chairman at Booz Allen states that the U.S. was not using its full capability because of privacy concerns [NYT 6/1013 "After profits defense contractor faces pitfalls of cybersecurity" David Sanger].

[Also quoted in The New York Times "Only Nixon hurt a free press more" 7/31/13] was the opinion of James C. Goodale, a First Amendment lawyer who previously worked for The Times: "…no reporter had ever been successfully prosecuted on a conspiracy charge but that recent actions, like the investigation of a Fox News reporter, James Rosen, was evidence that the government was "moving toward criminalizing the reporting process."

Mr. Snowden has been charged with violating the espionage act and stealing. This is the seventh case under president Obama in which a government official has been criminally charged with leaking classified information to the news media. Under all previous presidents, just three such cases have been sought Max Frankel writing in the New York Times [6/23/13 "Where did our inalienable rights go?"], notes: "What ought to compound our skepticism is the news that there is money to be made in the mass approach. We are learning that much of the snooping is farmed out to profit-seeking corporations that have great appetites for government contacts, secured through executives who enrich themselves by shuttling between agency jobs and the contractors' board rooms."

According to documents provided by whistle-blower Edward Snowden and obtained by The Guardian, "Microsoft helped the NSA bypass encryption"7/11/13 by Glen Greenwald, Microsoft collaborated closely with U.S. intelligence over three years to allow users' communications to be intercepted, including allowing N.S.A. to circumvent the company's own encryption. Skype video calls collected by Prism were shared with the F.B.I. and C.I.A. One N.S.A. document described the program as a "team sport." N.S.A. had direct access to Microsoft, Skype, Apple, Google, Facebook and Yahoo. Top secret N.S.A. programs allows analysts to search with no prior authorization through vast databases containing emails, online chats, and the browsing history of millions of individuals. "Xkeyscore details how analysts can use it and other systems to mine enormous agency data bases by filling in a simple on-screen form giving only a broad justification for the search." The request is not reviewed by a court.

An editorial by The New York Times [8/9/13] highlights a revelation by Charles Savage that N.S.A. copies virtually all overseas messages that Americans send or receive, then scans them to see if they contain references to people or subjects the agency thinks might have a link to terrorists, however innocent the exchange of ideas might otherwise be. This is a violation of the Fourth Amendment's protection against illegal searches. The Obama administration justified this unwarranted expansion of surveillance powers by claiming that the messages are not stored "even if every message is analyzed by supercomputers as it is sent."

Edward Snowden, as reported in an editorial of The New York Times, released documents that show that the N.S.A. collaborated with big software companies and cipher authors, getting hidden access built right into their systems. The agency has access to the codes that protect commerce, banking, trade secrets, medical records, and everyone's email and internet chat messages.

The secret opaque courts routinely approve and expand N.S.A. requests to collect data. The chairman of the Senate Judiciary Committee, Patrick Leahy of Vermont, as reported in The New York Times, noted that the surveillance court has no adversarial process. There is no due process. Judge Reggie B. Walton, involved in some of the cases, pointed out that the court "is forced to rely upon the accuracy of the information provided" to it.

Stalin and Hitler also set up courts but they served the political goals of the party, not democracy.

The symbiotic and mutually rewarding convergence of Silicon Valley profits and government spy agencies

[James Risen and Nick Wingfield; "Quest for Pools of Data Binds Silicon Valley and Spy Agency"; NYT 6/20/13]: "When Max Kelly, the chief security officer for Facebook, left the social media company in 2010, he did not go to Google, Twitter or a similar Silicon

Valley concern. Instead the man who was responsible for protecting the personal information of Facebook's more than one billion users went to work for another giant institution that manages and analyses large pools of data: the National Security Agency."

"To get their hands on the latest software technology to manipulate and take advantage of large volumes of data, United States intelligence agencies invest in Silicon Valley start-ups, award classified contracts and recruit technology experts like Mr. Kelly." Ray Wang, a technology analyst and chief executive of Constellation Research, states: "There are a lot of connections now because the data scientists and the folks who are building these systems have a lot of common interests."

Contrary to claims by the companies geared for public consumption, "current and former industry officials say the companies sometimes secretly put together teams of in-house experts to find ways to cooperate more completely with the N.S.A. and to make their customers' information more accessible to the agency. The companies do so, the officials say, because they want to control the process themselves."

Skype, the internet-based calling service, began its own secret program, Project Chess, to explore the technical issues in making Skype calls readily available to intelligence agencies and the police. Microsoft owns Skype. Mr. Snowden says Skype joined Prism on Feb. 6, 2011.

Gen. Keith B. Alexander, the agency's director and the chief of the Pentagon's Cyber Command, in a T-shirt and jeans, gave the keynote speech at one of the world's largest hacker conferences, Delcon, to recruit hackers for his spy agency.

Snowden is currently among the nominees for a European Human Rights Prize as well as The Nobel Peace Prize.

Emulating Big-Brother-Power lures and fascinates the unthinking as they race toward self-effacement, puppetry, and mutual paranoia

Thrilled with the available technology that allows one to play-act Little-Big-Brother, average citizens are equipping themselves with devices that allow them to surreptitiously record private conversations on their cellphones, secretly photograph strangers with Goggleglasses and instantaneously globalize their snooping across the planet on You-tube, Twitter etc., Your privacy and your true identity becomes the grist of millions of strangers for gossip, ridicule and character assassination. NOW THAT'S REAL POWER.

The plutocracy will be laughing up their sleeve as privacy, personal identity, and all opposing organized power-blocks will succumb to their homogenizing brainwashing machine and all individuality will be sucked into the black hole of a "post human species".

20

Psychiatry Dehumanized

My investigation explores the current state of dehumanization in psychiatry and of our culture in general. Bureaucrats take their cue from corporate and governmental interests. The Psychiatric Times, the official newspaper of the American Psychiatric Association, has a rather sad history when it comes to standing up for the individual. In the December 5, 2003 edition, coverage is given to the agenda of the Institute of Medicine and their report "Research Training in Psychiatry Training: Strategies for Reform." Officials of The National Institute of Mental Health, a governmental agency, asked the IOM to study the problem of reversing "the severe shortage of psychiatric researchers" "in an era when scientific knowledge about brain and behavior is exploding." This quasi-governmental body, the IOM, routinely rubber stamps political agendas. It solemnly advises that there is too much emphasis on clinical treatment of patients especially on psychotherapy training: which is "Hindering research career development" (strange, because psychotherapy training in psychiatric residency programs doesn't exist anymore). They want to tell The Psychiatry Residency Review Committee which accredits residency training programs that the current standards of achievement of competency in five broad areas of psychotherapy training could be reduced to merely "knowledge" in those areas, plus, "traditional nine months inpatient service could be reduced to six months." "This will be achieved by encouraging university presidents, hospital CEO's and medical deans to advance mental health through greater investment in research oriented faculty and psychiatry department's research training infrastructure" ("research faculty," of course, can be counted on to bring with them tens of millions of dollars of corporate industry and government grant money. Needless to say they will also be beholden to corporate and governmental interests).The wisdom of the IOM further suggests "remote network training when on-site mentoring is not possible."

The IOM also addresses "money matters" etc.. The 12 member IOM was chaired by a pediatrician. Six members are psychiatrists, one being Michelle Riba M.D. the then APA President-elect. She deems the report "a bold step" "toward insuring a healthy future for psychiatric research." It is incredible to me that the then future president of the American Psychiatric Association could demonstrate such an appalling disregard for patient welfare and jeopardize even further the relevance of psychiatrists in patient treatment. Promoting "research" sounds unassailable but brain research in its current form is corrupted by corporate financial interests that seek to eliminate the doctor-patient relationship. The pharmaceutical industry encourages the belief that treatment is simply a matter of prescribing the right psychoactive drugs for emotional problems. For those knowledgeable in the use of psychiatric medications, nothing could be further from the truth. Medication may be necessary to treat symptoms but only understanding can shed light on the origin of symptoms and lead to meaningful resolution. There is no magic pill. President Obama recently authorized $100 million for "brain research. This "research" will ignore the environment of human to human relationships, the foundation of reality.

[WebSleuths 10/31/05 David Maust "Young male victims," the news story of a serial killer responsible for the deaths of a number of adolescent boys. He killed a boy while in the army and was discharged on a manslaughter conviction. Subsequently he killed two more "friends." In the one trial he was found not guilty after lying on the witness stand. "The judge said to me you should not be throwing knives around other people and I told the judge I would not throw any more knives around." In 1981 he picked up a 15-year-old boy whom he knifed and left to drown: "I can still hear Donald Jones saying to me I am only 15 years old please do not kill me." The killer served only 16 years for that murder (less time than many serve for tax evasion) along with two years in Texas for injuring a child. In 1999 he was released. Now the bodies of three teenagers were found under concrete in his basement.

His history reveals that at age 13 he went from a state mental hospital to a children's home in Chicago: "I had sex with Steve maybe three times and there were two more boys that I did this with….. because all I wanted was to have someone to love me." The Chicago Sun-Times reports: at 16 he remembers "going back and forth between Chicago and Georgia,….[he] recalled his mother being abusive." "She got a knife and was coming at me with the knife, telling me to get out of her house right now or she was going to stab me with the knife so my stepfather got up and stopped her." "I helped my mother and stepfather around the house, it made me feel like a son for the first time in my life."

This is a story of a tragedy. Childhood abuse and rejection created a killer. The poor boys he murdered were also himself, doing to others what had been done to him. Life did this to all of them and irresponsible authorities in a barbaric society are guilty. The tragedy could have been averted had this man as a child or adolescent or adult received real help, help without a deadline, in a humane hospital setting. Suffering can cause people to do horrendous things to others and to themselves.

We do not live in a civilized world. Where is common decency when an 18 year old "with profound mental disabilities" was sentenced to 100 years in prison after pleading guilty to charges of "fondling" his six year old neighbor. The offender has an I.Q. of 47 and was diagnosed as mentally disabled as a child. He can neither read nor write. Didn't he suffer too? Wasn't he the abused child too?

None of this comes as a surprise to decent people but, then again, the average decent person isn't in charge of anything. Most politicians, administrators and bureaucrats aren't interested in what happens to other people. They are only interested in expanding their empires big and small because their priority is power and control. The IOM is surely aware of the realities of life and how life experiences affect people. Yet they talk of brain research as if brain phenomena had nothing to do with human relationships. Being physicians instructed in the art of healing, they surly must acknowledge that there is a desperate need for the human bond. The 12 members of the IOM should question their politics and leave brain-talk to the molecular biologists.

Increasing societal violence parallels the increasing abandonment of the mentally ill

A society fashioned by plutocratic billionaire priorities where the individual is nothing, will descend into chaos. The alternative plutocratic solution is a controlling totalitarian state of puppets. The Nation's refusal to spend dollars on long term intensive treatment, both inpatient and outpatient, of the mentally ill, is leading to increasingly desperate behavior on the part of those struggling with mental illness. Dehumanizing human beings by labeling them "diseased brains," will only aggravate the overwhelming emotional deprivation and repressed rage they experienced growing up in a sick family.

So-called experts solemnly intone that violent behavior cannot be predicted. Yet recent cases gave ample warning that these mentally ill individuals were about to take action.

Harris and Klebold, the Columbine killers, were given antidepressants and enrolled in "anger management classes." Did such patently worthless (but cheap) measures solve the issues of rage and dehumanization that consumed these individuals? A realistic treatment plan would have necessitated long term analytically oriented psychotherapy, several times a week, no managed care interference, no deadlines, court mandated if necessary, and/or hospitalization, conducted by a psychiatrist who understood the mind.

[NYT 11/21/14, "Adam Lanza's mental problems completely untreated before Newton.." by Alison Leigh Cowan] Adam Lanza, the Sandy Hook Elementary School killer, who murdered 20 schoolchildren and six adults, was categorized as suffering from "brain disease" by a psychiatrist in his letter to The New York Times. Nowhere in the newspaper write-ups or media accounts of this tragedy was parenting considered to be an important causal factor.

What are the facts?: His parents were divorced. His mother collected guns, took him to target practice on a regular basis, and bought him the very gun he used to kill her and the others. He had been delusional, probably for years, yet there is no indication that she made any attempt to get him serious psychiatric help. He and the mother communicated only by email although they lived in the same house. His online obsessions revolved around violence. The scene of the tragedy was the same school that employed his mother as a teacher. There can be no other conclusion but that the quality of the mother-child relationship engendered his psychosis. The children he killed were himself.

In another mass shooting in a Chicago suburb, the killer had been psychotic for years, had attempted suicide, threatened homicide. His Father equipped him with assault rifles yet said he had no idea why his son could resort to such behavior. When a swat team visited the parent's home, the Mother flew into a rage. The newscaster was in disbelief that the parents lwere the ones who caused his psychosis. The killer, in the past, had contact with "mental heath professionals." One can only imagine how ignorant they were.

The unfolding dictatorship

The billionaire puppet-masters have betrayed America. The individual's identity and our ability to care about one another is being supplanted by their agenda that will make puppets of us all. Valuing the intrinsic worth of every individual is the foundation of true civilization, not the State or "the greater good." Every major psychiatric disorder (depression, schizophrenia, sociopathy etc.) has its origins in a corrupt culture and a sick, dysfunctional family where the child was not treated as a person in their own right.

"Already long ago, from when we sold our vote to no man, the People have abdicated our duties; for the People who once upon a time handed out military command, high civil office, legions, everything, now restrains itself and anxiously hopes for just two things: bread and circuses." Juvenal, Roman poet.

www.ingramcontent.com/pod-product-compliance
Lightning Source LLC
LaVergne TN
LVHW080035210926
848481LV00011B/3197
* 9 7 9 8 3 4 9 2 6 0 4 7 6 *